Atlas of Human Infectious Diseases

Atlas of Human Infectious Diseases

EDITED BY

Heiman F.L. Wertheim MD PhD

Wellcome Trust Major Overseas Program, Oxford University Clinical Research Unit,
National Hospital of Tropical Diseases, Hanoi, Vietnam; Centre for Tropical Medicine,
Nuffield Department of Clinical Medicine, University of Oxford, Oxford, UK

Peter Horby MBBS FFPH

Wellcome Trust Major Overseas Program, Oxford University Clinical Research Unit,
National Hospital of Tropical Diseases, Hanoi, Vietnam; Centre for Tropical Medicine,
Nuffield Department of Clinical Medicine, University of Oxford, Oxford, UK

John P. Woodall MA PhD

ProMED-mail co-founder and Associate Editor; Institute of Medical Biochemistry,
Centre for Health Sciences, Federal University of Rio de Janeiro, Brazil (retired)

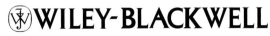

WILEY-BLACKWELL

A John Wiley & Sons, Ltd., Publication

Library of Congress Cataloging-in-Publication Data

Atlas of human infectious diseases / edited by Heiman F.L. Wertheim, Peter Horby, John P. Woodall.
p. ; cm.
Includes bibliographical references and index.
ISBN-13: 978-1-4051-8440-3 (hard cover : alk. paper)
ISBN-10: 1-4051-8440-X (hard cover : alk. paper)
1. Communicable diseases–Atlases. I. Wertheim, Heiman F. L. II. Horby, Peter. III. Woodall, John P.
[DNLM: 1. Communicable Diseases–Atlases. 2. Parasitic Diseases–Atlases. 3. Topography, Medical–Atlases. 4. Virus Diseases–Atlases. WC 17]
RC113.2.A85 2012
616.90022′3–dc23   2011027411

A catalogue record for this book is available from the British Library.

Wiley also publishes its books in a variety of electronic formats. Some content that appears in print may not be available in electronic books.

Set in 8.75/12pt Palatino by Thomson Digital, Noida, India
Printed and bound in Malaysia by Vivar Printing Sdn Bhd

1   2012

Contents

Editors, viii

Contributors and Reviewers, ix

Foreword, xv

Preface, xvii

User's Guide, xix

Abbreviations, xxi

The World, xxii

Section 1: Infectious Disease Drivers, 1

1 Emerging Infectious Diseases, 3

2 Population, 5

3 Urbanization, 7

4 Global Connectivity, 9

5 Human Development, 11

6 Global Peace Index, 13

7 Life Expectancy and Child Mortality, 15

8 Water and Sanitation, 17

9 Undernutrition, 19

10 Climate, 21

11 Forest Cover Change, 23

12 Natural Disasters, 25

13 Antibiotic Use, 27

14 Inherited Blood Disorders and Duffy Antigen, 29

15 Immunization Coverage – DTP3, 31

16 *Aedes aegypti* and *Aedes albopictus*, 33

17 Malaria Vectors, 35

18 Livestock Density, 37

19 Bird Migration, 39

Section 2: Bacterial Infections, 41

20 Anthrax, 43

21 Bartonellosis, *Bartonella bacilliformis*, 45

22 Bartonellosis, *Bartonella quintana*, 47

23 Botulism, 49

24 Brucellosis, 51

25 Buruli Ulcer, 53

26 Cholera, 55

27 Diphtheria, 57

28 Donovanosis, 59

29 Ehrlichioses, 61

30 Endemic Treponematosis, 63

31 *Haemophilus influenzae* Type b, 65

32 Leprosy, 67

33 Leptospirosis, 69

34 Listeriosis, 71

35 Lyme Disease, 73

36 Melioidosis, 75

37 Meningococcal Meningitis, 77

38 Noma, 79

39 Pertussis, 81

40 Plague, 83

41 Pneumococcal Disease, 85

42 Q Fever, 87

43 Rat Bite Fever, 89

44 Relapsing Fever, 91

45 Rickettsioses, Tick-borne, New World, 93

46 Rickettsioses, Tick-borne, Old World, 95

47 Scrub Typhus, 97

48 *Streptococcus suis*, 99

49 Tetanus, 101

50 Trachoma, 103

51 Tuberculosis, 105

52 Tularemia, 107

53 Typhoid Fever, 109

Section 3: Fungal Infections, 111

54 Blastomycosis, 113

55 Coccidioidomycosis, 115

56 Histoplasmosis, 117

57 Mycetoma, 119

58 Paracoccidioidomycosis, 121

59 Penicilliosis, 123

Section 4: Parasitic Infections, 125

60 Amebiasis, *Entamoeba histolytica*, 127

61 Anisakidosis, 129

62 Babesiosis, 131

63 Capillariasis, Intestinal, 133

64 Clonorchiasis, 135

65 Cysticercosis, 137

66 Diphyllobothriasis, 139

67 Dracunculiasis, 141

68 Echinococcosis, *Echinococcus multilocularis*, 143

69 Eosinophilic Meningitis, *Angiostrongylus cantonensis*, 145

70 Fascioliasis, 147

71 Fasciolopsiasis, 149

72 Filariasis, 151

73 Hookworm, 153

74 Leishmaniasis, Cutaneous and Mucosal, New World, 155

75 Leishmaniasis, Cutaneous and Mucosal, Old World, 157

76 Leishmaniasis, Visceral, 159

77 Loiasis, 161

78 Malaria, *Plasmodium falciparum*, 163

79 Malaria, *Plasmodium knowlesi*, 165

80 Malaria, *Plasmodium ovale*, 167

81 Malaria, *Plasmodium vivax*, 169

82 Onchocerciasis, 171

83 Opisthorchiasis, 173

84 Paragonimiasis, 175

85 Schistosomiasis, Africa & Americas, 177

86 Schistosomiasis, Asia, 179

87 Strongyloidiasis, 181

88 Trypanosomiasis, African, 183

89 Trypanosomiasis, American, 185

Section 5: Viral Infections, 187

90 Avian influenza (A/H5N1), 189

91 Barmah Forest & Ross River Virus Disease, 191

92 Bunyamwera Viral Fever, 193

93 Bunyavirus Group C Disease, 195

94 California Group Virus Disease, 197

95 Chikungunya Fever, 199

96 Colorado Tick Fever, 201

97 Crimean–Congo Hemorrhagic Fever, 203

98 Dengue, 205

99 Eastern Equine Encephalitis, 207

100 Ebola and Marburg Virus Disease, 209

101 Hantaviral Disease, New World, 211

102 Hantaviral Disease, Old World, 213

103 Hendra and Nipah Virus, 215

104 Hepatitis A, 217

105 Hepatitis B, 219

106 Hepatitis C, 221

107 Hepatitis E, 223

108 Human Immunodeficiency Virus, 225

109 Human T-Lymphotropic Virus 1, 227

110 Japanese Encephalitis, 229

111 Lassa Fever, 231

112 Mayaro Fever, 233

113 Measles, 235

114 Monkeypox, 237

115 Mumps, 239

116 O'nyong-nyong Virus Disease, 241

117 Oropouche Virus Disease, 243

118 Poliomyelitis, 245

119 Rabies, 247

120 Rift Valley Fever, 249

121 Rotaviral Enteritis, 251

122 Rubella, 253

123 Severe Acute Respiratory Syndrome, 255

124 Sindbis Fever, 257

125 Tacaribe Complex Virus Disease, 259

126 Tick-borne Encephalitis, 261

127 Variant Creutzfeldt–Jakob Disease, 263

128 Venezuelan Equine Encephalitis, 265

129 Western Equine Encephalitis, 267

130 West Nile Fever, 269

131 Yellow Fever, 271

132 Zika Fever, 273

Index, 275

Editors

Contributors and Reviewers

David Addiss, MD MPH
Kalamazoo College, Kalamazoo, Michigan, USA

Tamuna Akhvlediani, MD
Clinical Research Unit, Technology Management Company, Tbilisi, Georgia

Cornelis W. Ang, MD PhD
Department of Medical Microbiology and Infection Control, VU University Medical Center, Amsterdam, The Netherlands

Kingsley B. Asiedu, MD
World Health Organization, Geneva, Switzerland

Kevin Baird, PhD
Eijkman Oxford Clinical Research Unit, Jakarta, Indonesia; Centre for Tropical Medicine, Nuffield Department of Clinical Medicine, University of Oxford, Oxford, United Kingdom

María-Gloria Basáñez, MSc PhD FRES
Department of Infectious Disease Epidemiology, Faculty of Medicine, Imperial College London, London, United Kingdom

Maria T. A. Berasategui, PhD
Department of Allergy and Immunology, Santiago Apostol Hospital, Vitoria–Gasteiz, Spain

Eric Bertherat, MD MPH
Epidemic Readiness and Intervention, EPR/CDS, World Health Organization, Geneva, Switzerland

Tiffany Bogich, PhD
EcoHealth Alliance, New York, USA

Michel Boussinesq, MD PhD
Institut de Recherche pour le Développement, Montpellier, France

Monica Brackney, MSc
HIV and Hepatitis Epidemiology Program, Infectious Disease Bureau, Epidemiology and Response Division, New Mexico Department of Health, New Mexico, Santa Fe, USA

Itzhak Brook, MD MSc
Department of Pediatrics, Georgetown University School of Medicine, Washington DC, USA

Simon Brooker, PhD
London School of Hygiene and Tropical Medicine, London, United Kingdom; Kenya Medical Research Institute-Wellcome Trust Research Programme, Nairobi, Kenya

Remi Charrel, MD PhD HDR
Uniteé des Virus Emergents, UMR190 'Emèergence des Pathologies Virales, Faculté de Medecine, Marseille, France

James Chin, MD MPH
Department of Epidemiology, School of Public Health, University of California at Berkeley, California, USA

Bruno B. Chomel, PhD
Department of population Health and reproduction, School of Veterinary Medicine, University of California, Davis, USA

Archie C. Clements, PhD
School of Population Health, University of Queensland, Herston, Queensland, Australia

Sally Cuttler, PhD
School of Health & Bioscience, University of East London, London, United Kingdom

Andrew A. Cunningham, BVMS PhD Dip ECZM MRCVS
Institute of Zoology, Zoological Society of London, United Kingdom

Alje P. van Dam, MD PhD
Department of Medical Microbiology, Onze Lieve Vrouwe Gasthuis Hospital, Amsterdam, The Netherlands

David Dance, MB ChB MSc FRCPath
Wellcome Trust-Mahosot Hospital-Oxford Tropical Medicine Research Collaboration, Mahosot Hospital, Vientiane, Laos

Peter Daszak, PhD
EcoHealth Alliance, New York, USA

Jeremy Day, MD PhD
Wellcome Trust Major Overseas Program, Oxford University
Clinical Research Unit, Hospital of Tropical Diseases,
Ho Chi Minh City, Vietnam; Centre for Tropical Medicine,
Nuffield Department of Clinical Medicine, University of
Oxford, Oxford, United Kingdom

David T. Dennis, MD MPH
Senior Associate Research, Duke-National University of
Singapore Graduate Medical School, Singapore;
Department Microbiology, Immunology and Pathology,
Colorado State University, Fort Collins,
Colorado, USA

Peter Deplazes, PhD
Institute of Parasitology, University of Zurich, Zurich,
Switzerland

Michael S. Diamond, MD PhD
Departments of Medicine, Molecular Microbiology,
Pathology & Immunology. Washington University School of
Medicine; Midwest Regional Center for Excellence in
Biodefense and Emerging Infectious Disease Research,
St. Louis, Missouri, USA

Arjen Dondorp, MD PhD
Mahidol Oxford Research Unit, Faculty of Tropical Medicine,
Mahidol University, Bangkok, Thailand; Centre for Tropical
Medicine, Nuffield Department of Clinical Medicine,
University of Oxford, Oxford, United Kingdom

Rogier van Doorn, MD PhD
Wellcome Trust Major Overseas Program, Oxford University
Clinical Research Unit, Hospital of Tropical Diseases,
Ho Chi Minh City, Vietnam; Centre for Tropical Medicine,
Nuffield Department of Clinical Medicine, University of
Oxford, Oxford, United Kingdom

J. Stephen Dumler, MD
Division of Medical Microbiology, Department of Pathology,
The Johns Hopkins University School of Medicine, Baltimore,
Maryland, USA

John M. Dye Jr., PhD
Virology Division, US Army Medical Research Institute of
Infectious Diseases (USAMRIID), Fort Detrick, Maryland,
USA

Sean P. Elliott, MD
Infection Prevention – UMC, AHSC-Pediatrics, Tucson,
Arizona, USA

Hubert P. Endtz, MD PhD
Laboratory Sciences Division, ICDDR, B, Dhaka, Bangladesh;
Department of Medical Microbiology and Infectious
Diseases, ErasmusMC, Erasmus University Medical Center,
Rotterdam, The Netherlands

Cyril O. Enwonwu, MDS PhD
Department of Biomedical Sciences, School of Dentistry,
University of Maryland, Baltimore, USA

Ryan Fagan, MD MPH
US Public Health Service, National Surveillance Team,
Centers for Disease Control and Prevention, Atlanta, Georgia,
USA

Elisabeth Fichet-Calvet, PhD
Bernhard-Nocht Institute of Tropical Medicine, Hamburg,
Germany

Hume Field, PhD
Queensland Centre for Emerging Infectious
Diseases, Biosecurity Queensland, Department of
Employment, Economic Development and Innovation,
Health & Food Science Precinct, Coopers Plains,
Queensland, Australia

Gerard Fitzsimmons, MD
Zoonoses, Foodborne and Emerging Infectious Diseases,
Communicable Diseases and Surveillance Branch, Office of
Health Protection, Australian Government Department of
Health and Ageing, Canberra, Australia

Agnes Fleury, MD PhD
Instituto de Investigaciones Biomédicas, UNAM/Instituto
National de Neurologia y Neurocirugia, Mexico City,
Mexico

Annette Fox, PhD
Wellcome Trust Major Overseas Program, Oxford University
Clinical Research Unit, National Hospital of Tropical
Diseases, Hanoi, Vietnam

Bernard Fried, PhD
Department of Biology, Lafayette College, Easton,
Pennsylvania, USA

Kenneth L. Gage, PhD
Bacterial Diseases Branch, Division of Vector-Borne
Infectious Diseases, Centers for Disease Control and
Prevention, Atlanta, Georgia, USA

Jeff Gilbert, MB BCh BVM&S
International Livestock Research Institute, Vientiane,
Lao People's Democratic Republic

Denise U. Gonçalves, MD PhD
Federal University of Minas Gerais, Postgraduate Program in Infectious Diseases and Tropical Medicine, Brazil

Carlos Graeff-Teixeira, PhD
Laboratório de Biologia Parasitária, Faculdade de Biociências, Pontifícia Universidade Católica do Rio Grande do Sul, Porto Alegre, Brazil

Marina Gramiccia, PhD
Reparto di Malattie Trasmesse da Vettori e Sanità Internazionale, Dipartimento di Malattie Infettive, Parassitarie e Immunomediate, Instituto Superiore di Sanità, Rome, Italy

Kevin Griffith, MD MPH
National Center for Emerging and Zoonotic Infectious Diseases, Division of Vector-Borne Diseases, Centers for Disease Control and Prevention, Fort Collins, Colorado, USA

Carlos Guerra, MD PhD
Spatial Ecology and Epidemiology Group, Department of Zoology, University of Oxford, Oxford, United Kingdom

Chadi A. Hage, MD
Pulmonary-Critical Care and Infectious Diseases, Indiana University, Roudebush VA Medical Center, Indianapolis, Indiana, USA

Kristin N. Harper, PhD
Robert Wood Johnson Health & Society Scholar, Columbia University, New York, New York, USA

John Hayman, MD PhD
Department of Anatomy and Cell Biology, Monash University, Victoria, Australia

Richard Hector, MD JD
UCSF, Global Health Sciences, San Francisco, California, USA

Brian Hjelle, MD
Departments of Pathology, Biology, and Molecular Genetics & Microbiology, Center for Infectious Diseases and Immunity, Health Sciences Center, University of New Mexico, Albuquerque, New Mexico, USA

Wim van der Hoek, MD MSc
RIVM, National Institute for Public Health and the Environment, Epidemiology and Surveillance Unit, Bilthoven, The Netherlands

Bethany Hoye, BSc
Department of Animal Ecology, Wageningen University, the Netherlands

Zdeněk Hubálek, DrSc
Institute of Vertebrate Biology, Academy of Sciences, Department of Medical Zoology, Valtice, Czech Republic (Sindbis virus map)

Lars Hufnagel, PhD
Cell Biology and Biophysics & Developmental Biology Programmes, European Molecular Biology Laboratory – EMBL, Heidelberg, Germany

Martin Hugh-Jones, PhD
Department of Environmental Sciences, School of the Coast and Environment, Louisiana State University, Baton Rouge, Louisiana, USA

Nnaemeka C. Iriemenam, MD
Department of Medical Microbiology & Parasitology, College of Medicine of the University of Lagos, Idi-araba, Lagos, Nigeria

Kathryn H. Jacobsen, MPH PhD
Department of Global & Community Health, George Mason University, Fairfax, Virginia, USA

Susan Jacups, MSc
School for Environmental Research, Charles Darwin University, Darwin, Australia

Paul Johnson, MD PhD
Infectious Diseases Department, Austin Health, Melbourne, Australia

Menno D. de Jong, MD PhD
Department of Medical Microbiology, Academic Medical Center, University of Amsterdam, Amsterdam, The Netherlands

Valerie Kapos, PhD
UNEP- World Conservation Monitoring Centre, Cambridge, United Kingdom

Jennifer Keiser, PhD
Department of Medical Parasitology and Infection Biology, Swiss Tropical and Public Health Institute, Basel, Switzerland

Charles H. King, BS MD MS
Center for Global Health and Diseases,
Department of Epidemiology and Biostatics,
Case Western University, Cleveland,
Ohio, USA

Anthony Kiszewski, ScD
Department of Natural and Applied Sciences, Bentley
University, Waltham, Massachusetts, USA

Boris Klempa, PhD
Institute of Virology, Slovak Academy of Science, Bratislava,
Slovakia; Institute of Virology, Helmut-Ruska-Haus, Charité
University Hospital, Berlin, Germany

Keith P. Klugman, MB BCh PhD FRCP
Hubert Department of Global Health Epidemiology,
Rollins School of Public Health, and Division of Infectious
Diseases, School of Medicine, Emory University, Atlanta,
Georgia, USA

Roman Kuchta, RNDr PhD
Department of Helminthology, Institute of Parasitology,
Ceské Budejovice, Czech Republic

Kiersten J. Kugeler, MPH
National Center for Emerging and Zoonotic Infectious
Diseases, Division of Vector-Borne Diseases,
Centers for Disease Control and Prevention, Fort Collins,
Colorado, USA

Jens H. Kuhn, MD PhD MS
Integrated Research Facility at Fort Detrick
(IRF-Frederick), NIH/NIAID/DCR, Fort Detrick,
Frederick, MD, USA

Satu Kurkela, MD PhD
Haartman Institute, University of Helsinki, and
Div Clinical Microbiology,
Helsinki University Hospital Laboratory, Finland

Ramanan Laxminarayan, PhD
Center for Disease Dynamics, Economics & Policy,
Washington DC, USA

Lisette van Lieshout, PhD
Department of Parasitology, Leiden University Medical
Center, Leiden, The Netherlands

Len J.A. Lipman, PhD
Division of Public Health and Food Safety, Institute for Risk
Assessment Sciences, Utrecht University, Utrecht, The
Netherlands

Rolf Luyendijk, MSc MPH
UNICEF, New York, USA

John S. Mackenzie, PhD
Australian Biosecurity Cooperative Research Centre for
Emerging Infectious Diseases, Division of Health Sciences,
Curtin University of Technology, Perth, Australia

Klaas W. Marck, MD PhD
Dutch Noma Foundation, Leeuwarden, The Netherlands

Luis A. Marcos, MD
Infectious Diseases Division, Washington University, Barnes-
Jewish Hospital, St. Louis, Missouri, USA

Santiago Mas-Coma, MD PhD
Departamento de Parasitologia, Facultad de Farmacia,
Universidad de Valencia, Valencia, Spain

Jolyon Medlock, FRES
Medical Entomology & Zoonoses Ecology group, MRA,
Emergency Response Department, Health Protection Agency,
Salisbury, United Kingdom

Andrew Mellinger
MDA Information Systems, Rockville, USA

Anna M. Molesworth, MSc PhD
National CJD Surveillance Unit, Edinburgh, United Kingdom

Kristy Murray, DVM PhD
Center for Infectious Diseases & Center for Emergency
Preparedness, The University of Texas Health Science Center
at Houston, School of Public Health, Houston, Texas, USA

Paul Newton, BM BCh DPhil MRCP DTM&H
Wellcome Trust – Mahosot Hospital – Oxford Tropical
Medicine Research Collaboration, Mahosot Hospital,
Vientiane, Laos

Maurício L. Nogueira, MD PhD
Laboratório de Pesquisas em Virologia,
Departamento de Doen as Dermatológicas,
Infecciosas e Parasitárias, Faculdade de Medicina de
São José do Rio Preto – FAMERP, Brazil

Peter Odermatt, PhD MPH
Swiss Tropical and Public Health Institute, Basel,
Switzerland

Gene G. Olinger Jr., PhD MBA
US Army Medical Research Institute of Infectious Diseases,
Virology Division, Fort Detrick, Frederick, Maryland, USA

Philippe Parola, MD PhD
Infectious Diseases & Tropical Medicine Unit, North
University Hospital, Marseille, France; WHO Collaborative
Centre for Rickettsioses and other Arthropod-Borne Bacterial
Diseases

Adalberto Pérez de León, DVM MS PhD
Knipling-Bushland U.S. Livestock
Insects Research Laboratory, United States
Department of Agriculture - Agricultural Research Service,
Kerrville, Texas, USA

Leon Peto, MD
Wellcome Trust Major Overseas Program,
Oxford University Clinical Research Unit,
National Hospital of Tropical Diseases,
Hanoi, Vietnam

William A. Petri, Jr, MD PhD
Division of Infectious Diseases and International Health,
University of Virginia Health System, Charlottesville,
Virginia, USA

Frederic B. Piel, PhD
Spatial Ecology and Epidemiology Group,
Department of Zoology, University of Oxford, Oxford,
United Kingdom

Sarah Polack, PhD
Department of Infectious and Tropical Diseases, London
School of Hygiene and Tropical Medicine, London,
United Kingdom

Ann M. Powers, PhD
Alphavirus Laboratory, Division of Vector-Borne
Diseases, Centers for Disease Control and Prevention,
Fort Collins, Colorado, USA

Ric Price, MD PhD
Global Health Division, Menzies School of Health Research,
Casuarina, Darwin, Australia

Gary W. Procop, MD MS
Department of Molecular Pathology, Cleveland Clinic,
Cleveland, Ohio, USA

Sarah Randolph, PhD
Department of Zoology, University of Oxford, Oxford,
United Kingdom

Richard Reithinger, MD PhD
Department of Infectious and Tropical Diseases, London
School of Hygiene and Tropical Medicine, London,
United Kingdom

Mary Reynolds, PhD
Poxvirus and Rabies Branch,
Centers for Disease Control and Prevention,
Atlanta, Georgia, USA

David J. Rogers, PhD
Spatial Ecology & Epidemiology Group (SEEG),
Department of Zoology, University of Oxford, Oxford,
United Kingdom

Gustavo C. Roman, MD
Alzheimer & Dementia Center, Methodist Neurological
Institute, Houston, Texas, USA

Thomas Romig, PhD
Department of Parasitology, University of Hohenheim,
Stuttgart, Germany

Charles E. Rupprecht, VMD MS PhD
CDC Rabies Program, Centers for Disease Control and
Prevention, Atlanta, Georgia, USA

Wendy W.J. van de Sande, PhD
Department of medical microbiology, Erasmus MC,
Erasmus University Medical Center, Rotterdam,
The Netherlands

Lance Sanders, PhD
Zoonoses, Food-borne and Emerging Infectious
Diseases Section, Communicable Diseases &
Surveillance Branch, Office of Health Protection,
Australian Government Department of Health and
Ageing, Canberra, Australia

Tomas Scholz
Department of Helminthology, Institute of Parasitology,
Ceské Budejovice, Czech Republic

Pere P. Simarro, MD
World Health Organization, Control of Neglected Tropical
Diseases, Innovative and Intensified Disease Management,
Geneva, Switzerland

Fabrice Simon
Department of Infectious Diseases and Tropical Medicine,
Laveran Military Teaching Hospital, Marseille, France

Marianne E. Sinka, PhD
Spatial Ecology and Epidemiology Group, Department of
Zoology, University of Oxford, Oxford, United Kingdom

Anthony Solomon, MRCP PhD DTM&H PGCAP
Hospital for Tropical Diseases/UCH, London, United
Kingdom

Mark Taylor, PhD
Molecular and Biochemical Parasitology Group,
Liverpool School of Tropical Medicine, Liverpool,
United Kingdom

Michael J. Turell, MD PhD
Virology Division, US Army Medical Research Institute of
Infectious Diseases, Fort Detrick, Maryland, USA

Annemarie van 't Veen, MD PhD
Department of Medical Microbiology, University Medical
Center Utrecht, Utrecht, The Netherlands

Paulo E.N.F. Velho, MD PhD
Department of Dermatology, Medical School, Campinas
University, Campinas, Brazil

Joseph M. Vinetz, MD
Division of Infectious Diseases, Department of Medicine,
University of California, San Diego School of Medicine,
La Jolla, California, USA

Henry J.C. de Vries, MD PhD
Department of Dermatology,
Academic Medical Center, University of Amsterdam,
Amsterdam, The Netherlands

Scott C. Weaver, PhD
Institute for Human Infections and Immunity,
Galveston National Laboratory, University of Texas
Medical Branch, Galveston National Laboratory,
Galveston, Texas, USA

Chris Whitehouse, MS PhD
U.S. Army Medical Research Institute of Infectious Diseases,
Fort Detrick, Maryland, USA

Rodney E. Willoughby, MD
Department of Pediatric Infectious Diseases,
Medical College of Wisconsin, Milwaukee,
Wisconsin, USA

Foreword

Maps have magical properties. They convert all kinds of data into colors, shades, shapes, and figures, and display them in a spatial framework. Map-making involves planting data on drawings of contours of land masses or representations of geographic regions. Maps are an ancient and common form of communication. Maps enable us to see where we are and identify many attributes of people, places – really any characteristic of the biosphere – by geographic location. Maps can convey large volumes of information, tell stories, and help to answer questions. Here we have an atlas, a collection of maps. As someone with in inordinate fondness for maps, I take great pleasure in this book.

The topic of the spatial distribution of diseases – and how and why this changes – has been one of endless fascination for me. Thus it was a joy for me to be contacted by someone else who also has a passion for this topic – for 'understanding the special preferences of infectious agents for specific niches and hosts.' Even better, Heiman Wertheim, who has led this project, has had the energy, creativity, and vision to pull together a book that assembles material that is essential for trying to make sense of the patchwork of infectious diseases globally. It is not an easy task to do even the first part – to create maps showing where diseases exist – or rather, where they have been reported in the past. Most maps showing disease distributions found in textbooks are old, based on incomplete data, and often out-of-date by the time they are printed. Disease distribution is dynamic because of the inherent properties of life and its interaction with the abiotic environment, and it is difficult to provide maps that accurately capture the current situation

Important as it is, it is not enough just to know where diseases have been if one is trying to understand why diseases exist in some locations or populations and not in others. Under- standing disease distribution requires input from multiple disciplines – and knowledge of microbiology and pathology is only a part of this. For this atlas, the authors have identified many of the critical environmental, ecoclimatic, and economic factors that influence the distribution of diseases. Some diseases can be transmitted only in focal areas because of the need for specific ecoclimatic conditions or a specific arthropod vector or an intermediate or reservoir host. But even pathogens with a global distribution are spread unevenly among regions or populations. For these diseases it is useful to know the geographic areas or populations at highest risk for infection. By also studying maps of features

called 'drivers of disease' – or by superimposing locations of cases on maps that display other characteristics, such as rainfall, for example – one can begin to identify some factors that may limit exposure or may predispose to specific infections. These maps provide important tools for spatial analysis to characterize risks of exposures or of outbreaks. Maps in this volume include ones showing features of the human population (e.g. size, urbanization, economic status, access to clean water and sanitation, nutrition, genetic factors), ecoclimatic conditions (e.g. climate, elevation, mountain ranges, rainfall, type of land cover or terrain), other life (e.g. arthropod vectors, livestock). Other important drivers or combinations may emerge that are relevant for future analyses. The current maps show key attributes of people and places that influence the likelihood of exposure and vulnerability to infection or to poor outcome.

Even a casual review of the distribution of many of the diseases leads to the conclusion that areas that share two attributes, hot and poor, are disproportionately affected by infectious diseases. Species diversity (including that of organisms pathogenic for humans) increases at lower latitudes and decreases at higher latitudes (i.e. at greater distance from the Equator), also known as the species' latitudinal gradient. Many developing countries are also found in low latitude areas, which are regions of particularly high risk for infectious diseases, and poverty increases contact between pathogens and people through multiple mechanisms. Much of the global population growth today, and projected for the future, is in developing countries in low latitude areas.

Even if we have maps that perfectly depict the global situation today, things change. The pace of change in new infectious disease events has increased in recent decades. We are finding known diseases in new geographic areas (e.g. chikungunya virus infections); the spread of pathogens that are more antibiotic resistant (e.g. MDR-and XDR-TB), virulent, or transmissible; and the identification of new pathogens (e.g. SARS coronavirus). We humans are changing the epidemiology of infectious diseases at a brisk rate. Humans transport other life – macroscopic and microscopic — and change the Earth in ways that create fertile soil for the sustenance of microbes and their transmission. We have also created conduits for expanded and novel transmission events – transmission of cryptosporidium to large populations through municipal water supplies; transmission of prions, viruses, such as West Nile virus, protozoa such as *Trypanosoma cruzi* (the cause of Chagas disease), and other microbes through organ and tissue transplantation. Old diseases change – especially in becoming resistant to antimicrobials – in large part because of our inappropriate application of drugs for treatment. There are many reasons to believe that these changes in infectious disease events will continue and perhaps increase, driven by global travel and trade, high population size and density (humans and farmed animals), extensive contact between animals and humans, including markets in bushmeat, farms raising wild animals in large numbers for food and other products, the massive global market in exotic pets, and expansion of human populations into new geographic areas.

This magnificent book helps to show where diseases are and helps us to start to understand factors associated with that location. The authors reviewed an extraordinary amount of material to create these maps, many for diseases for which no maps or only crude ones existed. Many of the maps are unique and draw on data not previously used to develop maps.

This book provides a wonderful structure, the scaffold on which to add more data – or from which to jettison outdated material. The maps reflect the best available information, but the available databases are incomplete. The book provides a framework and an impetus for researchers and public health workers to add data to fill in the gray areas. The current collection is an excellent beginning. Even in geographic areas where good data is available, distributions may expand and contract, therefore maps will require continual updating. The maps also provide a useful research tool that will allow investigators to test a variety of hypotheses with respect to factors that drive disease location. This may allow projections about where a disease might appear, because of the constellation of attributes of the people, place, and other species present, even if cases have not been documented in that area. The sheer volume of data required is daunting because it is relevant to have knowledge of vectors, reservoir hosts for many diseases as well as data about the physicochemical and ecoclimatic environment. Maps of other drivers can be added, as they are found to be relevant for specific pathogens.

This first edition is an auspicious start to a project that will never be finished. The maps can be improved and will change over time, but will never be final.

Mary E. Wilson

Preface

Understanding the special preferences of infectious agents for specific niches and hosts has been the basis for my career as a clinical microbiologist. During my training I encountered Mary Wilson's book *A World Guide to Infections: Diseases, Distribution, Diagnosis* and realized that in order to render infectious diseases easily understandable, one has to display the overwhelming amount of available data using concise presentations, like maps. *A World Guide to Infections* was an eye-opener, as it comprehensively displayed the distribution of infectious diseases using tables, texts, and several maps

Since then, whenever I see a world map of the distribution of an infectious disease, I wonder who made it, what data was used to make it, and, most importantly, why the disease is confined to specific regions. Digging deeper, I often find that it is difficult to discover the sources for the maps, and inaccuracies are not uncommon (please let me know if you find any in this atlas). There is a pressing need for good maps with verifiable sources, and collecting all of these infectious disease maps together in one book allows the reader to leaf through and discover similarities between diseases and ecological niches, which helps an understanding of their distribution.

It took many years to go from idea to proposal, to secure funding and find a publisher, and, of course, to do the actual work. The map-making process began in 2007, and several maps made at that time needed an update by the end of 2010. As the distribution of infectious diseases adjusts to a shifting environment (war, deforestation, flooding, and other changes), maps will need periodic updates. Therefore, this atlas should be seen as a starting point and a living document. Besides showing the status of infectious diseases through 2010, the atlas also helps to explain why diseases occur where they do by showing the driving forces behind them.

It is my hope that this atlas will inspire health professionals to submit their own epidemiological data when they notice it has not been included. In particular, data from Africa is often absent owing to the lack of good diagnostics or of any incentive to publish findings. It is worrying that most countries on this vast continent are regularly depicted in the gray scale of 'No data,' except when it concerns HIV, malaria, poverty, or lack of sanitation. We hope this will change in the near future with the help of this atlas. Too often the etiology of disease syndromes is based on 'developed' world data, although data from Asia shows that this is often misleading. For instance, *Streptococcus suis* is a common cause of adult bacterial meningitis in several Southeast Asian countries, where it is more frequent than *Streptococcus pneumoniae* or *Neisseria meningitidis* that typically cause the disease in western countries. This kind of information has important consequences for treatment.

It has been a wonderful experience to assemble this atlas with Jack Woodall and Peter Horby. Jack is a walking encyclopedia with regard to arboviruses. His historical knowledge of infectious diseases and his network of well-known virologists are of tremendous value. Peter and I have been working together for four years for the Oxford University Clinical Research Unit in Hanoi. Apart from making the atlas, doing research with Peter on tropical diseases in Vietnam has been one of the most rewarding working experiences of my career

Many people have made important contributions to this atlas, but as they are all listed in the contributors section, I will not repeat them here. We are grateful to all those researchers who make their data available to the scientific community for use in other works, like this atlas. I want to thank the board members of the Infectious Disease Research Foundation who enabled us to obtain funding and to manage this project: Wim Ang, Maarten Merkus, Annemarie van 't Veen, Bernard Jan Verkoren, and Jaap Wertheim. The Malaria Atlas Project group has been a wonderful source of data, maps, and inspiration. Their rigorous method of map-making will hopefully be copied or, even better, improved by others for other diseases. Disease mapping is a rapidly evolving field and many more good maps are yet to come.

I am indebted to the Vietnamese colleagues with whom I work daily in Hanoi: Nguyen Van Kinh (Director of the National Hospital of Tropical Diseases), Bui Huyen Trang (Chi Trang), and Le Thu Thuy (Em Thuy) for their wonderful and patient administrative support. I am also very grateful to Jeremy Farrar, director of our research unit in Vietnam, for providing me with the opportunity and the freedom to assemble this atlas as part of our research program in Hanoi.

Finally, I am honored that Mary Wilson has written the Foreword for this atlas, as it was her book that set all this in motion.

This Atlas was made possible with funds from: MusartE Continuendo Foundation (The Netherlands); Infectious Disease Research Foundation (The Netherlands); and the Wellcome Trust (United Kingdom).

Heiman Wertheim
Hanoi

User's Guide

The atlas is divided into five sections: (1) Infectious Disease Drivers, (2) Bacterial Infections, (3) Fungal Infections, (4) Parasitic Infections, and (5) Viral Infections. Disease maps are ordered alphabetically within their section by the most commonly used name for the particular disease. In general, these are the names also used by the *Control of Communicable Diseases Manual* (CCDM, 19th edition). Synonyms for diseases are stated and diseases may be found by these other names using the index

Each disease map is accompanied by a fact sheet that provides key information on the pathogen, disease transmission, incubation time, clinical findings, prevention, treatment, epidemiology, main sources for the map, and key references. The definitions of each heading in the fact sheet are as follows:

- **Classification**: International Classification of Diseases codes (ICD-9 and ICD-10) are provided for each disease
- **Syndromes and synonyms**: Other names by which the disease may be known or types of diseases caused by the agent. Diseases are indexed by common name, syndromes, and synonyms.
- **Agent**: The disease-causing pathogen(s) with key characteristics. Agents are indexed.
- **Reservoir**: The main animal host or environmental niche where the pathogen is predominantly found and from where it can be transmitted.
- **Vector**: The living carrier that predominantly transmits the infectious agent to humans.
- **Transmission**: The mechanism(s) by which the pathogen is transmitted to humans
- **Cycle**: A summary of the lifecycle of the pathogen.
- **Incubation period**: Time period between the exposure to the pathogen and disease onset.
- **Clinical findings**: Key symptoms of the disease(s). A single pathogen may cause more than one disease syndrome.
- **Diagnostic tests**: Standard laboratory tests used to identify the infection.
- **Therapy**: Treatments commonly recommended for the disease. No specific recommendations are given for pregnant women or children.
- **Prevention**: Strategies to prevent infection and disease transmission.

- **Epidemiology**: Information on the determinants, distribution, and burden of the disease. Groups at risk of disease are also identified in this section.
- **Map sources:** Key sources used for the map are mentioned here.
- **Key references**: Key references relating to the disease are listed here.

The fact sheets for the maps in Section 1 'Infectious Disease Drivers' have a different format than those for the diseases. This section includes maps that illustrate some of the principal driving forces of infectious disease distribution, ranging from poverty and sanitation, to climate, forest cover, and antibiotic use. We acknowledge that for some factors shown in this section the relationship is two-way, with the factor being both a cause and a consequence of infection, e.g. poverty and undernutrition. Life expectancy and under-5 mortality are shown since infectious diseases remain a leading preventable cause of death and disability, especially in children and the poor. The fact sheets in this section provide a **definition**, the **trends** and the **relation to infections**. Also **map sources** and **key references** are included in these fact sheets.

We have utilized many different sources to compile this atlas, including review papers, primary research papers, maps produced by others, key reference texts such the *Control of Communicable Diseases Manual* (CCDM, 19th edition), and the websites of the World Health Organization and Centers for Disease Control and Prevention, USA.

The starting point for each map was to seek the most recent review on the disease and to establish whether a map of disease distribution was already available. Based on available information, the editorial team decided how the disease distribution should be visualized and with what data source(s). Where high-quality maps were already available we would use these unchanged (e.g. *P. falciparum* endemicity map) or modified and updated as needed, and permissions were obtained when necessary. Where there was no existing map, a literature search strategy was developed in order to gather information on disease distribution. The mapping team prepared draft maps for review and comment by the editors. Finally, the maps and fact sheets were sent for external peer review to check for accuracy and completeness.

DISCLAIMER

Although extensive effort has been made to produce accurate and up-to-date information, all geographic information has limitations due to the scale, resolution, date, and interpretation of the original source materials. The information shown on our maps is compiled from numerous sources and may not be complete. The authors are not responsible for any errors, omissions, or deficiencies in these maps. The maps are intended for illustrative and educational purposes. Medicine is a constantly changing field and huge amounts of new data emerge on a daily basis. Therefore, the contents of this work may not be up-to-date and should not be used as a guide to patient treatment, or as medical or travel advice.

This work does not imply the expression of any opinion on the part of the authors, the University of Oxford, or their or its sponsors concerning the legal status of any country or territory or concerning the delimitation of frontiers or boundaries.

Abbreviations

AFB	acid fast bacilli		IF	immunofluorescent assay
AMR	antimicrobial resistance		IgM	immunoglobulin class M
ARBO	arthropod-borne		IgG	immunoglobulin class G
AIDS	acquired immunodeficiency syndrome		im	intramuscular
BSL	biosafety level		iv	intravenous
CAR	Central African Republic		IVDU	intravenous drug user
CDC	Centers for Disease Control and Prevention, USA		MDR	multidrug resistant
CFR	case fatality rate		MSM	men who have sex with men
CFT	complement fixation test		ORS	oral rehydration solution
CSF	cerebrospinal fluid		PCR	polymerase chain reaction
DIC	disseminated intravascular coagulation		PEP	post-exposure prophylaxis
DNA	deoxyribonucleic acid		po	oral
DRC	Democratic Republic of Congo		RNA	ribonucleic acid
EIA	enzyme-immunoassay		RT-PCR	reverse transcriptase polymerase chain reaction
ELISA	enzyme-linked immunosorbent assay		SAE	severe adverse event
FAO	Food and Agricultural Organization		STD	sexual transmitted disease
GAVI	Global Alliance for Vaccines and Immunization		TB	tuberculosis
GDP	gross domestic product		UN	United Nations
GI	gastrointestinal		UNDP	United Nations Development Program
GIS	geographic information system		USA	United States of America
HAART	highly active antiretroviral therapy		WHO	World Health Organization
ICD	international classification of diseases			

The World

This section contains maps of five world regions: (1) Africa, (2) Americas, (3) Asia, (4) Europe, and (5) Oceania. Considering that this is an atlas of human infectious diseases and that most humans live on land, the oceans, the seas and the polar regions will therefore be outside the scope of this atlas. The Russian Federation has been split: the area west of the Ural Mountains is part of the map of Europe and the eastern side is part of the map of Asia. In 2011, Sudan was split into two seperate states: Sudan and South Sudan. Most maps in this atlas were made before this split and most maps will therefore still show Sudan and South Sudan as one country.

As the infectious disease maps do not always contain names of countries, the maps in this section can be used as a reference to locate a certain disease or disease driver. These maps show both landcover and elevation and may aid in identifying typical ecological environments for some of the infectious disease distributions included in this atlas.

WHO uses a different classification of world regions for their activities: (1) Africa, (2) Americas, (3) Southeast Asia, (4) Europe, (5) Eastern Mediterranean, and (6) Western Pacific (see below). Each region has its own WHO regional office and activities.

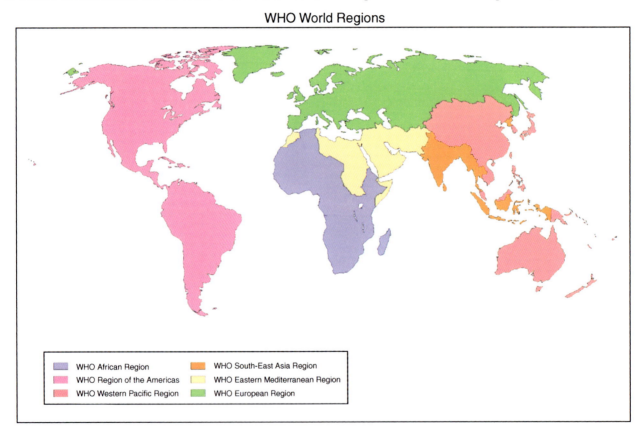

WHO World Regions

- WHO African Region
- WHO Region of the Americas
- WHO Western Pacific Region
- WHO South-East Asia Region
- WHO Eastern Mediterranean Region
- WHO European Region

MAP SOURCES

The world maps were made with landcover and shaded relief data created by Tom Patterson (and are available at http://www.shadedrelief.com/natural/index.html or http://www.naturalearthdata.com/), and were modified by ArcGIS software (Version 10, ESRI, California, USA).

Africa

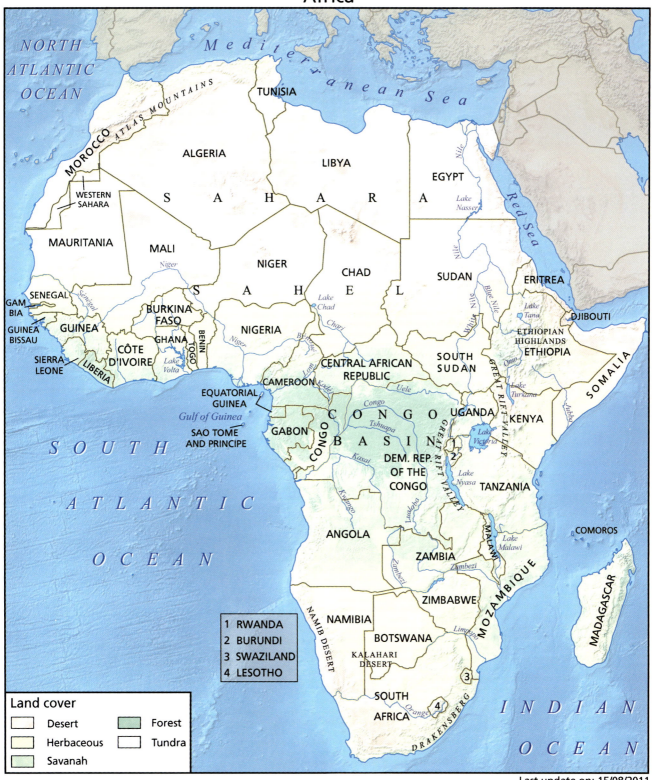

Land cover

- Desert
- Herbaceous
- Savanah
- Forest
- Tundra

1 RWANDA
2 BURUNDI
3 SWAZILAND
4 LESOTHO

Last update on: 15/08/2011

Americas

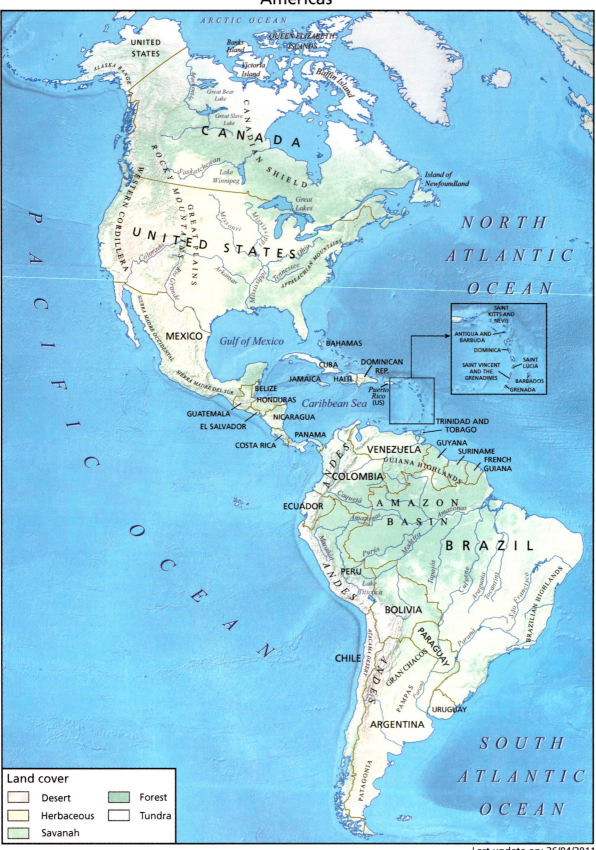

Land cover

- Desert
- Herbaceous
- Savanah
- Forest
- Tundra

Last update on: 26/04/2011

Asia

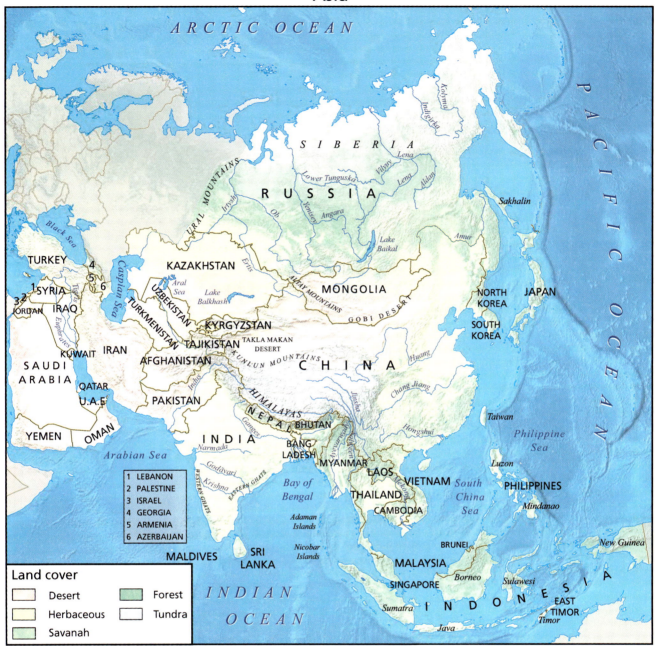

ARCTIC OCEAN

PACIFIC OCEAN

SIBERIA

Kolyma

Indigirka

RUSSIA

Lena

Lower Tunguska

Vilyuy

Lena

Aldan

Ob

Yenisey

Angara

Sakhalin

Irtysh

Ural Mountains

Lake Baikal

Amur

TURKEY

Black Sea

4
5
6

1 SYRIA

Caspian Sea

KAZAKHSTAN

Aral Sea

Lake Balkhash

MONGOLIA

GOBI DESERT

NORTH KOREA

JAPAN

3 2

JORDAN

IRAQ

Tigris

UZBEKISTAN

TURKMENISTAN

ALTAY MOUNTAINS

SOUTH KOREA

Euphrates

KYRGYZSTAN

TAJIKISTAN

TAKLA MAKAN DESERT

KUWAIT

IRAN

AFGHANISTAN

KUNLUN MOUNTAINS

C H I N A

Huang

SAUDI ARABIA

QATAR

Indus

Chang Jiang

Jinsha

Taiwan

U.A.E.

PAKISTAN

HIMALAYAS

NEPAL

BHUTAN

Hongshui

Philippine Sea

YEMEN

OMAN

Ganges

Narmada

INDIA

BANG LADESH

Ayeyarwady

MYANMAR

Luzon

Arabian Sea

Godavari

Salween

Mekong

LAOS

VIETNAM

South China Sea

PHILIPPINES

WESTERN GHATS

Krishna

EASTERN GHATS

Bay of Bengal

THAILAND

CAMBODIA

Mindanao

1 LEBANON
2 PALESTINE
3 ISRAEL
4 GEORGIA
5 ARMENIA
6 AZERBAIJAN

Adaman Islands

Nicobar Islands

MALDIVES

SRI LANKA

BRUNEI

New Guinea

MALAYSIA

Borneo

Sulawesi

INDONESIA

SINGAPORE

INDIAN OCEAN

Sumatra

EAST TIMOR

Java

Timor

Land cover

☐ Desert	☐ Forest
☐ Herbaceous	☐ Tundra
☐ Savanah	

Last update on: 26/04/2011

Europe

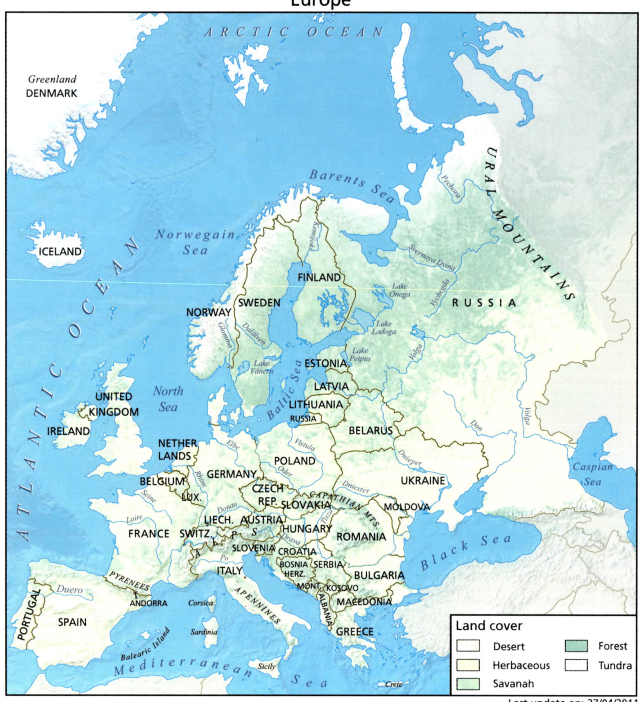

Last update on: 27/04/2011

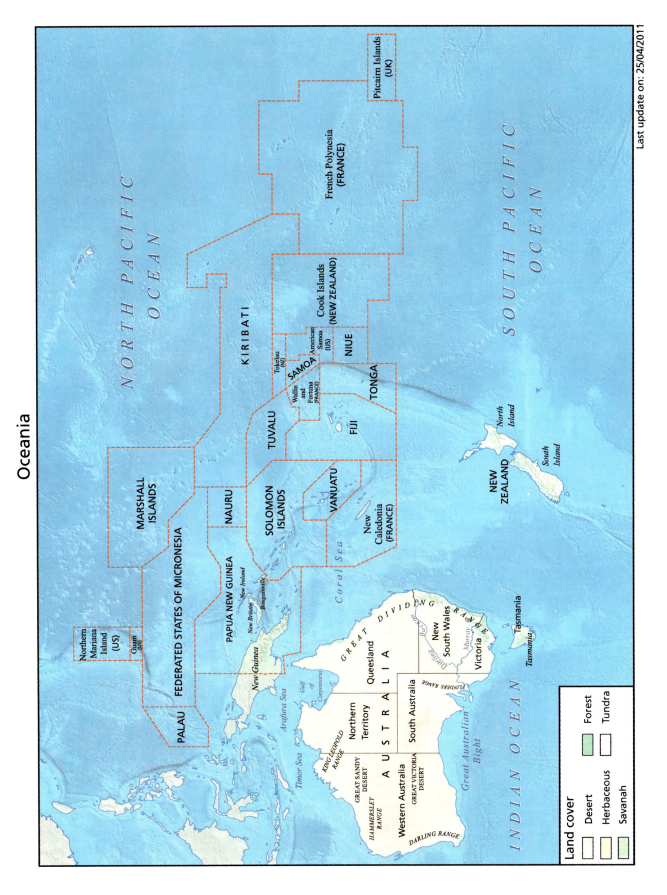

Oceania

Last update on: 25/04/2011

NORTH PACIFIC OCEAN

SOUTH PACIFIC OCEAN

INDIAN OCEAN

Pitcairn Islands (UK)

French Polynesia (FRANCE)

Cook Islands (NEW ZEALAND)

KIRIBATI

Tokelau (NZ)

American Samoa (US)

NIUE

SAMOA

Wallis and Fortuna (FRANCE)

TONGA

TUVALU

FIJI

MARSHALL ISLANDS

NAURU

SOLOMON ISLANDS

VANUATU

New Caledonia (FRANCE)

NEW ZEALAND

North Island

South Island

Coral Sea

Northern Mariana Island (US)

Guam (US)

FEDERATED STATES OF MICRONESIA

PALAU

PAPUA NEW GUINEA

New Ireland

New Britain

Bougainville

New Guinea

Gulf of Carpentaria

Arafura Sea

Timor Sea

GREAT DIVIDING RANGE

Queesland

New South Wales

Victoria

Tasmania

Tasmania

Murray

Darling

FLINDERS RANGE

Northern Territory

South Australia

AUSTRALIA

Western Australia

KING LEOPOLD RANGE

GREAT SANDY DESERT

HAMMERSLEY RANGE

GREAT VICTORIA DESERT

DARLING RANGE

Great Australian Bight

Land cover

☐ Desert		☐ Forest
☐ Herbaceous		☐ Tundra
☐ Savanah		

Infectious Disease Drivers

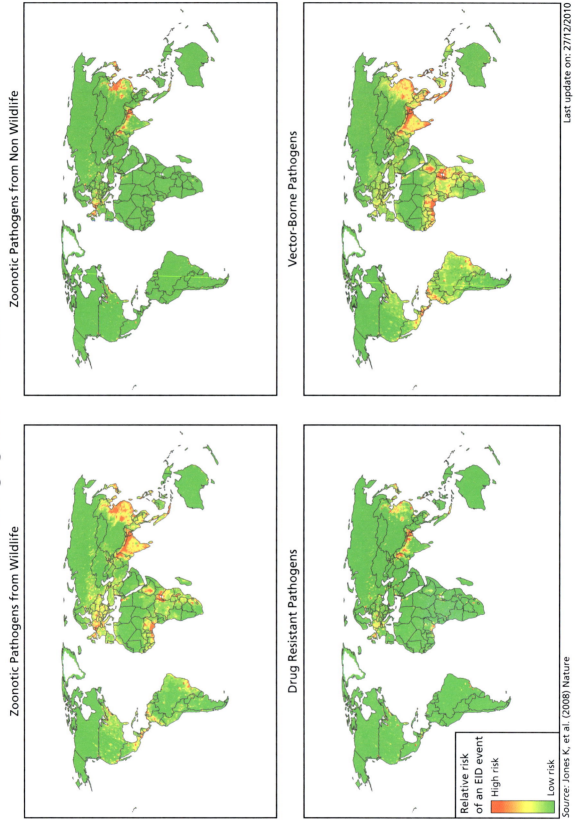

Emerging Infectious Diseases

Zoonotic Pathogens from Non Wildlife

Vector-Borne Pathogens

Zoonotic Pathogens from Wildlife

Drug Resistant Pathogens

Relative risk
of an EID event

High risk

Low risk

Source: Jones K, et al. (2008) Nature

Last update on: 27/12/2010

Subject: Emerging Infectious Diseases

Definition: According to a report by the Institute of Medicine (USA), emerging infectious diseases (EIDs) are diseases of infectious origin whose incidence in humans has increased within the past two decades or threatens to increase in the future. The maps opposite show the spatial distribution of the predicted relative risk of various categories of emerging infectious disease (EID) events, with green representing lower risk of an EID and red higher risk. The maps are based on an analysis of 335 EID events identified between 1940 and 2004, and the distribution of selected 'drivers' of EID events, such as population growth, latitude, and the richness of wildlife species. For this analysis an EID event was defined as 'the first temporal emergence of a pathogen in a human population which was related to the increase in distribution, increase in incidence, or increase in virulence or other factors that led to that pathogen being classed as an emerging disease'. The maps have been corrected for geographical reporting bias by adjusting for the frequency of the country listed for the affiliation of authors in each article in the *Journal of Infectious Diseases* from 1973 to 2004.

Patterns and trends: An analysis of the published literature suggests that the frequency of EIDs has increased since the 1940s, peaked in the decade 1980–1990, and declined slightly in the 1990s. The peak in the 1980s can be attributed to the HIV pandemic and the associated identification of a range of opportunistic infections. Another significant proportion of EID events is attributable to known pathogens with new antimicrobial resistance patterns. It is probable that the dissemination of diagnostic technologies and the development of more discriminatory and efficient methods for describing pathogen diversity (e.g. genotyping) has played an important role in the temporal increase in reports of EID events. There is also geographic heterogeneity in the reporting of EID events, with a preponderance of reports from North America, western Europe, Japan, and Australia. Undoubtedly this pattern is largely attributable to better funding and facilities for diagnosis, surveillance, and research, and of a culture of publication. The maps opposite are an attempt to identify future hot-spots of infectious disease emergence based on the distribution of 'drivers' that are associated with previous EID events whilst correcting for the geographic bias in reporting of events.

Significance: Emerging infections, whether they are entirely new pathogens, a resurgence of known pathogens, or new drug-resistant patterns, are a serious health and economic threat. HIV is a testimony to the possible health effects of a new pathogen, whilst SARS and influenza A/H5N1 are good examples of emerging diseases with limited health impacts but enormous economic impacts. Antimicrobial resistance is possibly the most significant emerging infectious disease problem now facing us. The health and economic impacts are not well characterized but there are indications that the situation is deteriorating as humans and animals are exposed to an ever-increasing volume and diversity of antimicrobial agents. It is now well recognized that the emergence of new infections is predominantly driven by human activities, whether that be increased contact with wild animals, changes in farming practices, drug pressure, or through disturbance of ecological balances. Biodiversity loss frequently increases disease transmission. In contrast, areas of naturally high biodiversity can serve as a source pool for new pathogens. Much of the research on EIDs is therefore now focused on identifying the specific conditions that drive EID events, monitoring pathogen ecology in putative 'hot-spots,' and developing interventions to mitigate the risk of EID events.

Map sources: The Emerging Infectious Diseases map is reproduced with the original data from Jones et al. (2008), with permission.

Key references

Committee on Emerging Microbial Threats to Health, Institute of Medicine Report (1992) Emerging Infections: Microbial Threats to Health in the United States.

Jones KE, et al. (2008) Global trends in emerging infectious diseases. *Nature* **451**:990–994.

Keesing F, et al. (2010) Impacts of biodiversity on the emergence and transmission of infectious diseases. *Nature* **468**(7324):647–652.

Morens DM, et al. (2001) The challenge of emerging and re-emerging infectious diseases. *Nature* **430** (6996):242–249.

Wolfe ND, et al. (2005) Bushmeat hunting, deforestation, and prediction of zoonoses emergence. *Emerg Infect Dis* **11**(12):1822–1827.

4

World Population

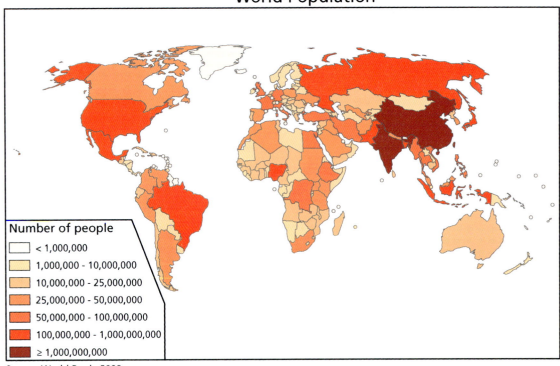

Number of people
- ☐ < 1,000,000
- ☐ 1,000,000 - 10,000,000
- ☐ 10,000,000 - 25,000,000
- ☐ 25,000,000 - 50,000,000
- ☐ 50,000,000 - 100,000,000
- ☐ 100,000,000 - 1,000,000,000
- ☐ ≥ 1,000,000,000

Source: World Bank, 2009

Population Density

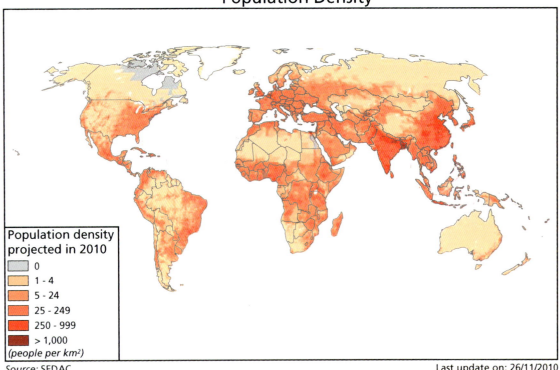

Population density
projected in 2010
- ☐ 0
- ☐ 1 - 4
- ☐ 5 - 24
- ☐ 25 - 249
- ☐ 250 - 999
- ☐ > 1,000

(people per km²)

Source: SEDAC

Last update on: 26/11/2010

Subject: Population

Definition: The maps opposite show the estimated number of people living within national boundaries in 2007 (top) and the number of people per square kilometer of land, the population density (bottom). National populations are generally estimated through intermittent national censuses, which attempt to enumerate all people alive and living in the country on a specified day. The United Nations recommends a census every 10 years. Between censuses, estimates of population are derived by extrapolation, using birth, death, and migration statistics and other survey data. The reliability of population estimates varies considerably, with, at one extreme, Iceland maintaining a full population register, while Somalia last conducted a national census in 1987. Population density at national level hides a great degree of internal heterogeneity, with populations more or less concentrated in cities.

Trends: The population growth rate is closely linked to the level of economic development, with growth rates in the poorest countries being twice that of the developed world. The world population is expected to increase from the current 6.8 billion to over 9 billion by 2050. Most of this increase (roughly the population of Italy every year) will occur in developing countries, with the population of developed countries remaining fairly stable. Over the same period the population living in urban areas is expected to increase by around 2.9 billion; therefore urban areas will absorb all of the predicted population growth over the next 4 decades and also pull in people from rural settings (see Urbanization map). Although rural populations are expected to decline somewhat over coming decades, it is important to note that in Africa and Asia 6 out of every 10 people still live in rural areas.

Population aging is also a significant phenomenon and although the populations of developing countries remain predominantly young, globally the fastest growing age group is those aged 60 years and over and many developing countries face a significant increase in the proportion of their population that is elderly.

Significance for infectious diseases: It has long been argued that war, famine, and disease are the inevitable consequences when population density exceeds the natural carrying capacity of the ecosystem.

> "The power of population is so superior to the power of the earth to produce subsistence for man, that premature death must in some shape or other visit the human race. The vices of mankind are active and able ministers of depopulation. They are the precursors in the great army of destruction, and often finish the dreadful work themselves. But should they fail in this war of extermination, sickly seasons, epidemics, pestilence, and plague advance in terrific array, and sweep off their thousands and tens of thousands."
>
> Malthus TR (1798) *An Essay on the Principle of Population,*. Chapter VII, p. 61

Malthus failed, however, to predict the ability of technological, commercial, and social advances to sustain ever-increasing population densities. Although the size and demographic profile of populations influence the infectious diseases that thrive, densely populated countries can be healthy. For health policy makers, a distinction is needed between the risk of infection, which may be greatest in poor rural areas, and the overall burden, which may be greatest in densely populated areas.

Map sources: World Population 2009 data obtained from World Bank and population density data from *Gridded Population of the World*, version 3 (GPWv3) by the Center for International Earth Science Information Network (CIESIN), available at Socioeconomic Data and Applications Center (SEDAC), at: http://sedac.ciesin.columbia.edu/gpw/credits.jsp.

Key references

United Nations, Department of Economic and Social Affairs, Population Division (2008): *World Population Prospects: The 2008 Revision.* New York.

United Nations, Department of Economic and Social Affairs, Population Division (2010) *World Urbanization Prospects: The 2009 Revision: Highlights.* New York.

Atlas of Human Infectious Diseases, First Edition. Heiman F.L. Wertheim, Peter Horby and John P. Woodall.
© 2012 Blackwell Publishing Ltd. Published 2012 by Blackwell Publishing Ltd.

Urbanization

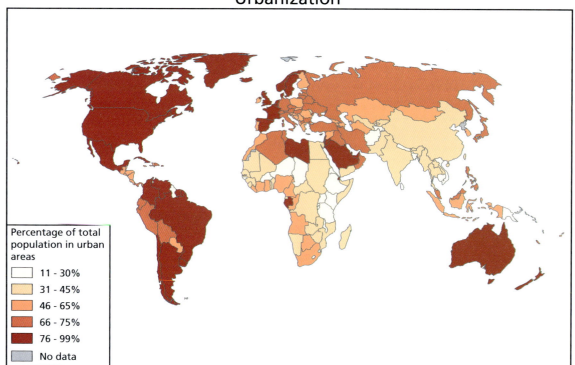

Percentage of total population in urban areas

- 11 - 30%
- 31 - 45%
- 46 - 65%
- 66 - 75%
- 76 - 99%
- No data

Population in Urban Slums

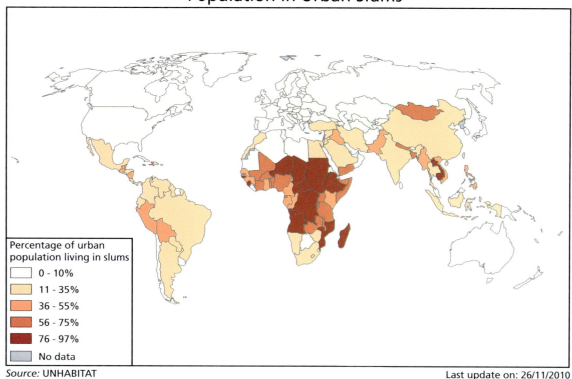

Percentage of urban population living in slums

- 0 - 10%
- 11 - 35%
- 36 - 55%
- 56 - 75%
- 76 - 97%
- No data

Source: UNHABITAT

Last update on: 26/11/2010

Subject: Urbanization

Definition: Urbanization is an increase in the *proportion* of people living in urban settings. Urban growth is an increase in the *number* of people living in cities. If population growth rates are equal in rural and urban areas, urban growth can occur without urbanization. Most changes in urbanization are due to the migration of people into or out of urban areas. Urbanization can also occur if areas become newly defined as urban because of changes in administrative boundaries or definitions of 'urban'.

Trends: We live in a predominantly urban world: in 2009 the proportion of the global population living in urban settings exceeded 50% for the first time, with an estimated 3.4 billion people living in urban areas, more than the entire global population in 1960. This trend is expected to continue, with urban areas absorbing all of the expected population growth over the next four decades. By 2050 the world urban population is predicted to have increased 84% compared to 2009, with 69% of the population living in urban settings. Most of the world's urban population is now concentrated in low- or middle-income countries: Asia now has half the world's urban population and Africa's urban population is larger than that of North America. Asia and Africa have three-quarters of the world's 100 fastest-growing large cities, whereas Europe has none. Although megacities (cities with at least 10 million inhabitants) receive a lot of attention, they are home to less than 10% of the world urban population, whilst over half of urban residents live in towns and cities of less than half a million inhabitants, and one third in towns of less than 100,000 people. Although the proportion of the urban population living in slums in the developing world has declined from 39% in 2000 to 32% in 2010, the absolute numbers have increased and an estimated 1 billion people (1 in 3 urban dwellers) live in slums or informal settlements.

Significance for infections: Urbanization is a feature of stronger economies, and higher levels of urbanization are associated with higher per capita incomes and with better health. Urban areas usually have a better provision of drinking water, sanitation, education, and healthcare than rural areas of the same country, and consequently urban populations have better health. Cities are, however, home to great inequalities and the health of the urban poor can be as bad, or even worse, than that of the rural poor. Slum dwelling is associated with increased risks of diarrhea, typhoid, respiratory diseases, and tuberculosis. Vector born diseases such as malaria and dengue may also flourish in slum settings. Historically, cities have been closely associated with epidemics and the increased mixing, mobility, and consumer demands of urban populations means that urban centers continue to drive disease epidemiology. Cities may act as 'pace-makers' of local epidemiology (e.g. dengue), hubs for national and global spread (e.g. SARS and influenza), or as a bridge between people and ecosystems (e.g. H5N1). Urban life is also associated with a heterogeneous landscape of social behaviors and a patchwork of subcultures and communities. Consequently, cities will contain subpopulations with increased risk of sexually transmitted infections, infections associated with injecting drug use (e.g. blood-borne viruses, anthrax), imported infections, and tuberculosis. The concentration of healthcare services, people, and wealth in cities provides abundant opportunities for the generation and transmission of healthcare-associated infections and antimicrobial resistance. The multitude and magnitude of food production and distribution systems, including extensive urban and peri-urban farming in low-income countries, may result in favorable conditions for food-borne infections.

Key references

Patel RB (2009) Urbanization – an emerging humanitarian disaster. *NEJM*, **361**, 8.

Saker L et al. (2004) *Globalization and Infectious Diseases: A Review of the Linkages*. UNICEF/UNDP/World Bank/WHO.

Satterthwaite D (2007) *The Transition to a Predominantly Urban World and its Underpinnings*. International Institute for Environment and Development.

United Nations Department of Economic and Social Affairs/ Population Division (2009) *World Urbanization Prospects: The 2009 Revision*.

United Nations Human Settlements Programme (2008) *State of the World's Cities 2010/2011. Bridging the Urban Divide*.

Atlas of Human Infectious Diseases, First Edition. Heiman F.L. Wertheim, Peter Horby and John P. Woodall.
© 2012 Blackwell Publishing Ltd. Published 2012 by Blackwell Publishing Ltd.

Global Connectivity

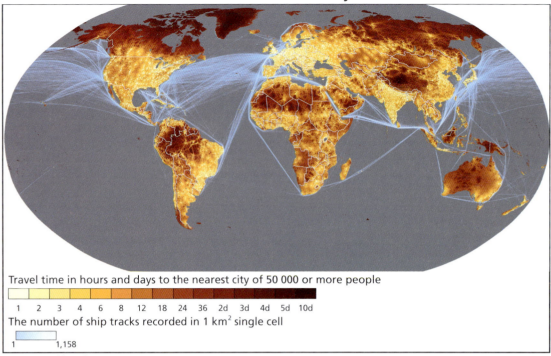

Travel time in hours and days to the nearest city of 50 000 or more people

1 2 3 4 6 8 12 18 24 36 2d 3d 4d 5d 10d

The number of ship tracks recorded in 1 km² single cell

1   1,158

Source: World Bank, 2009

Air Travel

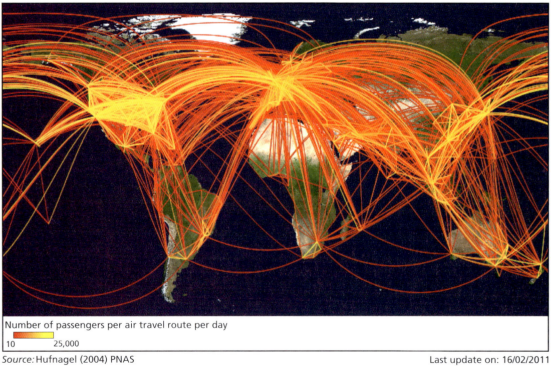

Number of passengers per air travel route per day

10   25,000

Source: Hufnagel (2004) PNAS   Last update on: 16/02/2011

Subject: Global Connectivity

Definition: Globalization has been defined as a change *'in the nature of human interactions across a wide range of spheres, including the economic, social, political, technological, and environmental.'* Increased connectedness of people in space and time is one dimension of globalization that is especially relevant for infectious diseases. The accessibility map (top) shows the estimated travel time in hours and days to the nearest town with a population of at least 50,000 and was produced by integrating a variety of data sources, including road and rail networks, waterways, national borders, and terrain (land cover, slope, and elevation). The top map also shows the major shipping routes. The bottom map shows major air travel routes.

Trends: Human interactions on a physical and intellectual level have been increasing for centuries but we are now more connected than ever. The dominant force behind this increasing connectedness has been economic, with individuals, corporations, and nations seeking ever-greater opportunities to exploit resources and new markets. New technologies have facilitated this contraction of space and time and now only 10% of the world is remote (defined as more than 48 hours' travel time to a big city). As well as improved methods of transport and communication, we have also witnessed a contraction of the space in which we live. The space that we choose to inhabit is now predominantly urban and in 2009 it was estimated that 95% of the world's population live on 10% of the land (see world population density map).

Significance for infections: Globalization has both positive and negative consequences for health. Increased accessibility to information, diagnosis and care, and preventive health services – such as immunization – have a very positive impact on health, as does access to education and, most importantly, the economic benefits of global integration. On the other hand, people and goods carry diseases and there are sobering historic examples of the devastating effect of the introduction of new diseases to vulnerable populations. Severe Acute Respiratory Syndrome (SARS) is perhaps the most dramatic modern equivalent, where air travel rapidly disseminated a highly virulent infection. More recently, a novel influenza A/H1N1 subtype emerged in Central America in 2009 and rapidly spread around the globe. However, the immediate and frightening impact of globally transmitted epidemic diseases such as SARS and influenza perhaps diverts attention from the importance of more insidious infections. The spread of HIV has been less rapid but much more damaging than any other contemporary epidemic and has undoubtedly been expedited by globalization, with HIV transmission associated with economic migrants, the commercial sex trade, and changes in sexual behaviors. Dengue is another globalizing disease: the precise reasons for the geographic expansion of dengue over the past 50 years are not clear but factors may include the dissemination of vectors through global trade and the movement of viruses by infected travelers. This demonstrates how increased connectivity links previously separated ecological systems and offers new opportunities for pathogens to extend beyond their traditional niche.

Map sources: Global accessibility map is obtained from World Bank Development Report 2009 and the Aviation map from Hufnagel L, et al. (2004), with permission.

Key references

Dollar D (2001) Is globalization good for your health? *WHO Bulletin* **79**(9).

Hufnagel L, et al. (2004) Forecast and control of epidemics in a globalized world. *PNAS* **101**(42).

Lee K (2003) *Globalization and Health; An Introduction*. London: Palgrave Macmillan.

Saker L, et al. (2004) *Globalization and Infectious Diseases: A Review of the Linkages*. UNICEF/UNDP/World Bank/WHO.

Tatem AJ, et al. (2006) Global traffic and disease vector dispersal. *PNAS* **103**(16).

World Bank (2009) *World Development Report 2009 'Reshaping Economic Geography.'*

Atlas of Human Infectious Diseases, First Edition. Heiman F.L. Wertheim, Peter Horby and John P. Woodall.
© 2012 Blackwell Publishing Ltd. Published 2012 by Blackwell Publishing Ltd.

Human Development

Gross Domestic Product per Capita

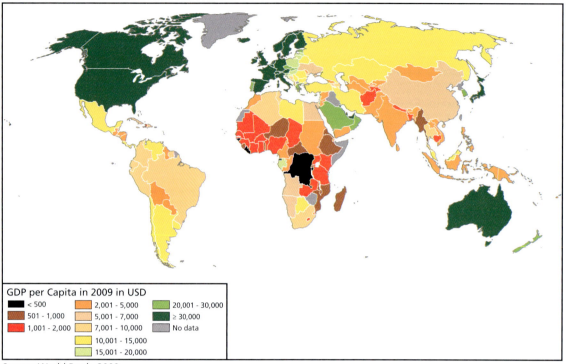

GDP per Capita in 2009 in USD

■ < 500	■ 2,001 - 5,000	■ 20,001 - 30,000
■ 501 - 1,000	■ 5,001 - 7,000	■ ≥ 30,000
■ 1,001 - 2,000	■ 7,001 - 10,000	■ No data
	■ 10,001 - 15,000	
	■ 15,001 - 20,000	

Source: World Bank, 2009

Human Development Index

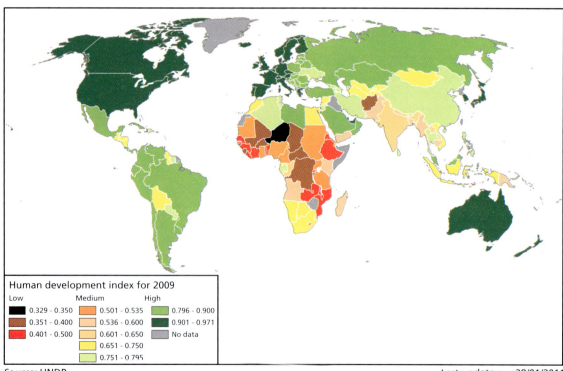

Human development index for 2009

Low	Medium	High
■ 0.329 - 0.350	■ 0.501 - 0.535	■ 0.796 - 0.900
■ 0.351 - 0.400	■ 0.536 - 0.600	■ 0.901 - 0.971
■ 0.401 - 0.500	■ 0.601 - 0.650	■ No data
	■ 0.651 - 0.750	
	■ 0.751 - 0.795	

Source: UNDP

Last update on: 28/01/2011

Subject: Human Development

Definition: Gross Domestic Product (GDP) is a measure of a nation's economic output and is defined as the total monetary value of all goods and services produced by a country in one year. The top map shows GDP per capita adjusted for purchasing power. The GDP per capita is simply the GDP divided by the number of people in the country. Purchasing power parity (PPP) is a method for adjusting for differences in the price of everyday items between countries by adjusting the GDP for the relative cost in US dollars of a common 'basket of goods.'

The Human Development Index (HDI) is a composite measure developed by the United Nations Development Program (UNDP) and introduced in 1990 to provide a single metric for comparing the level of socioeconomic development of countries. It is a derived from measures of life expectancy at birth, GDP per capita, and educational attainment. HDI is expressed as a value from 0 (lowest) to 1 (highest).

Trends: Economic development is a global phenomenon, and between 1999 and 2005 the number of people living on $1.25 per day or less fell by 325 million. The speed of development has not, however, been equal and Sub-Saharan Africa has lagged behind other regions. Following independence from colonial rule in the mid 1970s, Sub-Saharan Africa has been characterized by low growth with a long period of stagnation, and even declines in GDP, between the 1970s and mid-1990s; but from around 1995 growth has taken off.

GDP is strongly correlated with health indices such as life expectancy and infant mortality, and as national income increases, poverty falls and health increases. However, some countries have better health indices than expected from their GDP, whereas others have lower than expected health indices (see Gapminder: http://www.gapminder.org/). A comparison of the two maps opposite reveals areas where HDI is relatively high for the GDP (e.g. Vietnam and Cuba). Snapshots of GDP and HDI do not encompass trends in the difference in income and health status between the richest and poorest people or countries. Although the direction and extent of inter- and intra-country income inequalities has been argued, it remains that 40% of the world's wealth is owned by just 1% of the population, and around 2 billion people live on less than $2 a day.

Significance for infectious diseases: Poverty is the single most important global determinant of infectious disease risk. Poverty is a marker of a constellation of vulnerabilities that includes environmental, sanitary, nutritional, behavioral, and healthcare access components. But poverty is also both the result and a cause of poor governance structures, a condition that is accompanied by weak preventive and curative health systems, food insecurity, and internal social disruption. In general, infectious diseases remain a significant health problem in countries with low GDP, whereas non-communicable diseases dominate the illness landscape of richer nations. The combined causal effects of infectious diseases on poverty and poverty on infectious diseases results in a positive feedback system, leading to 'poverty traps.' The epidemiological transition, from infectious diseases to non-communicable diseases, is not, however, always smooth and many countries experience a period of a 'double-burden' where infectious diseases predominate in certain risk groups while non-communicable diseases begin to burden more affluent sectors of society. Achieving continued reductions in poverty is probably the most effective intervention to reduce the global burden of infectious diseases. This should include simultaneous improvement of public health systems for disease prevention in areas of extreme poverty.

Map sources: The Human Development map is derived from the UNDP Human Development Report 2009 and the data relate to 2007.

Key references

Bonds MH, et al. (2010) Poverty trap formed by the ecology of infectious diseases. *Proc Biol Sci* **277**(1685):1185–1192.

Human Development Report (2009) *Overcoming Barriers: Human Mobility and Developement*. UNDP. ISBN 978-0-230-23904-3.

Regional Economic Outlook (2008) *Sub-Saharan Africa*. World Economic and Financial Summaries. International Monetary Fund 2008. ISBN 978-1-58906-763-9.

World Economic Outlook. *Rebalancing Growth*. ISBN 978-1-58906-915-2.

World Bank (2010) *World Development Indicators*. ISBN 978-0-8213-8232-5.

Atlas of Human Infectious Diseases, First Edition. Heiman F.L. Wertheim, Peter Horby and John P. Woodall.
© 2012 Blackwell Publishing Ltd. Published 2012 by Blackwell Publishing Ltd.

Global Peace Index

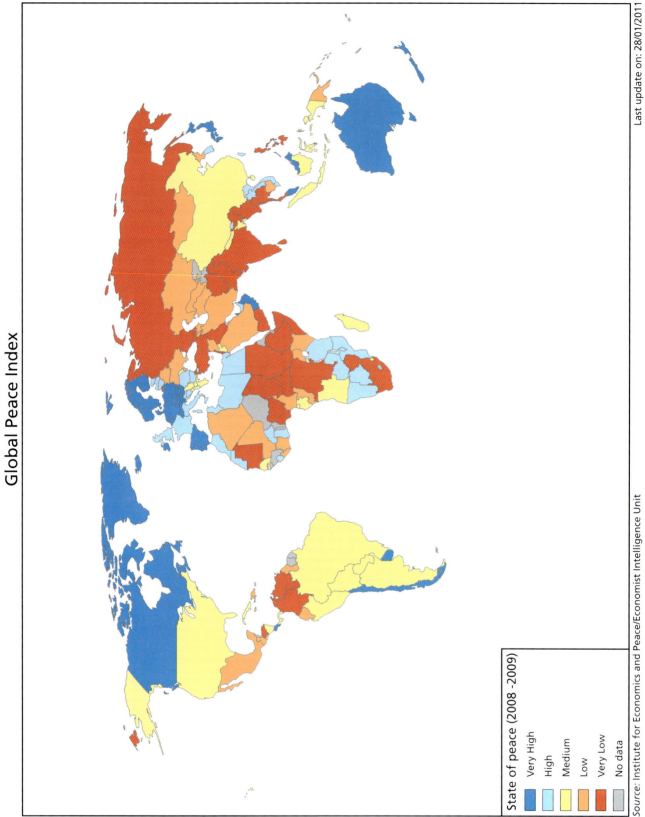

State of peace (2008 - 2009)

Very High
High
Medium
Low
Very Low
No data

Source: Institute for Economics and Peace/Economist Intelligence Unit

Last update on: 28/01/2011

Subject: Global Peace Index

Definition: The Global Peace Index (GPI) is a composite measure of 23 different quantitative and qualitative measures intended to give an overall, relative measure of *peacefulness*. The measures are broadly categorized into (a) societal safety and security (internal peace), such as violent crime, political, stability respect of human rights, displaced persons; and (b) militarization (external peace). The 2010 GPI ranks 149 countries using data from 2008 and 2009.

Trends: Western Europe (and Scandinavia in particular) is the most peaceful region; followed by North America and then central and eastern Europe. Sub-Saharan Africa is the region least at peace while nations in a chronic state of war or internal conflict – such as Iraq, Afghanistan, Somalia, and Sudan – are, unsurprisingly, the lowest ranked. Although the GPI has only been in existence for four years, it suggests that over this period the world has become slightly less peaceful. Over a longer time-scale the overall level of conflict has declined since the end of the Cold War in the early 1990s but there are predictions that climate change, population growth, resource scarcity, ideological movements, and shifts in global power will result in an increase in conflicts in the coming decades.

Significance for infectious diseases: Health security is one dimension of human security that is adversely affected by violence, conflict, and societal instability. Good governance and political stability leads to societal security, wealth, and health; whereas conflict results in poverty, degraded infrastructure, dysfunctional systems, poor living condition, under nutrition, anxiety, and ultimately illness and death.

Acutely, war kills people through violence, but may also increase the burden of infections through sexual violence and the transmission of sexually transmitted infections, and through the displacement of large numbers of people who, gathered together, are at risk of diseases that flourish in crowded and unsanitary conditions, such as cholera, dysentery, measles, and respiratory infections. Displacement is also associated with acute food insecurity, leading to under-nutrition and an increased risk of infection and a more severe illness as a result of infection (see under-nutrition map).

Acute and chronic humanitarian crises result in a breakdown of preventive and curative healthcare systems. Poor healthcare infrastructure and a lack of infection control is repeatedly associated with outbreaks of blood-borne viruses such as Ebola hemorrhagic fever and a low GPI is correlated with shorter life expectancy and increased infant mortality. Poorly functioning immunization programs lead to inadequate control of vaccine preventable diseases such as polio, diphtheria, pertussis, measles, and yellow fever, while a breakdown of vector control can lead to resurgences of vector-borne diseases such as malaria. Conflict also results in disrupted public health surveillance systems, making it difficult to quantify the impact of conflict on infectious disease risks. However, specific studies of the health impacts of chronic crises, such as those in Darfur, Sudan, and the Democratic Republic of Congo, have shown that, following an initial peak in violent deaths, more deaths are caused by preventable, largely infectious, diseases than violence.

On an international scale, war spreads disease, with historical examples including influenza, typhus, and dysentery. Unconventional global conflict by non-state actors and the specter of the deliberate release of pathogens, such as anthrax and smallpox, have in the past decade added a new dimension to the international infectious risks of conflict.

Map sources: The Global Peace Index map was made with data from the Institute for Economics and Peace/Economist Intelligence Unit (2010). More detailed data on conflicts can be obtained from the Uppsula Conflict Data Program, available at: www.pcr.uu.se.

Key references

Coghlan B, et al. (2006) Mortality in the Democratic Republic of Congo: a nationwide survey. *Lancet* **367**(9504):44–51.

Degomme O, et al. (2010) Patterns of mortality rates in Darfur conflict. *Lancet* **375**(9711):294–300.

Gayer M, et al. (2007) Conflict and emerging infectious diseases. *Emerg Infect Dis* **13**(11):1625–1631.

Institute for Economics and Peace. (2010) *Global Peace Index* (available online from: http://www.visionofhumanity.org/info-center/media-pack/2010-global-peace-index/)

Zapor MJ, Moran KA (2005) Infectious diseases during wartime. *Curr Opin Infect Dis* **18**(5):395–399.

Atlas of Human Infectious Diseases, First Edition. Heiman F.L. Wertheim, Peter Horby and John P. Woodall.
© 2012 Blackwell Publishing Ltd. Published 2012 by Blackwell Publishing Ltd.

Life Expectancy

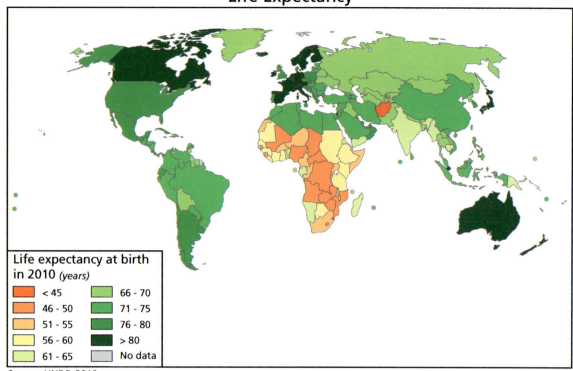

Life expectancy at birth
in 2010 *(years)*

▮	< 45	▮	66 - 70
▮	46 - 50	▮	71 - 75
▮	51 - 55	▮	76 - 80
▮	56 - 60	▮	> 80
▮	61 - 65	▮	No data

Source: UNDP, 2010

Child Mortality

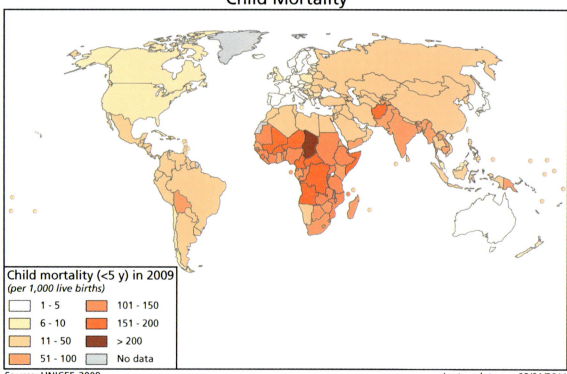

Child mortality (<5 y) in 2009
(per 1,000 live births)

▮	1 - 5	▮	101 - 150
▮	6 - 10	▮	151 - 200
▮	11 - 50	▮	> 200
▮	51 - 100	▮	No data

Source: UNICEF, 2009

Last update on: 09/01/2011

Subject: Life Expectancy and Child Mortality

Definition: *Life expectancy at birth* (top panel) is the number of years that a person can expect to live from birth. It is an average measure for the whole population and therefore obscures a great deal of nuance in the risk of death over the life course. A low-average life expectancy for a population may be due to a high child mortality (bottom panel) rate followed by a reasonable life span among those who manage to survive childhood. Life expectancy is a widely used measure of health because it is both sensitive to broad influences on health and is a simple measure that allows temporal and geographic comparisons. *Child mortality rate* (bottom panel) is the number of children who die before the age of 5 years per 1,000 live births.

Trends: Life expectancy has generally been increasing in most regions of the world, but some areas have gone through dips, the most notable examples being: (1) Sub-Saharan Africa where the HIV/AIDS epidemic has dramatically reduced life expectancy at birth in high prevalence countries, such that it is now less than 50 years for the southern Africa sub-region; (2) the USSR and post-Soviet countries which experienced rising mortality from the mid-1960s, especially among males. What is striking in the map opposite is the low life expectancy throughout most of Sub-Saharan Arica. HIV has contributed heavily to this in some countries but comparison with the Gross Domestic Product map shows how the distribution of poverty closely matches low life expectancy. In all regions the life expectancy of males is considerably shorter than that of females, mainly due to an excess risk of deaths between the ages of 15 and 60 years.

The under-5 mortality rate per 1,000 live births in 2009 was 60: ranging from 6 for industrialized countries to 150 for West and Central Africa. Seventy percent of under-5 deaths occur in the first year of life. Under-5 mortality has fallen by around one-third since 1990 and the rate of decline has increased in the period 2000–2009 compared to the 1990s. Despite this, only 9 of the 64 countries with high under-5 mortality rates (≥40 per 1000) are on track to achieve Millennium Development Goal 4 (to reduce by two-thirds the mortality rate among children under 5) by 2015, and in 2009 an estimated 8.1 million children died before their fifth birthday: an average of more than 22,000 deaths every day. Under-5 mortality is geographically concentrated; with 99% of all deaths in children under 5 occurring in developing countries, mostly in Africa (50%) and Asia (42%). Half of child deaths occur in five countries: India, Nigeria, Democratic Republic of the Congo, Pakistan, and China. In Sub-Saharan Africa 1 in 8 children die before their fifth birthday. The adverse effects of chronic war can be clearly observed in the low life expectancy and high childhood mortality in Afghanistan.

Significance for infectious diseases: Globally infectious diseases are the second commonest cause of death after cardiovascular disease, and in low-income countries infectious diseases remain the leading cause, with HIV/AIDS the leading cause of adult mortality in Africa. Additionally, approximately 18% of all cancers are caused by infections, e.g. liver cancer and hepatitis B and C, *H. pylori* and stomach cancer, cervical cancer and papilloma viruses, bladder cancer and flukes. However, infections that kill in childhood have a much greater influence on life expectancy figures than infections that kill older people. In 2008 pneumonia, diarrhea, malaria, and HIV/AIDS accounted for 43% of all deaths in children under 5 worldwide. This effect is especially marked in Africa, which contributes 9 out of every 10 childhood deaths from malaria, 9 out of every 10 childhood deaths from HIV/AIDS, and half of all childhood deaths from pneumonia and diarrhea. Although the contribution of infectious diseases to overall mortality has been declining infections remain a leading preventable cause of death and disability, especially in children and the poor.

Map sources: The Life Expectancy map was made with data obtained from the UNDP (available at: http://unstats.un.org) and the Child Mortality map with data from UNICEF (available at: www.childinfo.org).

Key references

Black RE, et al. (2010) Global, regional, and national causes of child mortality in 2008: a systematic analysis. *Lancet* **375**(9730):1969–1987.

Parkin DM (2006) The global health burden of infection-associated cancers in the year 2002. *Int J Cancer* **118**(12): 3030–3044.

Rajaratnam JK, et al. (2010) Neonatal, postneonatal, childhood, and under-5 mortality for 187 countries, 1970–2010: a systematic analysis of progress towards Millennium Development Goal 4. *Lancet* **375**(9730):1988–2008.

Report (2010) Levels and Trends in Child Mortality. Estimates Developed by the UN Inter-agency Group for Child Mortality Estimation.

World Health Organization (2008) *The Global Burden of Disease: 2004 Update*.

World Health Organization (2009) *Global Health Risks: Mortality and Burden of Disease Attributable to Selected Major Risks*.

Atlas of Human Infectious Diseases, First Edition. Heiman F.L. Wertheim, Peter Horby and John P. Woodall.
© 2012 Blackwell Publishing Ltd. Published 2012 by Blackwell Publishing Ltd.

Water and Sanitation

Access to Clean Water

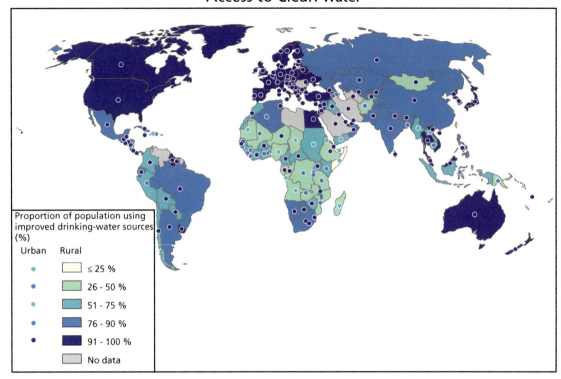

Proportion of population using improved drinking-water sources (%)

Urban | Rural
- | ≤ 25 %
- | 26 - 50 %
- | 51 - 75 %
- | 76 - 90 %
- | 91 - 100 %
| No data

Access to Sanitation

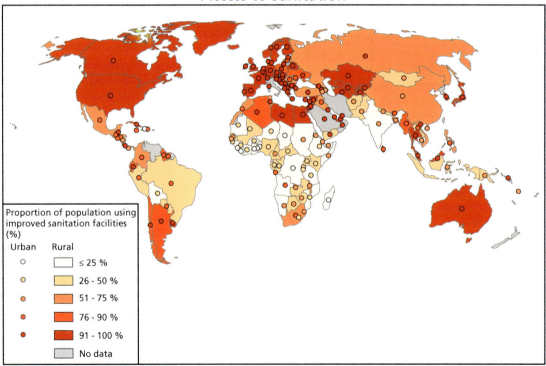

Proportion of population using improved sanitation facilities (%)

Urban | Rural
○ | ≤ 25 %
○ | 26 - 50 %
● | 51 - 75 %
● | 76 - 90 %
● | 91 - 100 %
| No data

Source: WHO / UNICEF Joint Monitoring Programme (JMP) for Water Supply and Sanitation   Last update on: 25/10/2010

Subject: Water and Sanitation

Definition: Millennium Development Goal 7, target 7c is to "Halve, by 2015, the proportion of people without sustainable access to safe drinking-water and basic sanitation." The two monitoring indicators to assess progress toward achieving this goal are (shown opposite) the *Proportion of population using an improved drinking water source* and *Proportion of population using an improved sanitation facility*. An *improved drinking-water source* is defined as one that is protected from outside contamination, in particular from contamination with fecal matter. An *improved sanitation facility* is defined as one that hygienically separates human excreta from human contact.

Trends: In 2008 an estimated 2.6 billion people do not have access to an improved sanitation facility and at the current rate of progress it is unlikely that the global sanitation target 7c of the Millennium Development Goals will be reached. Most countries in Sub-Saharan Africa and Asia are not on track to meet the sanitation target. The world is, however, on track to meet the drinking-water target. But that still leaves an estimated 884 million people (in 2008) without an improved drinking-water source, with Sub-Saharan Africa accounting for 37% of that number. Increasing water scarcity, as a result of population growth, urbanization, and climate change may challenge future progress in access to adequate water and sanitation.

Significance for infections: It is estimated that around 2.4 million deaths could be prevented annually if everyone had access to good water and sanitation and practiced good hygiene. Most of these deaths are of young children in developing countries from diarrhea or as a consequence of undernutrition related to diarrhea (see Undernutrition map). Infections associated with poor quality or volume of water can be categorized in to *water-borne*, *water-based*, and *water-washed* infections. Water-borne infections include: amebiases, typhoid, cholera, hepatitis A and E, campylobacter, rotavirus, *E. coli*, giardiasis, and cryptosporidiosis. Water-based infections include dracunculiasis and schistosomiasis. Water-washed infections are those, such as trachoma and scabies, where poor access to water for basic hygiene increases the risk of infection. Around 1 in 5 people in the world defecate in the open and in addition to the feco-orally transmitted infections already mentioned above, exposure to feces also results in a cycle of infection with intestinal nematode infections (Ascariasis, Trichuriasis, and hookworm disease). These intestinal parasites impair nutrition, growth, and cognitive function.

The distinction between water-borne or water-washed infections, and between water- or sanitation-related infections, is however somewhat artificial since the process of transmission of feco-oral infections involves unsafe disposal of feces and the vehicle for transmission may be unclean water, unclean hands, or contaminated food. Poor water and sanitation also contribute to the burden of non-diarrheal diseases, particularly respiratory infections. There are two main mechanisms for this: first, enteric disease increases susceptibility to non-enteric diseases such as pneumonia, and second, the risk of respiratory infections can be reduced by hand washing with soap and water.

It is estimated that 19% of deaths in children are associated with inadequate hygiene, water, or sanitation. This burden could be substantially reduced by the implementation of proven and cost-effective interventions to improve accessibility, quality, and reliability of basic water and sanitation services, and to improve hygiene practices.

Map sources: Data for the Water and Sanitation map was obtained from the WHO/UNICEF Joint Monitoring Programme (JMP) for Water Supply and Sanitation, available at: www.wssinfo.org/datamining/tables.html.

Key references

Bartram J, et al. (2010) Hygiene, sanitation, and water: forgotten foundations of health. *PLoS Med* **7**(11):e1000367.

Hunter PR, et al. (2010) Water supply and health. *PLoS Med* **7**(11):e1000361.

Mara D, et al. (2010) Sanitation and health. *PLoS Med* **7**(11): e1000363.

Prüss-Üstün A, et al. (2008) *Safer Water, Better Health: Costs, Benefits and Sustainability of Interventions to Protect and Promote Health*. World Health Organization: Geneva.

WHO and UNICEF (2010). *Progress on Sanitation and Drinking Water; 2010 update*. Joint Monitoring Programme for Water Supply and Sanitation.

18

Undernutrition

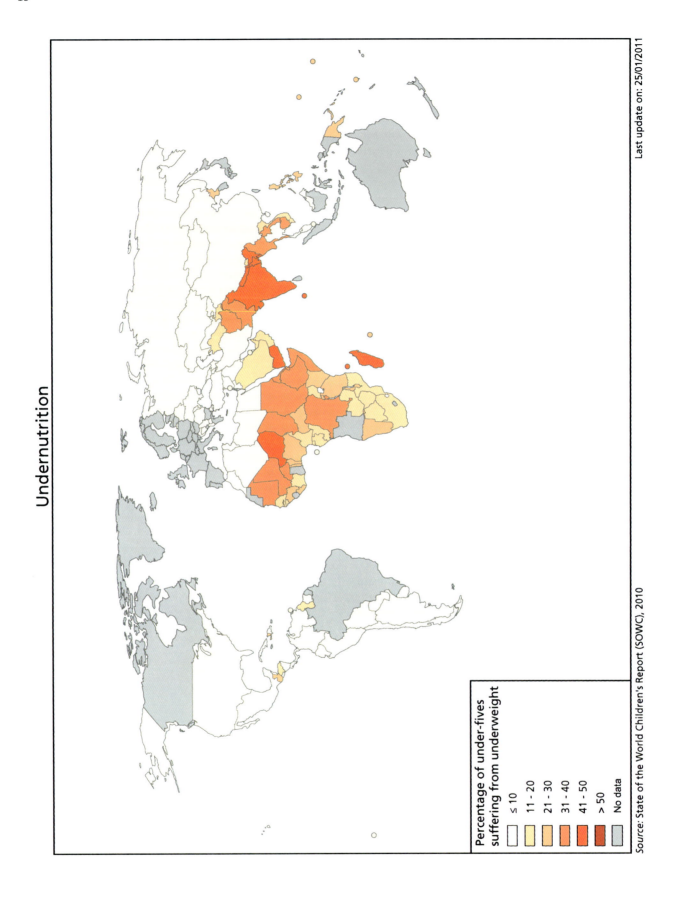

Percentage of under-fives
suffering from underweight

≤ 10
11 - 20
21 - 30
31 - 40
41 - 50
> 50
No data

Source: State of the World Children's Report (SOWC), 2010

Last update on: 25/01/2011

Subject: Undernutrition

Definitions: A person has *undernutrition* if his or her diet does not contain sufficient protein and calories for growth or maintenance, or if he or she is not able to absorb sufficient protein and calories because of ill health. Undernutrition manifests as low weight for age (underweight), low weight for height (wasted), or low height for age (stunted). The prevalence of stunting is a good measure of chronic undernutrition. A person has *overnutrition* if his or her diet supplies more calories and protein than he or she requires, leading to unhealthy weight gain. The term *malnutrition* encompasses both undernutrition and overnutrition.

Trends: Among children under the age of 5 in developing countries, an estimated 129 million are underweight and 195 million are stunted: more than 90% of the developing world's stunted children live in Africa and Asia. An even larger number of children suffer the effects of undernutrition in the womb and micronutrient deficiencies. One indicator of progress toward achieving Millennium Development Goal 1, the eradication of poverty and extreme hunger, is the proportion of children aged under 5 who are underweight. Progress toward this goal has been limited in Africa, with 28% of children under 5 years old being underweight around 1990, compared with 25% around 2008. Progress has been slightly better in Asia, with 37% underweight prevalence around 1990 and 31% around 2008.

Significance for infectious diseases: Undernutrition, including micronutrient deficiency (such as vitamin A and zinc), compromises mucosal integrity and impairs both innate and acquired immunity. This leads to both an increased risk of infection and an increased risk of severe disease and death. Common infections recognized to be associated with undernutrition include diarrhea, pneumonia, measles, malaria, and TB. Since these infections are widespread in less-developed countries, the impact of undernutrition on childhood deaths from infection is large, and undernutrition is estimated to contribute to one-third of all deaths in children under the age of 5 years.

Conversely, infection itself can increase macro- and micronutrient requirements, impair nutrient uptake and increases loses. Intestinal parasites in particular have a large impact on childhood nutrition as a result of loss of appetite, malabsorption, and chronic blood loss, which in turn lead to physical and intellectual growth retardation. Pneumonia, diarrhea, malaria, and HIV/AIDS are all recognized as direct causes of undernutrition.

Undernutrition and infection are therefore a deadly coalition, whereby undernutrition increases susceptibility to infection and infection exacerbates undernutrition. In a speech to at the World Food Summit in 2002, the Deputy Executive Director of UNICEF said,

> *"The world produces enough food to feed every man, woman and child on earth. Hunger and malnutrition therefore are not due to lack of food alone, but are also the consequences of poverty, inequality and misplaced priorities."*

Map sources: Data for the Child Undernutrition map was obtained from the State of the World Children's Report, UNICEF (2010), available at: www.unicef.org. Subnational level maps are available from the Center for International Earth Science Information Network (CIESIN), available at: http://sedac.ciesin.columbia.edu/povmap.

Key references

Black RE, et al. (2008) Maternal and child undernutrition: global and regional exposures and health consequences. *Lancet* **371**(9608):243–260.

Katona P, et al. (2008) The interaction between nutrition and infection. *Clin Infect Dis* **46**(10):1582–1588.

Schaible UE, et al. (2007) Malnutrition and infection: complex mechanisms and global impacts. *PLoS Med* 4(5):e115.

UNICEF Report. (2009) *Tracking Progress on Child and Maternal Nutrition. A Survival and Development Priority.*

Sen A (1981) *Poverty and Famines: An Essay on Entitlement and Deprivation.* Clarendon Press/Oxford University Press, Oxford, UK.

Atlas of Human Infectious Diseases, First Edition. Heiman F.L. Wertheim, Peter Horby and John P. Woodall.
© 2012 Blackwell Publishing Ltd. Published 2012 by Blackwell Publishing Ltd.

Climate

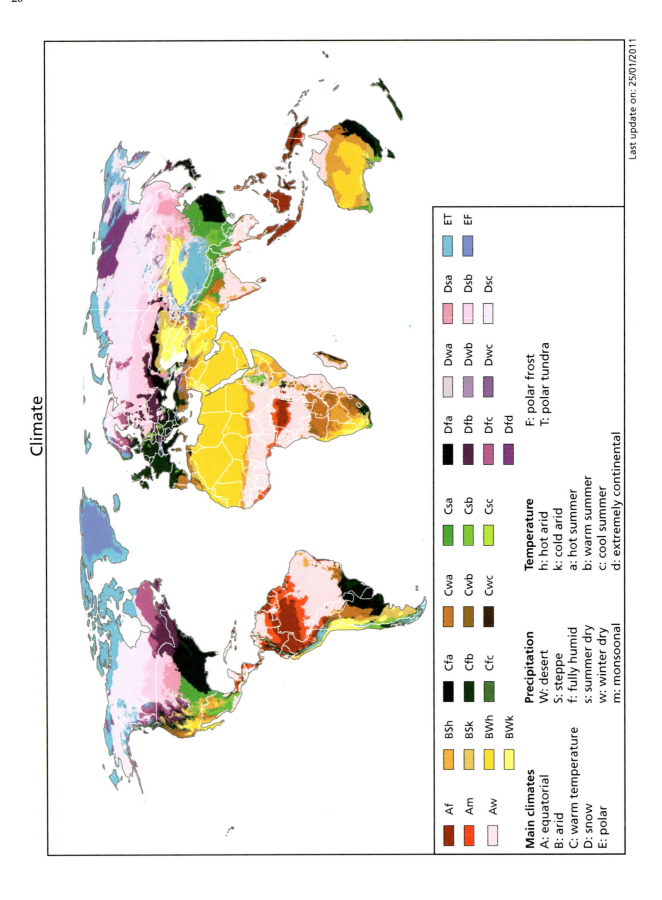

Last update on: 25/01/2011

Af
Am
Aw

BSh
BSk
BWh
BWk

Cfa
Cfb
Cfc

Cwa
Cwb
Cwc

Csa
Csb
Csc

Dfa
Dfb
Dfc
Dfd

Dwa
Dwb
Dwc

Dsa
Dsb
Dsc

ET
EF

Main climates
A: equatorial
B: arid
C: warm temperature
D: snow
E: polar

Precipitation
W: desert
S: steppe
f: fully humid
s: summer dry
w: winter dry
m: monsoonal

Temperature
h: hot arid
k: cold arid
a: hot summer
b: warm summer
c: cool summer
d: extremely continental

F: polar frost
T: polar tundra

Subject: Climate

Definition: Climate can be considered to be the "average weather." The map opposite shows climate zones based on the system developed by Wladimir Köppen and Rudolf Geiger in the early 1900s. The system classifies land surface into five major climate zones (designated by uppercase letters) based on annual and monthly mean temperature and precipitation. Further subdivisions (designated by lowercase letters) are based on seasonal patterns of temperature and precipitation. The data used to derive the map covers the period 1950–2000. The Köppen classification and variations on it remain widely popular.

Trends: The map opposite is based on annual and monthly climate data over a 50-year period and does not consider non-seasonal trends in climate. Climate change is a controversial subject and despite general consensus about the existence of global warming, future trends and impacts on local climate and weather is less easily agreed. However, attempts to model the effect of global warming on climate using the Köppen classification have estimated a shift between major climate classes of around 3% during the 21st century. Prediction of how these changes might affect infectious diseases is also difficult, as discussed below.

Significance for infectious diseases: Climate has a major influence on infectious disease epidemiology that is both spatial (affecting the geographic distribution of disease) and temporal (affecting the timing of transmission peaks). Temporal patterns are typically seasonal but longer, non-annual, climate cycles, such as the El Niño Southern Oscillation (ENSO), may also influence infectious disease epidemiology. ENSO has been linked to dengue, malaria, Rift Valley Fever, and cholera epidemiology. The effect of climate may be mediated by climate-dependent vector competence (e.g. malaria), climate-dependent pathogen survival, or by climatically determined habitat suitability for environmental pathogens (e.g. *Burkholderia pseudomallei, Coccidioides immi-*

tis), their vectors (e.g. mosquitoes, ticks, flies), or animal reservoirs (e.g. bats). In general, human pathogen diversity is associated with latitude, being maximum at the equator and decreasing with distance from the equator. Climate is also associated with temporal changes in social behaviors, such as the mixing of children during school terms, which influence disease epidemiology. Temperature, humidity, and perhaps sunlight may also directly affect individual susceptibility to infection by altering mucosal integrity or innate immunity. However, despite very clear spatial and seasonal patterns of many infections, the precise mechanism or interactions are rarely disentangled and usually remain a matter of speculation. Longer-term trends in climate and the effect on the distribution and prevalence of infectious diseases are even less easily identified, and this remains an area of controversy, particularly since trends in disease epidemiology may be confounded by many other concomitant changes, such as land use, disease control programs, and socioeconomic development.

Map sources: The Climate map was made by using climate data obtained from WorldClim – Global Climate Data, available at: www.worldclim.org.

Key references

Dunn RR, et al. (2010) Global drivers of human pathogen richness and prevalence. *Proc R Soc B*: doi: 10.1098.

Guernier V, et al. (2004) Ecology drives the worldwide distribution of human diseases. *PloS Biol* **2**(6):e141.

Hijmans RJ, et al. (2005) Very high resolution interpolated climate surfaces for global land areas. *Int J Climat* **25**:1965–1978.

Lafferty KD. (2009) The ecology of climate change and infectious diseases. *Ecology* **90**(4):888–900.

Rubel F, et al. (2010) Observed and projected climate shifts 1901–2100 depicted by world maps of the Köppen–Geiger climate classification. *Meteorol Z* **19**:135–141.

Forest Cover Change

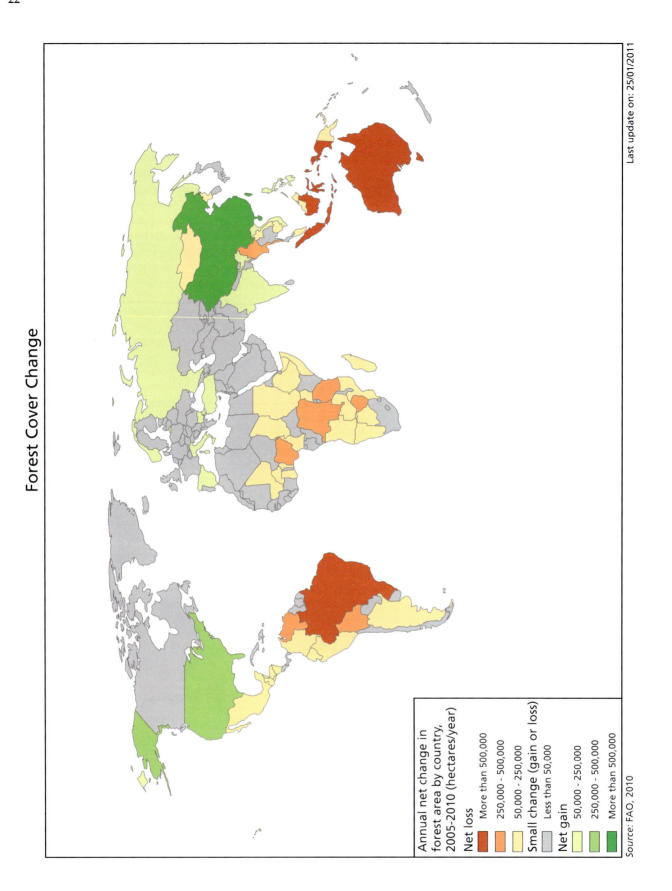

Annual net change in
forest area by country,
2005-2010 (hectares/year)

Net loss
More than 500,000
250,000 - 500,000
50,000 - 250,000
Small change (gain or loss)
Less than 50,000
Net gain
50,000 - 250,000
250,000 - 500,000
More than 500,000

Source: FAO, 2010

Last update on: 25/01/2011

Subject: Forest Cover Change

Definition: The Food and Agriculture Organization (FAO) conducts periodic questionnaire surveys through the Global Forest Resources Assessment (FRA) in which forest is defined as "Land spanning more than 0.5 hectare with trees higher than 5 meters and a canopy cover of more than 10%, or trees able to reach these thresholds *in situ*." The definition excludes agricultural production (e.g. fruit orchards) and urban parks, but includes commercial plantations (e.g. rubber or cork). The last FRA was conducted in 2010 and is the source of the forest cover change map opposite.

Trends: In 2010 an estimated 31% of total land area was forested and, of this, 36% was primary forest, 57% naturally regenerated forest, and 7% planted forest. Although the rate of deforestation has declined, it remains high, with an annual estimated loss of around 13 million hectares of forest per year (1 hectare = 10,000 m^2). The predominant cause of deforestation is the conversion of tropical forest to agricultural land. New forest planting and natural expansion of existing forests does, however, reduce net forest loss to an estimated 5.8 million hectares per year.

Significance for infections: Forests are habitats for animal reservoirs and vectors of a wide range of infectious diseases that may infect humans either opportunistically or as part of the pathogen's natural lifecycle. Forest associated infections where humans are the definitive host are rare, but notably include malaria transmitted by forest-associated *anopheles* species and Loa Loa. More commonly, forest-associated infections of humans are opportunistic zoonoses, where humans are not part of the natural pathogen lifecycle. These opportunistic infections may be vector borne (e.g. Chagas disease, mucocutaneous leishmanisasis, Kyasanur forest virus, Semliki forest virus, and *Plasmodium knowlesi*), the result of human predation on animals (e.g. Ebola, monkeypox), or from environmental sources (e.g. *Cryptococcus gattii*). Yellow fever has both a non-human primate transmission cycle that occasionally infects humans and an urban cycle in which humans are the reservoirs. Sometimes there may be limited human-to-human transmission that is either not sustained or is readily controlled (e.g. monkeypox, Ebola and Marburg viruses, Nipah virus). Occasionally these opportunistic transmission events are highly successful and the pathogen becomes fully adapted to the new host. It is likely that a large proportion of current human pathogens originated from animal pathogens: the best known of these is HIV, which probably originated from chimpanzees sometime prior to 1940.

Human activities have had an enormous impact on forests and will continue to do so as long as demand continues for hard wood, fire wood, pulp, agricultural and grazing land, living space, roads, minerals, and power. Deforestation can involve clearance or selected logging of high-value trees. Selected logging will bring workers into greater contact with zoonotic reservoirs and vectors, whereas clearance may increase or decrease contact with pathogens as the local ecology is disrupted. Transient outbreaks have occurred when deforestation activities have bought humans into close contact with animal reservoirs and vectors, e.g. Venezuelan hemorrhagic fever and Chagas disease (*Trypanasoma cruzi*) or when deforested areas have been colonized by pathogen-carrying vectors, e.g. black flies and onchocerciasis. The effects of deforestation and anthropogenic changes of ecology are not, however, easy to predict and may increase or decrease risks. An indirect effect of deforestation was observed when haze from forest clearance fires reduced fruit production, forcing fruit bats to encroach on domestic fruit orchards close to pig-rearing areas, leading to an outbreak of Nipah virus; thus demonstrating the complex interconnectedness of human activities, ecosystems, and infectious diseases.

Map sources: The Forest Cover Change map was made with data from FAO, available at: www.fao.org/forestry/.

Key references

Guerra CA, et al. (2006) A global assessment of closed forests, deforestation and malaria risk. *Ann Trop Med Parasitol* **100**(3):189–204.

Looi LM, et al. (2007) Lessons from the Nipah virus outbreak in Malaysia. *Malays J Pathol* **29**(2):63–67.

Teixeira AR, et al. (2001) Emerging Chagas disease: trophic network and cycle of transmission of Trypanosoma cruzi from palm trees in the Amazon. *Emerg Infect Dis* **7**(1):100–112.

Walsh JF, et al. (1993) Deforestation: effects on vector-borne disease. *Parasitology* **106**Suppl:S55–S75.

Wolfe ND, et al. (2005) Bushmeat hunting, deforestation, and prediction of zoonoses emergence. *Emerg Infect Dis* **11**(12):1822–1827.

Atlas of Human Infectious Diseases, First Edition. Heiman F.L. Wertheim, Peter Horby and John P. Woodall.
© 2012 Blackwell Publishing Ltd. Published 2012 by Blackwell Publishing Ltd.

Natural Disasters

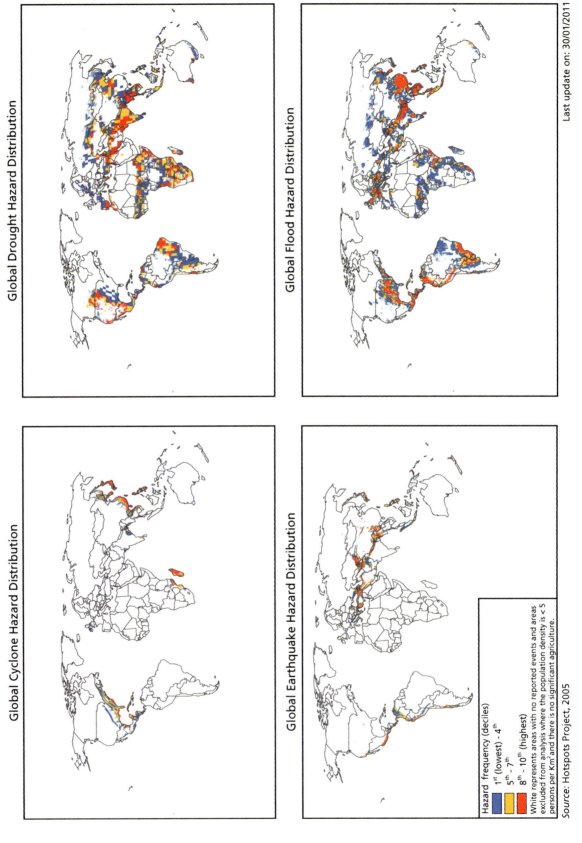

Global Drought Hazard Distribution

Global Flood Hazard Distribution

Global Cyclone Hazard Distribution

Global Earthquake Hazard Distribution

Hazard frequency (deciles)

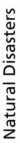

1st (lowest) - 4th

5th - 7th

8th - 10th (highest)

White represents areas with no reported events and areas excluded from analysis where the population density is < 5 persons per Km² and there is no significant agriculture.

Source: Hotspots Project, 2005

Last update on: 30/01/2011

Subject: Natural Disasters

Definition: The map shows the geographical distribution and frequency of natural hazards, based largely on historical data: cyclones 1980–2000, droughts 1980–2000, earthquakes 1976–2002, and floods 1985–2003. For the earthquake map, only events with a peak ground acceleration of greater than 2 meters per second were included. For each hazard the frequency within areas at risk has been classified into 10 categories (deciles) with 10 representing the highest frequency and 1 the lowest. White sections represent areas with no reported events and areas excluded from analysis because the population density is less than 5 persons per square kilometer and there is no significant agriculture.

Patterns and trends: The risk of natural disasters, especially cyclones and earthquakes, is highly geographically concentrated. The increasing concentration of people and economic activity in vulnerable coastal plains and urban centers may increase the impact of cyclone and flooding events. This may be further exacerbated if the predicted increase in the frequency and magnitude of extreme weather events, as a result of climate change, materializes.

Significance for infectious diseases: *Non-epidemic risks:* tetanus and wound infections are a concern for individual survivors with traumatic injuries. The pathogens responsible for wound infections will depend on the local microbial epidemiology and the nature of the disaster. Flooding increases the risk of skin infections, conjunctivitis, ear, nose, and throat infections, and aspiration pneumonia. Workers handling corpses need to protect themselves against the risk of blood-borne viruses, enteric pathogens, and tuberculosis. *Epidemic risks:* Large infectious disease outbreaks following natural disasters are uncommon, although leptospirosis cases may increase as a result of direct exposure to contaminated flood-waters. When outbreaks do occur they are usually in displaced populations living in crowded, temporary shelter with inade-quate infrastructure and healthcare. Contaminated drinking water and a lack of sanitation facilities can lead to epidemics of water-borne infections such as cholera. Overcrowding and poor living conditions result in a significant increase in morbidity and mortality from acute respiratory infections and, if vaccination coverage is low, vaccine preventable diseases such as measles. Disasters may also lead to an increase in suitable vector habitats, resulting in vector-borne disease outbreaks. Malaria outbreaks following flooding in endemic areas are well recognized and occur after a lag of six to eight weeks.

In the immediate aftermath of a natural disaster there is often great concern about the epidemic risk posed by dead bodies. There is, however, no evidence that dead bodies arising from natural disasters pose an epidemic risk. Most people who die as an immediate consequence of a natural disaster are killed by trauma or drowning. As most are not suffering from a communicable disease at the time of their death, and as pathogens do not survive long in the body after death, they do not pose an epidemic risk.

Map sources: The Natural Disasters map was made with data from the Hotspots project (a Worldbank and Columbia University initiative, 2005), available at: www.ldeo.columbia.edu.

Key references

Connolly MA (ed.) (2005) *Communicable Disease Control in Emergencies: A Field Manual.* World Health Organization, Geneva.

Dilley M, et al. (2005) *Natural disaster hotspots: a global risk analysis.* Synthesis Report.

Flooding and Communicable Diseases Fact Sheet (2005) WER **3**(80):21–28.

Morgan O (2004) Infectious disease risks from dead bodies following natural disasters. *Pan Amer J Publ Health* **15**(5): 307–312.

Atlas of Human Infectious Diseases, First Edition. Heiman F.L. Wertheim, Peter Horby and John P. Woodall.
© 2012 Blackwell Publishing Ltd. Published 2012 by Blackwell Publishing Ltd.

Antibiotic Use

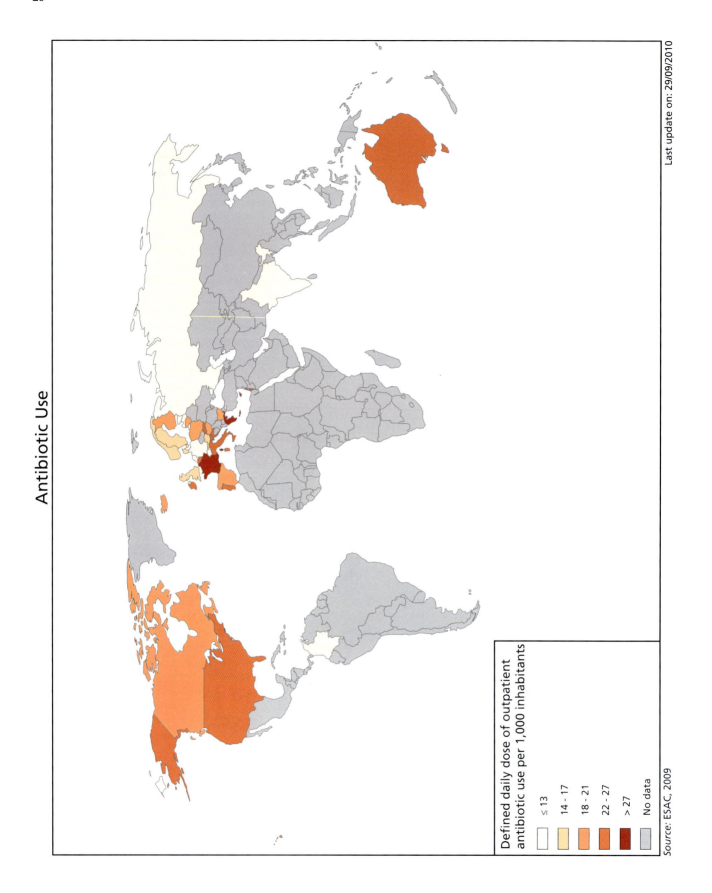

Defined daily dose of outpatient
antibiotic use per 1,000 inhabitants

≤ 13

14 - 17

18 - 21

22 - 27

> 27

No data

Source: ESAC, 2009

Last update on: 29/09/2010

Subject: Antibiotic Use

Definition: Antibiotic use in humans and animals is the main driver for the development of antibiotic resistance world wide. To be able to compare antibiotic consumption data, antibiotic use is expressed in defined daily doses, with the use of the Anatomic Therapeutic Chemical (ATC) classification system devloped by WHO. A defined daily dose is the assumed average maintenance dose per day for a drug used for its main indication in adults.

Trends: The more exposure bacteria have to an antibiotic, the more likely it is that strains resistant to that antibiotic will arise and spread. Antibiotic drug pressure is the most important factor promoting development of drug resistance in bacteria. However, reasons for drug pressure are multi-factorial. Although drug resistance is primarily a medical problem, the causes of resistance are ecological, epidemiological, sociocultural, and economic. Patients, physicians, veterinarians, farmers, hospitals, and pharmacies have little incentive to weigh the negative impact of their use of antibiotics on others, especially those in the future. Besides, there is little incentive for drug companies to develop new classes of antibiotics since that involves much greater risk and expense than producing new antibiotics that belong to existing drug classes.

Currently in- and outpatient antibiotic consumption data is available for Europe from the European Surveillance of Antimicrobial Consumption (ESAC) project. Countries outside Europe are now also reporting antibiotic consumption data with methods similar to ESAC. What can be seen is that several nordic European countries countries have lower outpatient antibiotic consumption as compared to mainly southern or eastern European countries. For instance, in the Netherlands, antibiotics are available only on precription and doctors are restrictive in prescribing antibiotics. European resistance data (EARSS) also show that countries with lower antibiotic use have lower antibiotic resistance levels. It is probable that differences in infection control practices in these countries also play a role. Hospital antibiotic consumption is approximately 10-fold lower than that used in ambulatory care.

The global problem of antimicrobial resistance is particularly pressing in developing countries, where the infectious disease burden is high and cost constrains the replacement of older antibiotics with newer, more expensive ones. Infections are leading causes of morbidity and mortality in the developing world, and management of all these conditions are critically compromised by the appearance and rapid spread of resistance. Though the antibiotic consumption in outpatients may still be lower in Asia as poverty prohibits access to these drugs, the absolute number of people exposed to antibiotics is very high due to high population density (see Population map).

Besides human use, antibiotics are commonly used in agriculture. The volumes of antibiotics used in agriculture are several magnitudes higher than in human use, but good data are not available. As antibiotics used in agriculture are often in the same class of antibiotics used in humans, this may lead to the emergence of human pathogens that are resistant to common antibiotics. In Europe, antibiotics are banned as a growth promotor.

Significance for infectious diseases: Like other shared resources, the effectiveness of antibiotics should be viewed as a precious global resource, to be protected and valued, not squandered through unnecessary use. The goal is that antibiotics are used only in people with bacterial infections that need to be cured by antibiotics. The agricultural use of antibiotics needs to be controlled. Failing to control antibiotic use and spread of resistance will likely lead to a higher burden of multiresistant bacteria with an increase in morbidity and mortality. Recent evidence of this is the spread of carbapenem-resistant bacteria (NDM-1) in several countries in Asia and Europe, including pan-resistant strains for which no antibiotics are available.

Map sources: Data for the Antibiotic Use map were obtained from the European Surveillance of Antimicrobial Consumption (ESAC) from 2000 to 2008, with additional data from references that reported outpatient antibiotic use. The ESAC database is available at: http://app.esac.ua.ac.be/public/.

Key references

Goossens H, et al. (2007) Comparison of outpatient systemic antibiotic use in 2004 between the United States and 27 European countries. *Clin Inf Dis* **44**:1091–1095.

Högberg LD, et al. (2010) The global need for effective antibiotics: challenges and recent advances. *Trends Pharmacol Sci* **31**(11):509–515.

Kumarasamy KK, et al. (2010) Emergence of a new antibiotic resistance mechanism in India, Pakistan, and the UK: a molecular, biological, and epidemiological study. *Lancet Infect Dis* **10**(9):597–602.

Livermore DM (2009) Has the era of untreatable infections arrived? *J Antimicrob Chemother* **64**(1):29–36.

Van de Sande-Bruinsma N, et al. (2008) Antimicrobial drug use and resistance in Europe. *Emerg Infect Dis* **14**(11):1722–1730.

Atlas of Human Infectious Diseases, First Edition. Heiman F.L. Wertheim, Peter Horby and John P. Woodall.
© 2012 Blackwell Publishing Ltd. Published 2012 by Blackwell Publishing Ltd.

Inherited Blood Disorders and Duffy Antigen

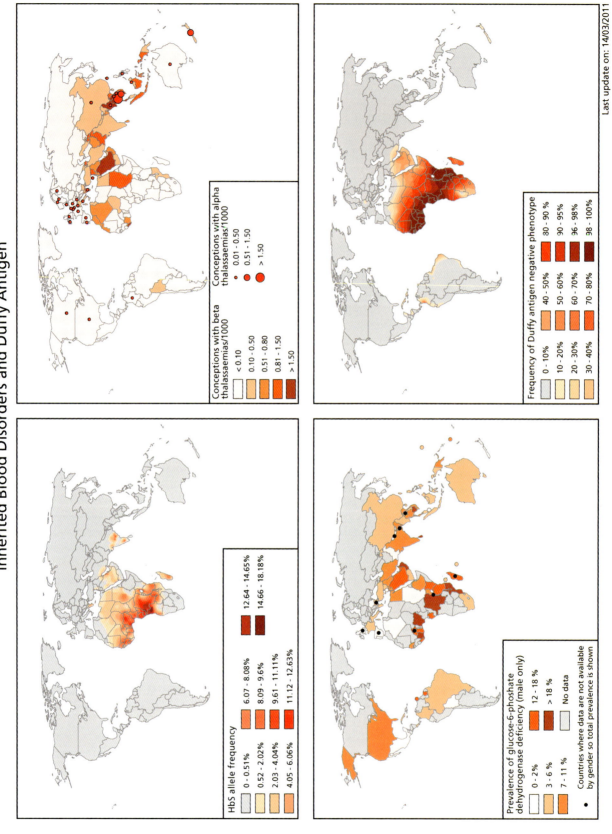

Conceptions with beta thalassaemias/1000
- < 0.10
- 0.10 - 0.50
- 0.51 - 0.80
- 0.81 - 1.50
- > 1.50

Conceptions with alpha thalassaemias/1000
- 0.01 - 0.50
- 0.51 - 1.50
- > 1.50

HbS allele frequency
- 0 - 0.51%
- 0.52 - 2.02%
- 2.03 - 4.04%
- 4.05 - 6.06%
- 6.07 - 8.08%
- 8.09 - 9.6%
- 9.61 - 11.11%
- 11.12 - 12.63%
- 12.64 - 14.65%
- 14.66 - 18.18%

Frequency of Duffy antigen negative phenotype
- 0 - 10%
- 10 - 20%
- 20 - 30%
- 30 - 40%
- 40 - 50%
- 50 - 60%
- 60 - 70%
- 70 - 80%
- 80 - 90 %
- 90 - 95%
- 96 - 98%
- 98 - 100%

Prevalence of glucose-6-phoshate dehydrogenase deficiency (male only)
- 0 - 2%
- 3 - 6 %
- 7 - 11 %
- 12 - 18 %
- > 18 %
- No data
- • Countries where data are not available by gender so total prevalence is shown

Last update on: 14/03/2011

Subject: Inherited Blood Disorders and Duffy Antigen

Definition: The term Inherited Blood Disorders (IBDs) encompasses a large number of genetically inherited disorders of the blood. Three IBDs are shown here: sickle hemoglobin (HbS), glucose-6-phosphate dehydrogenase (G6PD) deficiency, and thalassemia. They, along with Duffy antigen (see below), are of interest because of their relationship with malaria. HbS is a variant of normal adult hemoglobin that results in red blood cells (RBCs) taking on an abnormal sickle shape under conditions of low oxygen concentration or oxidative stress. When HbS is inherited from only one parent (genotype HbAS, sickle trait) the individual is usually asymptomatic, but if HbS is inherited from both parents (genotype HbSS), the individual suffers a severe disorder (sickle cell disease). The map opposite (top left) shows the estimated world-wide distribution of HbS allele frequency. G6PD is an enzyme that is essential in the metabolism of RBCs. G6PD deficiency is an X-linked genetic disorder and, although most people are asymptomatic, the most common clinical manifestation is neonatal jaundice or acute hemolytic anemia (AHA). The map opposite (bottom left) shows the estimated prevalence of G6PD deficiency in males (where male prevalence is not available, total prevalence is used). Thalassemia causes abnormal hemoglobin molecules and RBCs with a shortened life span. Their clinical symptoms range from asymptomatic to severe anemia and death. The two major forms of thalassemia are termed alpha and beta, based on the globin chain affected. The Duffy antigen is a protein on the surface of RBCs that acts as a receptor for several signaling proteins but which also binds certain malaria species. Duffy antigen status is inherited but it is not an IBD since Duffy status itself does not result in any medical condition.

Trends: The time frame of human gene selection is long (1000s of years), although geographic dispersion of mutations through migration may occur over shorter time periods.

Significance for infections: The three IBDs are of interest since their high prevalence in malarious areas is hypothesized to result from the mutations providing some protection against malaria. This hypothesis is supported by the spatial correlation of G6PD deficiency, HbS, and thalassemia with malaria risk, studies of the severity of malaria in individuals with these IBDs, and in-vitro studies. Sickle trait provides protection against severe *Plasmodium falciparum* malaria either by limiting the growth of the parasite in HbAS cells or by the more efficient removal of parasitized HbAS cells. The precise mechanisms by which alpha and beta thalassemia provide protection against malaria remain unresolved. G6PD deficiency is of particular interest because the antimalarial drug primaquine can cause AHA in G6PD-deficient individuals. Primaquine is an effective gametocide, and is the only drug clinically validated for eradicating the malaria hypnozoites. Addressing the problem of G6PD deficiency and the limited drug options for eradicating the hypnozoite reservoir is one the great challenges for malaria elimination. The Duffy antigen is a receptor for *P. vivax* and *P. knowlesi* parasites. People who do not express Duffy antigens (Duffy negative) are resistant in experimental studies to *P. vivax* infection and the high prevalence of Duffy negative status in Sub-Saharan Africa is postulated to explain the rarity of *P. vivax* malaria in that area. However, recent work has shown that *P. vivax* can infect RBCs and cause disease in Duffy negative individuals.

Map sources: The Inherited Blood Disorders and Duffy antigen map was made using various sources:

Thalassemias: CHIME's WHO Collaborating Centre for the Community Control of Hereditary Disorders, at: www.chime.ucl.ac.uk/work-areas/cab/
Sickle cell disorders: F.B. Piel et al. (2010).
G6PD deficiency: E.T. Nkhoma et al. (2009).
Duffy antigen: F.B. Piel et al. (2011).

Key references

Lopez C, et al. (2010) Mechanisms of genetically-based resistance to malaria. *Gene* **467**(1–2):1–12.
Nkhoma ET, et al. (2009) The global prevalence of glucose-6-phosphate dehydrogenase deficiency. *Blood Cells Mol Dis* **42**:267–278.
Piel FB, et al. (2010) Global distribution of the sickle cell gene and geographical confirmation of the malaria hypothesis. *Nat Commun* **1**(8):104.
Howes RE, et al. (2011) The global distribution of the Duffy blood group. *Nat Commun* (in press).
Tishkoff SA, et al. (2001) Haplotype diversity and linkage disequilibrium at human G6PD: recent origin of alleles that confer malarial resistance. *Science* **293**(5529):455–462.
Weatherall DJ. (2010) The inherited diseases of hemoglobin are an emerging global health burden. *Blood* **115**:4331–4336.

Atlas of Human Infectious Diseases, First Edition. Heiman F.L. Wertheim, Peter Horby and John P. Woodall.
© 2012 Blackwell Publishing Ltd. Published 2012 by Blackwell Publishing Ltd.

Immunization Coverage DTP3

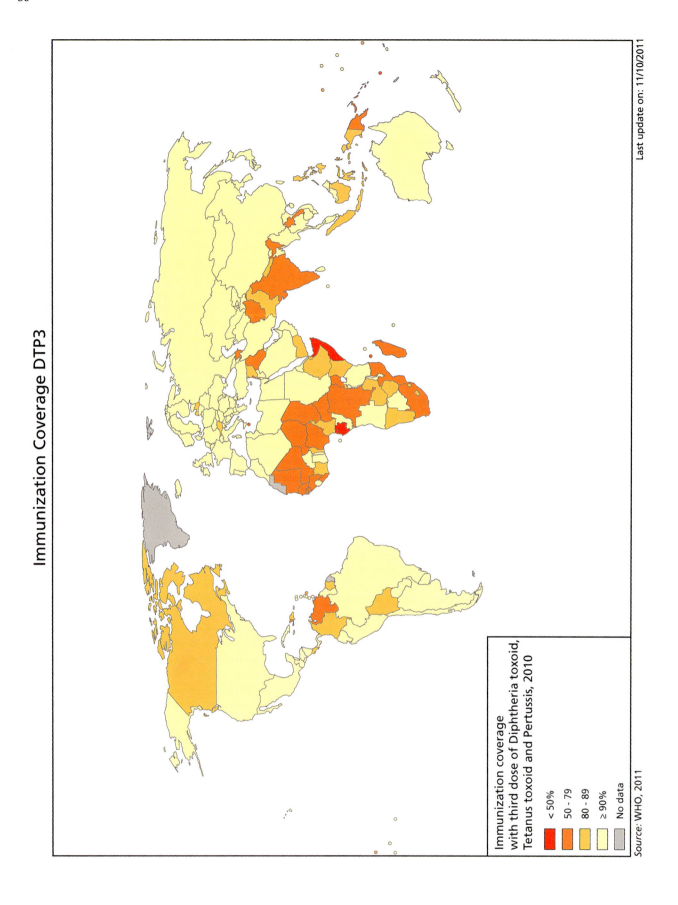

Immunization coverage
with third dose of Diphtheria toxoid,
Tetanus toxoid and Pertussis, 2010

	< 50%
	50 - 79
	80 - 89
	≥ 90%
	No data

Source: WHO, 2011

Last update on: 11/10/2011

Subject: Immunization Coverage – DTP3

Definition: The map shows the estimated coverage of the target population with three doses of the combined diphtheria, tetanus, and pertussis vaccine (DTP3). This vaccine is cheap, readily available and has been part of WHO recommended infant immunization schedule since the Expanded Program on Immunization began in 1974. Therefore, DTP3 coverage is often used to monitor the overall performance of national immunization programs.

Trends: In 2008 an estimated 106 million infants were vaccinated with DTP3, equivalent to a global coverage of infants with DTP3 of around 82%. This compared to 20%, 75%, and 73% in 1980, 1990, and 2000 respectively. Stagnation in coverage levels for basic childhood vaccines was observed in the 1990s and this resulted in the formation of the Global Alliance for Vaccines and Immunization (GAVI) as a public–private partnership to support vaccination programs in low- and middle-income countries. Global coverage rates for basic childhood vaccines have steadily risen during the past decade. In a few developed countries, coverage of some vaccines has slipped back slightly as a result of unproven concerns about side effects and the actions of antivaccine lobbyists.

Significance for infections: The world remains scarred by enormous health inequalities and for the impoverished, underserved children of the world, infectious diseases are the biggest killer and the biggest health burden. Around 9 million children under 5 die each year, mostly in developing countries. Immunization is one of the most effective life-saving interventions available to these children and is an essential tool for improving childhood survival. Every year vaccines prevent an estimated 2.5 million child deaths and an enormous burden of ill health, leading to strengthened human resources, greater economic productivity, improved socioeconomic development, and healthier and happier communities. Vaccination coverage is typically low in remote rural areas, deprived urban settings, mobile populations, and in regions affected by conflict or instability. In 2008 around 24 million children aged 1 year had not received three doses of DTP; 70% of these children lived in 10 countries: Chad, China, Democratic Republic of the Congo, Ethiopia, India, Indonesia, Iraq, Nigeria, Pakistan, and Uganda. While reaching these vulnerable children is not simple, better coverage with existing vaccines could prevent an additional 2 million deaths each year in children under 5.

Map sources: Data for the Vaccination Coverage DTP3 map were obtained from WHO, available at: www.who.int/immunization_monitoring/data/en/.

Key references

Andre FE (2008) Vaccination greatly reduces disease, disability, death and inequity worldwide. *Bull World Health Organ* **86**(2):140–146.

Lim SS, et al. (2009) Tracking progress towards universal childhood immunisation and the impact of global initiatives: a systematic analysis of three-dose diphtheria, tetanus, and pertussis immunisation coverage. *Lancet* **372**: 2031–2046.

WHO, UNICEF, World Bank. (2009) *State of the World's Vaccines and Immunization*, 3rd edn. Geneva: World Health Organization.

Atlas of Human Infectious Diseases, First Edition. Heiman F.L. Wertheim, Peter Horby and John P. Woodall.
© 2012 Blackwell Publishing Ltd. Published 2012 by Blackwell Publishing Ltd.

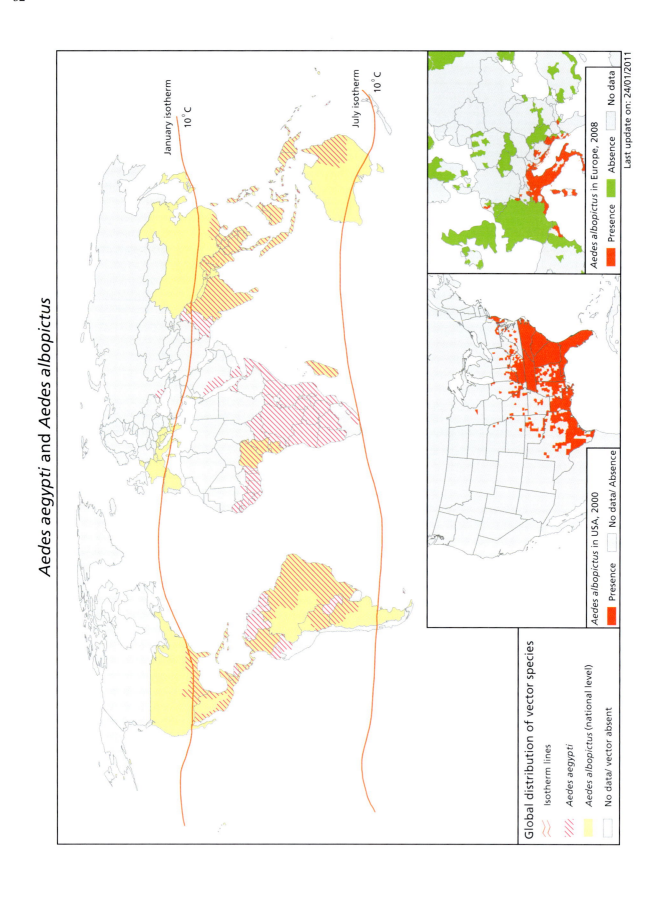

Aedes aegypti and Aedes albopictus

January isotherm 10° C

July isotherm 10° C

Aedes albopictus in Europe, 2008

- Presence
- Absence
- No data

Last update on: 24/01/2011

Aedes albopictus in USA, 2000

- Presence
- No data/ Absence

Global distribution of vector species

- Isotherm lines
- Aedes aegypti
- Aedes albopictus (national level)
- No data/ vector absent

Subject: *Aedes aegypti* and *Aedes albopictus*

Definition: *Aedes* is a genus of mosquito (*Order*: Diptera; *Family*: Culicidae) that includes over 900 species. The two most important species for man, *Aedes aegypti* and *Aedes albopictus* (Asian tiger mosquito), are members of the subgenus *Stegomyia* and transmit virus infections to humans. Female *Aedes* require blood meals to develop their eggs and feed predominantly during the day. *Ae. aegypti* feeds predominantly on humans and readily feeds indoors, whereas *Ae. albopictus* prefers humans but may feed on a wider range of animals and usually feeds outdoors. Female *Ae. aegypti* and *Ae. albopictus* lay their eggs in water-filled containers, preferably on rough, damp surfaces just above the water line, and the eggs hatch when submerged. The eggs may survive desiccation for several months. In urban areas *Aedes* use a wide range of water-filled containers, such as water storage containers, plant pots, discarded tires, building sites, and roof gutters. Natural sites where eggs may be laid include tree holes, leaf axils, and pools in riverbeds. Although *Aedes* species have a global distribution, *Ae. aegypti is a* tropical and subtropical species, and is uncommon in areas where the average winter temperature is 10 °C or less (10 °C winter isotherm) or at altitudes above 1,000 metres. *Ae. albopictus* is also historically a tropical species, but strains have evolved that are able to over-winter in temperate climates and become established at higher latitudes than *Ae. aegypti*.

Trends: *Ae. aegypti* originated in Africa and subsequently spread to the Americas, Asia, and the Pacific, probably through shipping routes during the 15th to 17th centuries. During the 20th century *Ae. aegypti* has retreated from southern Europe, North Africa, southern United States, and parts of Australia. Yellow fever eradication programs in South and Central America between the 1950s and 1970s saw large declines in *Ae. aegypti* abundance and even eradication in some countries, but *Ae. aegypti* has subsequently reinvaded large parts of Central and South America. *Ae. albopictus* is native to Asia and is highly invasive. Since 1980 *Ae. albopictus* has spread extensively, and is now established in many countries of the Americas, southern Europe, and in parts of West Africa, possibly through international trade in used tires. *Ae. albopictus* has recently been repeatedly found in the Netherlands associated with imported bamboo, but has not become established. While climate change might increase the range of climate suitability for *Ae. aegypti* and *Ae. albopictus*, the effects are difficult to predict, but it seems likely that temperate strains of *Ae. albopictus* will continue to expand their geographic range.

Significance for infections: *Ae. aegypti* is the main vector of yellow fever, dengue, and chikungunya. *Ae. albopictus* is an important vector of dengue and chikungunya, especially in areas where this species predominates. *Ae. aegypti* is a more efficient vector than *Ae. albopictus* partly, it is thought, because of its biting and habitat preferences, but also as a result of the mosquito's inherent susceptibility to infection and viral replication. Adult *Ae. aegypti* and *Ae. albopictus* mosquitoes spend their life in and around the place they emerged, rarely flying further than 100 meters (although up to 800 meters has been recorded). Thus it is mainly humans who are responsible for spreading dengue virus within and between communities. Anthropogenic transport of vectors over long distances and changes in habitat suitability drive the geographic expansion of arbovirus risk. *A. aegypti* and *A. albopictus* have been experimentally demonstrated to be potential vectors for a wide range of other arboviruses, including Japanese encephalitis, West Nile virus, Eastern Equine encephalitis, and La Crosse virus, but they are not thought to play an important role in the ecology or transmission of any of these viruses. However, pathogen and vector populations are not static, and adaptations of either may see the emergence of new arbovirus epidemiology associated with *Ae. aegypti* and *Ae. albopictus*.

Map sources: The *Aedes* map was made from various sources: CDC (www.cdc.gov/ncidod/dvbid/arbor/albopic_97_sm.htm; Accessed on: 02/12/2010) and the European Environment Agency (www.eea.europa.eu), and updated with recent literature.

Key references

Benedict MQ, et al. (2007) Spread of the tiger: global risk of invasion by the mosquito *Aedes albopictus*. *Vector Borne Zoonotic Dis* **7**(1):76–85.

Jansen CC, et al. (2010) The dengue vector *Aedes aegypti*: what comes next? *Microbes Infect* **12**(4):272–279.

Lambrechts L, et al. (2010) Consequences of the expanding global distribution of *Aedes albopictus* for dengue virus transmission. *PLoS Negl Trop Dis* **4**(5):e646.

Rogers DJ, et al. (2006) The global distribution of yellow fever and dengue. *Adv Parasitol* **62**:182–220.

Atlas of Human Infectious Diseases, First Edition. Heiman F.L. Wertheim, Peter Horby and John P. Woodall.
© 2012 Blackwell Publishing Ltd. Published 2012 by Blackwell Publishing Ltd.

Malaria Vectors

Distribution of Anopheles (Nysorhynchus) darlingi Root

Distribution of Anopheles (Cellia) gambiae Giles

Distribution of dominant or potentially important malaria vectors

Distribution of Anopheles (Cellia) dirus complex

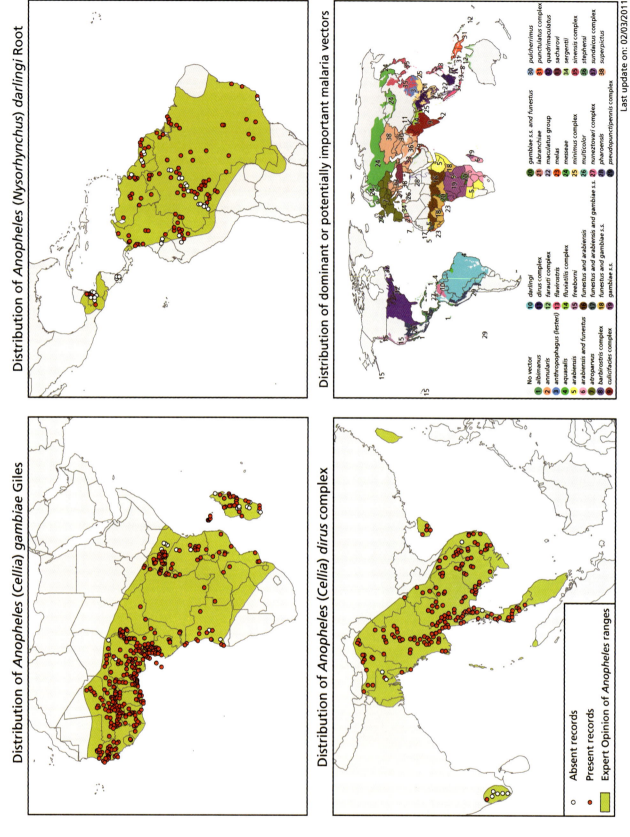

Last update on: 02/03/2011

No vector
10 darlingi
30 pulcherrimus
1 albimanus
11 dirus complex
20 gambiae s.s. and funestus
31 punctulatus complex
2 annularis
12 farauti complex
21 labranchiae
32 quadrimaculatus
3 anthropophagus (lesteri)
13 flavirostris
22 maculatus group
33 sacharovi
4 aquasalis
14 fluviatilis complex
23 melas
34 sergentii
5 arabiensis
15 freeborni
24 messeae
35 sinensis complex
6 arabiensis and funestus
16 funestus and arabiensis
25 minimus complex
36 stephensi
7 atroparvus
17 funestus and arabiensis and gambiae s.s.
26 multicolor
37 sundaicus complex
8 barbirostris complex
18 funestus and gambiae s.s.
27 nuneztovari complex
38 superpictus
9 culicifacies complex
19 gambiae s.s.
28 pharoensis
29 pseudopunctipennis complex

○ Absent records
● Present records
■ Expert Opinion of Anopheles ranges

Subject: Malaria Vectors

Definition: Malaria is transmitted to humans by female mosquitoes of the genus *Anopheles*. *Anopheles* are widely distributed and although there are over 450 formally identified species, only around 30–40 are considered important in the transmission of malaria to humans. The maps opposite show the distribution of some important *Anopheles* species (or species complexes). These maps encompass both expert opinions of species range and species occurrence records collected from searches of published literature. The bottom right panel shows the distribution of 34 dominant or potentially important *Anopheles* species (or species complexes). These maps depict areas of potential malaria receptivity rather than current malaria presence, since the socioeconomic development or malaria control may have eliminated malaria risk from some of the areas depicted. It is important to note that the species distribution and density of *Anopheles* is heterogeneous at relatively small spatial scales, and maps that attempt to show species distribution at large scales are an oversimplification.

Trends: Where transmission potential is marginal, general socioeconomic development – such as improvements in housing conditions and reduced proximity of humans and animals – is often sufficient to eliminate transmission. In higher risk areas, economic development combined with malaria control activities can substantially reduce transmission. Consequently, the spatial extent of malaria transmission has contracted substantially over the last century. Recent successes with malaria control have revived calls for malaria elimination and several initiatives are targeting national or regional elimination. Since vector longevity and the extrinsic incubation period are both temperature dependent, changes in temperature have a strong influence on malaria transmission risk. There has therefore been a lot of debate about the potential impact of climate change on the distribution of malaria risk. Some authors predict an increase in malaria as a result of climate change, while others argue that the effect of climate change will be entirely offset by decreased transmission resulting from socioeconomic development and malaria control efforts.

Significance for infections: Malaria is endemic in around 109 countries and although great progress has been made in malaria control in the past decade, WHO estimates that around 780,000 malaria deaths occurred in 2009. The intensity of malaria transmission is a function of: the susceptibility of the vector to the malaria parasite; vector density; vector longevity; the incubation time of the parasite in the vector (extrinsic incubation period); the prevalence of human infection; and vector biting behavior. Malaria transmission is most intense where there is a high density of a highly susceptible vector that likes to feed on humans (anthropophilic) and a climate that supports a short extrinsic incubation period and a long mosquito lifespan. An understanding of vector species distribution and their contribution to malaria epidemiology is critical for successful malaria control since the preferred feeding and resting behaviors of different species determine the relative efficacy of different control options. For instance, insecticide-treated mosquito nets (ITNs) are most effective against species that like to bite indoors (endophagic) and at night, while indoor residual insecticide spraying (IRS) is most effective against species that rest indoors (endophilic). Insecticide-treated hammocks may be helpful in areas where people work and sleep in forests that contain forest-adapted malaria vectors such as *An. dirus*.

Map source: The two top and the bottom left maps are derived from the Malaria Atlas Project and published by Sinka et al. in 2010 and 2011 (see key references). The bottom right map is modified with permission from Kiszewski et al. (2004).

Key references

Cohuet A, et al. (2010) Evolutionary forces on Anopheles: what makes a malaria vector? *Trends Parasitol* **26**(3):130–136.

Gething PW, et al. (2010) Climate change and the global malaria recession. *Nature* **465**(7296):342–345.

Hay SI, et al. (2010) Developing Global Maps of the Dominant Anopheles Vectors of Human Malaria. *PLoS Med* **7**(2): e1000209.

Kiszewski A, et al. (2004) A global index representing the stability of malaria transmission. *Am J Trop Med Hyg* **70**(5):486–498.

Patz JA, et al. (2006) Malaria risk and temperature: influences from global climate change and local land use practices. *Proc Natl Acad Sci USA* **103**(15):5635–5636.

Sinka ME, et al. (2010a). The dominant Anopheles vectors of human malaria in Africa, Europe and the Middle East: occurrence data, distribution maps and bionomic précis. *Parasites Vectors* **3**:117.

Sinka ME, et al. (2010b). The dominant Anopheles vectors of human malaria in the Americas: occurrence data, distribution maps and bionomic précis. *Parasites Vectors*, **3**:72.

Sinka ME, et al. (2011) The dominant Anopheles vectors of human malaria in the Asia Pacific region: occurrence data, distribution maps and bionomic précis. *Parasites Vectors* In press.

Livestock Density

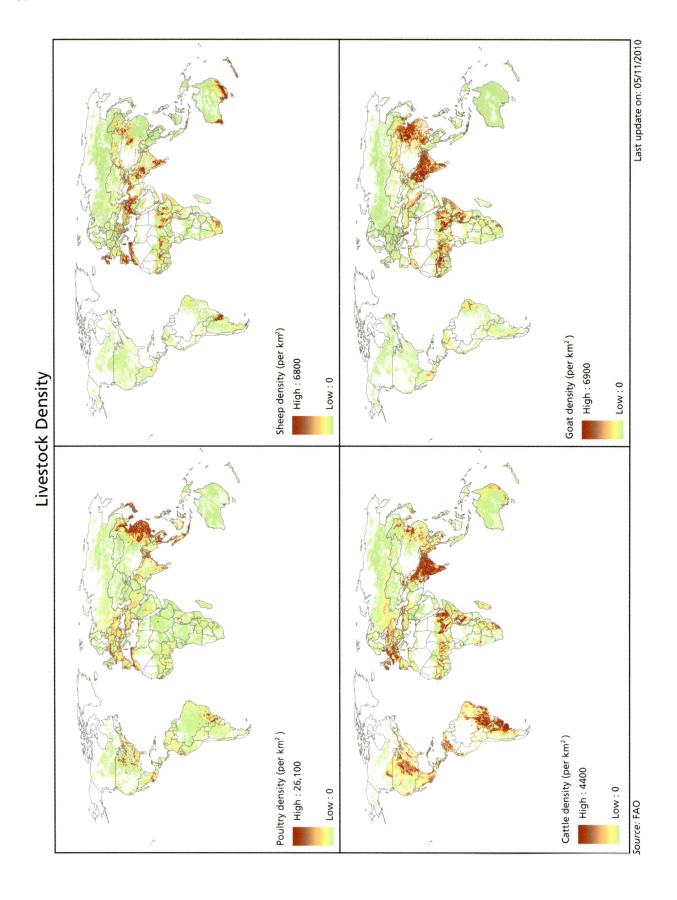

Poultry density (per km²)
High : 26,100
Low : 0

Sheep density (per km²)
High : 6800
Low : 0

Cattle density (per km²)
High : 4400
Low : 0

Goat density (per km²)
High : 6900
Low : 0

Last update on: 05/11/2010

Source: FAO

Subject: Livestock Density

Definition: The maps opposite show the global distribution of domesticated food production animals (cattle, poultry, sheep, and goats) per square kilometer. The distribution of pigs is shown on the *Streptococcus suis* map.

Trends: Global livestock production has increased markedly since the early 1980s and continued growth is expected. The demand for meat, eggs, and milk has been driven by population growth, increased incomes, and urbanization. Since the early 1960s the per capita consumption of meat in developing countries has more than tripled and egg consumption has increased five-fold. These trends have resulted in a more intensive and geographically concentrated production of livestock, especially pigs and poultry. The proportion of energy derived from livestock products has risen most dramatically in East and Southeast Asia, followed by Latin America and the Caribbean. The maps clearly show the heterogeneous distribution of livestock. For religious and cultural reasons there are few or no pigs in predominantly Islamic countries. Cattle are widespread but there are particularly high concentrations in India, northwest Europe, Brazil, and Argentina. Sheep are popular in the Near East, North Africa, Spain, the UK, and Australasia, while goats are more popular in north India, Pakistan, and north China. There are high numbers of poultry in China and Southeast Asia

Significance for infections: It has been proposed that the domestication of livestock around 10,000 years ago was a major factor behind the adaptation and emergence of many infections that are now well established in humans, e.g. measles. Today, livestock can be the source of a wide range of zoonotic infections. A non-exhaustive list includes: leptospirosis, trichinellosis, teniasis, and *Streptococus suis* from pigs; fascioliasis, bovine TB, brucellosis, African Trypanosomiasis, variant CJD, and leptospirosis from cattle; fascioliasis, brucellosis, orf virus, and Q fever (*Coxiella burnetii*) from sheep; and avian influenza from poultry. Buffaloes suffer similar diseases to cattle and there are large numbers in India and Southeast Asia. Bacterial pathogens that can infect a wide range of livestock species and be a source of infection for humans include non-typhoidal salmonellas, campylobacter, *Listeria monocytogenes*, and *E. coli*. Livestock may also act as amplifying hosts, e.g. Japanese encephalitis, anthrax, Nipah virus, Crimean-Congo Hemorrhagic fever, Rift Valley fever. Influenza is interesting since wild birds are the natural reservoir and it is also endemic in human populations, with livestock (pigs and poultry) acting as intermediary hosts and 'mixing vessels.. The widespread use of antimicrobials in animal production for the prevention and treatment of infection, and for growth promotion, presents a risk of the development and transfer of antimicrobial resistance. The intensification of livestock production systems can improve food safety but can also introduce new risks by increasing the interaction between livestock and wild animal reservoirs, while sophisticated production and distribution chains can increase opportunities for the rapid dispersal of pathogens.

Map sources: Data for the Livestock Density maps were obtained from the FAO, available at: www.fao.org/ag/againfo/resources/en/glw/home.html (accessed on: 15/05/2010).

Key references

Food and Agriculture Organization (2009) *The State of Food and Agriculture – Livestock in the Balance*. FAO Report.

Wint GRW, et al. (2007) *Gridded Livestock of the World 2007*. FAO Report.

38

Bird Migration

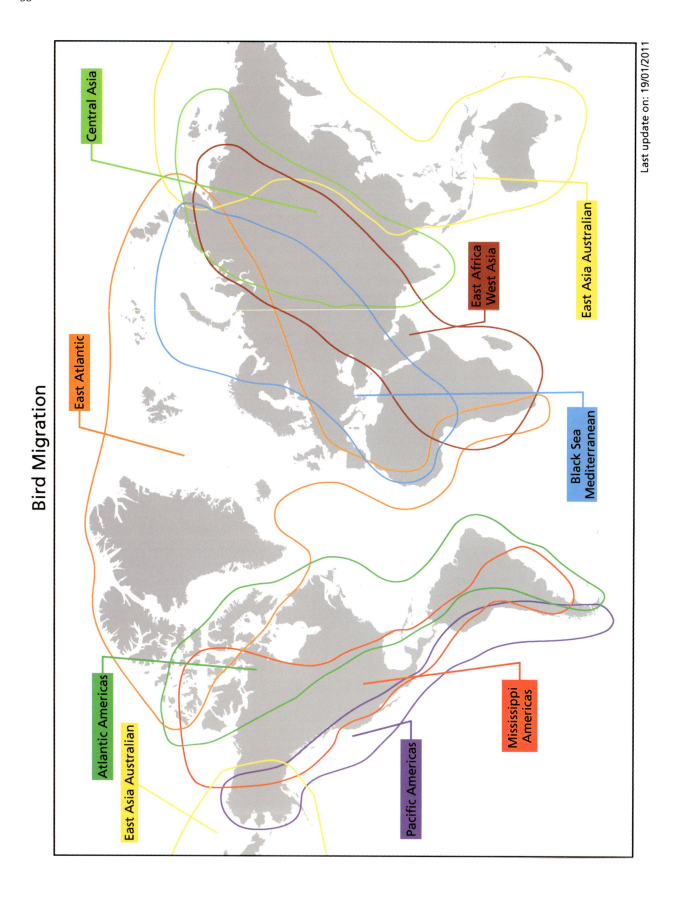

Central Asia

East Atlantic

East Africa
West Asia

East Asia Australian

Black Sea
Mediterranean

Atlantic Americas

East Asia Australian

Pacific Americas

Mississippi
Americas

Subject: Bird Migration

Definition: Each year, several billion birds migrate, and at any one point in time bird migration is occurring somewhere in the world. Migration is a seasonal event, in which certain species travel between breeding grounds and overwintering grounds in order to take advantage of seasonal changes in resource availability. Globally, around 40% of bird species migrate; however, the proportion of species that are migratory in any particular location increases with distance from the tropics. Since most of the global land mass is in the Northern hemisphere, the most common migratory pattern is a northward spring migration to breeding grounds, where young are raised, followed by a southward autumn migration in order to escape harsh northern winters. However, a wide range of alternative migratory patterns are common. Although a simplification, key migration routes, or flyways, can be identified, with some species migrating up to 35,000 miles annually. Birds rarely complete long-distance migration without several stops.

Trends: Bird populations and their migration patterns are to some extent dynamic, and changes in the timing and range of bird migrations have been observed over the past 20 years. There is some evidence that particular birds have shifted their ranges to higher latitudes, or altitudes; however, it is not possible to generalize about the impact of climate changes on bird distribution and movements since the effects are very species specific. Depending on the reproductive cycle and migration pattern of the species, both delays and advances in the timing of spring migrations have been observed in Europe in response to warmer springs.

Significance for infectious diseases: Birds may act as a source of infection to humans either as an asymptomatic reservoir host, a diseased host, or through the carriage of infected arthropod vectors (such as ticks). As a result, migration may both enhance the global spread of pathogens and facilitate cross-species transmission. Wild birds are well-recognized reservoirs for influenza A viruses, West Nile virus (WNV), Western equine encephalitis, St Louis encephalitis, and Japanese encephalitis. The 1999 outbreak of WNV in New York and the subsequent spread throughout North America has been attributed to the migratory movement of birds, but the evidence remains equivocal. Wild aquatic birds, primarily waterfowl and shorebirds, are the natural reservoir of influenza A viruses and are central to the ecology and dispersal of low pathogenic avian influenza viruses – the precursors of highly pathogenic strains. Although it is possible that the migratory movements of wild birds have played some role in the long-distance spread of A/H5N1. The regional spread of highly pathogenic avian influenza A/H5N1 in Asia is primarily the result of commercial movement of domestic poultry. Migrating birds have been shown to carry ticks infected with *Borrelia burgdoferi*, the cause of Lyme disease, and migration is thought to play a role in the spread and establishment of new foci of Lyme disease activity.

Wild birds commonly carry enteric bacteria that are a potential risk for humans but only a very small number of human cases have been directly attributed to wild birds. Antimicrobial-resistant enteric bacteria have been isolated from wild birds but the role of wild birds in the epidemiology of antimicrobial-resistant pathogens is unclear. The yeast *Cryptococcus neoformans* is found widely in the environment but is also commonly present in the feces of pigeons and other birds, and causes cryptococcal meningitis, especially in immune-compromised people. A wide range of other pathogens can be found in wild birds.

Bird migration is a potentially powerful mechanism for connecting diverse ecosystems, and may promote the transmission and emergence of infections through crowding of birds, mixing of species, and the stress of long-distance travel. Yet, if a pathogen causes disease in its avian host, this may seriously impair the ability of a bird to fly long distances. Migration has therefore also been suggested to allow uninfected birds to escape from infected habitats, reduce the level of disease in the population when infected birds do not migrate successfully, and even lead to the evolution of less-virulent pathogens. Further insight into the epidemiology of diseases in wild birds and their spread to humans is needed.

Map source: The Bird Migration map is modified from Olsen et al. (2006).

Key references

Olsen B, et al. (2006) Global patterns of influenza A virus in wild birds. *Science* **312**(5772):384–388.

Rappole JH, et al. (2000) Migratory birds and spread of West Nile virus in the western hemisphere. *Emerg Infect Dis* **6**(4):319–328.

Reed KD, et al. (2003) Birds, migration and emerging zoonoses: West Nile virus, Lyme disease, influenza A and enteropathogens. *Clin Med Res* **1**(1):5–12.

Ricklefs RS, et al. (2005) Migrants and their parasites. In Greenburg R and Marra P (eds). *Birds of Two Worlds: The Ecology and Evolution of Migration* (pp. 210–221). Johns Hopkins University Press, Baltimore.

Tsiodras S, et al. (2008) Human infections associated with wild birds. *J Infect* **56**(2):83–98.

Atlas of Human Infectious Diseases, First Edition. Heiman F.L. Wertheim, Peter Horby and John P. Woodall.
© 2012 Blackwell Publishing Ltd. Published 2012 by Blackwell Publishing Ltd.

Bacterial Infections

Anthrax

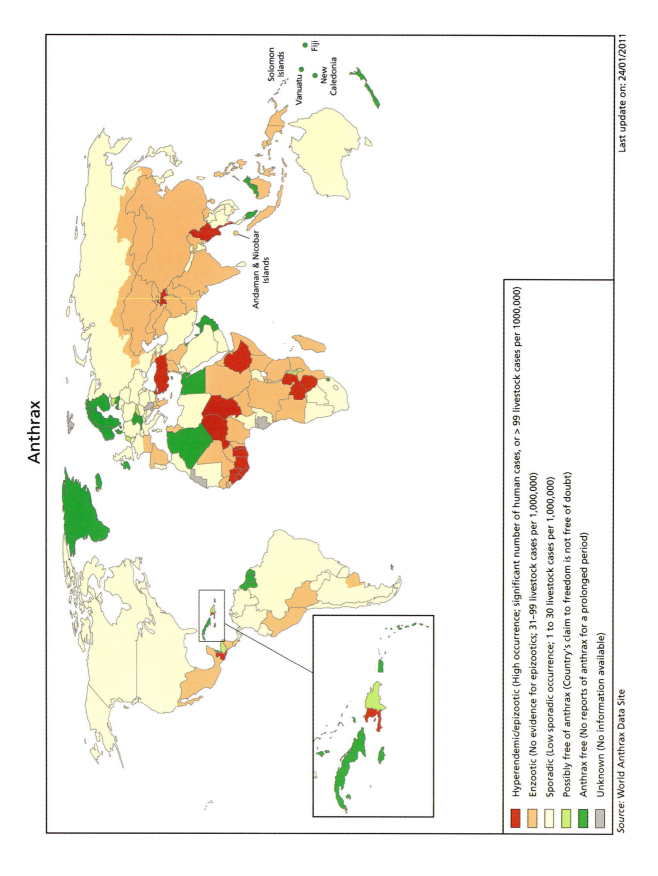

Solomon Islands

Fiji

Vanuatu

New Caledonia

Andaman & Nicobar Islands

Hyperendemic/epizootic (High occurrence; significant number of human cases, or > 99 livestock cases per 1000,000)

Enzootic (No evidence for epizootics; 31–99 livestock cases per 1,000,000)

Sporadic (Low sporadic occurrence; 1 to 30 livestock cases per 1,000,000)

Possibly free of anthrax (Country's claim to freedom is not free of doubt)

Anthrax free (No reports of anthrax for a prolonged period)

Unknown (No information available)

Source: World Anthrax Data Site

Last update on: 24/01/2011

Disease: Anthrax

Classification: ICD-9 022; ICD-10 A22

Syndromes and synonyms: Charbon, malignant pustule, malignant edema, woolsorter disease, tanner disease.

Agent: Spores of *Bacillus anthracis*, a Gram-positive, encapsulated, non-motile rod. The spores are resistant to desiccation, extremes of temperature and pH, ultraviolet radiation and many disinfectants, and can remain viable for 60 years. It is considered a biological warfare agent.

Reservoir: Soil, animal hair, wool or hides, particularly goat skins contaminated with soil. Spores can germinate outside an animal under appropriate conditions.

Vector: Tabanid and Stomoxys flies and mosquitoes can transmit, but are not epizootic vectors. Blow-flies can also spread the bacteria.

Transmission: Contact with infected animal tissue. *Cutaneous anthrax:* direct skin inoculation during processing of contaminated animal hides, hair, wool, or animal hide products. *Gastro-intestinal (GI) anthrax:* consuming meat from infected livestock. *Inhalation anthrax:* inhalation of anthrax spores by tanning/shearing sheep or processing contaminated hair/wool or intentional during a bioterrorist attack. Rare in IVDU from contaminated heroin. There is no direct person-to-person transmission.

Cycle: Herbivores become infected when they ingest spores during grazing on contaminated soil. When the animal dies, the soil under the carcase is contaminated. Omnivores and carnivores are infected by feeding on infected prey or carcases. Carnivores and humans are incidental hosts.

Incubation period: 1–7 days; up to 60 days in case of low inhaled dose.

Clinical findings: Depends on portal of entry. The skin lesion is a characteristic black eschar surrounded by edema, usually on the head, forearms or hands, accompanied by malaise and fever, in 80% of cases resolving spontaneously after 7–10 days, but if left untreated it may evolve into fatal septicemia. GI anthrax produces nausea, vomiting, abdominal pain, fever, hematemesis, occasionally bloody diarrhea and often fatal septicemia and shock. Inhalation anthrax is rapidly progressive and starts with fever, malaise and mild cough and chest pain, evolving to acute respiratory distress, diagnostic mediastinal widening, cyanosis and shock. Untreated cutaneous anthrax has a CFR of 5–20% (<1% with treatment), GI anthrax 25–60%, and inhalation anthrax 100% (75% with treatment).

Diagnostic tests: Microscopy (M'Fadyan stain) of lesion; bacterial culture of lesion, blood, or respiratory specimen; PCR; ELISA.

Therapy: Cutaneous anthrax: penicillin, ciprofloxacin or doxycycline po; severe anthrax (GI or inhalation): ciprofloxacin iv preferred. Clindamycin can inhibit toxin production.

Prevention: Vaccination of livestock and humans with occupational risk in endemic areas. Antibiotic prophylaxis when exposed and vaccination in case of inhalation anthrax. Infected animal carcases should be burned or deeply buried, preferably at the site of death.

Epidemiology: Anthrax has a worldwide distribution. Livestock vaccination, antibiotic treatment, and quarantaine regulations lead to a strong decline in anthrax infections in domestic lifestock. Anthrax occurs mainly in rural areas in countries where there is no livestock vaccination and no veterinary control of slaughtered animals. There is a seasonal variation in animal disease with an increase in cases during hot dry weather. Anthrax is an occupational hazard for people who process contaminated animal tissues. GI anthrax occurs when infected tissue is ingested. Of note is the terrorist distribution of anthrax powder by mail in the USA in 2001, which killed 5 people and produced sickness in 17.

Map sources: Modified from WHO World Anthrax Data Site, available at: www.vetmed.lsu.edu tropics (accessed Jan. 2011).

Key references

Dixon TC, et al. (1999) Anthrax. *N Engl J Med* **341**(11):815–826.

Hugh-Jones ME, et al. (2009) The ecology of *Bacillus anthracis*. *Mol Aspects Med* **30**(6):356–367.

Swartz MN (2001) Recognition and management of anthrax – An update. *N Engl J Med* **345**:1621–1626.

Atlas of Human Infectious Diseases, First Edition. Heiman F.L. Wertheim, Peter Horby and John P. Woodall.
© 2012 Blackwell Publishing Ltd. Published 2012 by Blackwell Publishing Ltd.

Bartonellosis, *Bartonella bacilliformis*

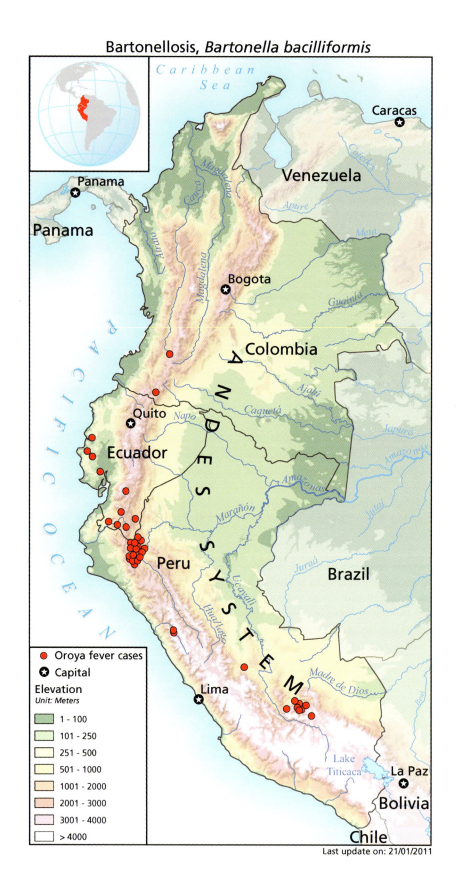

Last update on: 21/01/2011

Disease: Bartonellosis, *Bartonella bacilliformis*

Classification: ICD-9 088.0; ICD-10 A44

Syndromes and synonyms: Oroya fever, Carrión disease, verruga peruana (Peruvian wart).

Agent: *Bartonella bacilliformis*, a fastidious intracellular Gram-negative bacterium.

Reservoir: Humans are the only known reservoir host.

Vector: The sandfly *Lutzomyia verrucarum*. Preferred habitat: narrow river gorges at elevations between 500 and 3,200 meters.

Transmission: By bite of the female sandfly (usually at dusk and at sundown, often indoors); rarely by blood transfusion or transplacental. There is no direct person-to-person transmission.

Cycle: Human–sandfly–human. Humans can be bacteremic for many months. Period of infectivity in the sandfly is unknown.

Incubation period: 16–22 days, occasionally up to 7 months.

Clinical findings: There are two phases, divided into an acute phase (Oroya fever) followed after at least 2 weeks by a chronic phase (verruga peruana). Verruga peruana may occur without an evident acute phase. Oroya fever: fever, myalgia, arthralgia, headache, evolving to severe hemolytic anemia, generalized lymphadenopathy and hepatosplenomegaly; milder symptoms in children. The CFR for untreated Oroya fever is 40–88% and for treated disease is 1–9%. Survivors are immune. Mortality is associated with secondary infections (e.g. *Salmonella* and *Toxoplasma*). Verruga peruana: painless nodular rash, appearing as 'bleeding warts,' mainly on extensor surfaces of the limbs, face, trunk and mucous membranes; may last 3–6 months and is rarely fatal; relapses occur. Differences in clinical presentation and mortality may be due to strain heterogeneity.

Diagnostic tests: Giemsa stain of red blood cells or dermal biopsy; blood culture on special media (results take 3–6 weeks); PCR; serology.

Therapy: Oroya fever: penicillin, streptomycin, chloramphenicol and tetracyclines are all effective, with ampicillin for secondary infections, but the case may still evolve to verruga peruana, which is treatable with streptomycin or rifampicin. Severe cases: ceftriaxone iv is used and blood transfusion in case of severe anemia. Verruga peruana: rifampicin or streptomycin. *B. bacilliformis* is intrinsically resistant to quinolones.

Prevention: Sandfly control with residual insecticide; avoid endemic areas after sunset; use insect repellents and covering clothes; insecticide-treated bednets. Active case finding in households where cases occur. Vector-control efforts should target the homes of incident case patients. Patients should be kept in sandfly-proof wards.

Epidemiology: Bartonellosis due to *B. bacilliformis* was originally restricted to high, dry mountain valleys from 600 to 3,200 meters in the Andes of Colombia, Ecuador and Peru. Since 1997 it has expanded geographically to the Utcubamba river valley, Cusco, La Libertad and the low-lying hills below 600 meters in coastal Ecuador. The cause for this expansion is unknown. The disease incidence is increasing in Peru, particularly in children. In endemic areas attack rates of 12.7/100 person-years are found, with highest rates in children under 5. There is a decreasing incidence with increasing age due to acquired immunity. For each year of age, the risk of infection diminishes by 4%. Most cases cluster, with 70% occurring in only 18% of households in the community where the outbreak happens.

Map source: The *Bartonella bacilliformis* map was made by geocoding reported cases in the medical literature up to 2010. Elevation, rivers and lakes are also shown.

Key references

Chamberlin J, et al. (2002) Epidemiology of endemic *Bartonella bacilliformis*: a prospective cohort study in a Peruvian mountain valley community. *J Infect Dis* **186**(7):983–990.

Del Valle LJ, et al. (2010) *Bartonella bacilliformis*, endemic pathogen of the Andean region, is intrinsically resistant to quinolones. *Int J Infect Dis* **14**(6):e506–10.

Maguiña C, et al. (2009) Bartonellosis. *Clin Dermatol* **27**:271–280.

Atlas of Human Infectious Diseases, First Edition. Heiman F.L. Wertheim, Peter Horby and John P. Woodall.
© 2012 Blackwell Publishing Ltd. Published 2012 by Blackwell Publishing Ltd.

Bartonellosis, *Bartonella quintana*

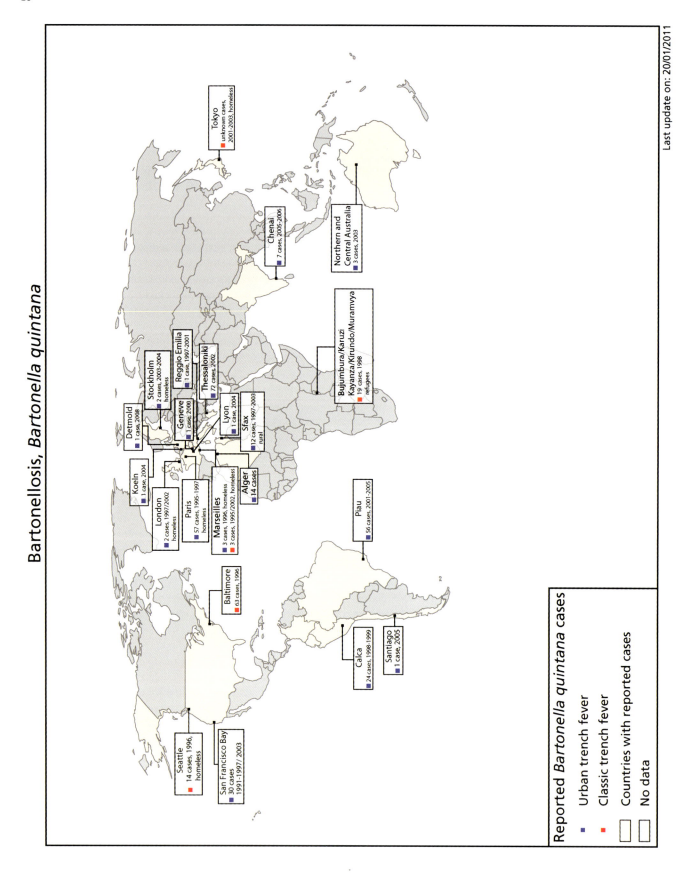

Tokyo
unknown cases,
2001-2003, homeless

Chenai
7 cases, 2005-2006

Northern and
Central Australia
3 cases, 2003

Stockholm
2 cases, 2003-2004
homeless

Reggio Emilia
1 case, 1997-2001

Thessaloniki
72 cases 2002

Detmold
1 case, 2008

Geneve
1 case, 2000

Lyon
1 case, 2004

Sfax
12 cases, 1997-2003
rural

Bujumbura/Karuzi
Kayanza/Kirundo/Muramvya
19 cases, 1998
refugees

Koeln
1 case, 2004

London
2 cases, 1997/2002
homeless

Paris
57 cases, 1995-1997
homeless

Marseilles
3 cases, 1996, homeless
3 cases, 1995/2002, homeless

Alger
14 cases

Piau
56 cases, 2001-2005

Baltimore
63 cases, 1996

Calca
24 cases, 1998-1999

Santiago
1 case, 2005

Seattle
14 cases, 1996,
homeless

San Francisco Bay
30 cases
1991-1997/ 2003

Reported *Bartonella quintana* cases

- Urban trench fever
- Classic trench fever
- Countries with reported cases
- No data

Last update on: 20/01/2011

Disease: Bartonellosis, *Bartonella quintana*

Classification: ICD-9 083.1; ICD-10 A79.0

Synonyms: Trench fever, quintana fever, quintan fever, shinbone fever, shank fever, His-Werner disease, and Wolhynia fever.

Agent: *Bartonella quintana* (formerly *Rochalimaea quintana* and *Rickettsia quintana*), a fastidious intracellular Gram-negative bacterium.

Reservoir: Humans and possibly cats.

Vector: The principle vector is the human body louse (*Pediculus humanus corporis*), which lives in clothes. *B. quintana* has also been detected in cat and monkey fleas.

Transmission: Transmission to humans occurs by rubbing infected louse feces into abraded skin or into the conjunctivae.

Cycle: *B. quintana* multiplies in the louse's intestine and is excreted in the feces. Body lice feed several times per day that leads to itchiness and scratching, by which the skin is inoculated with louses' contaminated feces. Chronic *B. quintana* bacteremia facilitates infection in lice and further spread.

Incubation period: 5–20 days, with a median of 8 days.

Clinical findings: 'Classic' trench fever is characterized by febrile attacks that last 1 to 3 days, with headache, shin pain, and dizziness. The attacks recur every 4 to 6 days, with succeeding attacks being less severe; no deaths have been reported. 'Urban' trench fever generally occurs generally in homeless people and clincal features are highly variable, including severe disease with endocarditis, non-specific symptoms with or without fever, and chronic asymptomatic bacteremia. Infection with *B. quintana* (or *B. henselae*) may also cause bacillary angiomatosis, usually in patients with HIV.

Diagnostic tests: Blood culture with prolonged incubation (42 days); lysis centrifugation blood culture systems or subculture of blood culture bottles onto fresh chocolate agar enhances sensitivity. Several serological assays are available (CFT, ELISA, IFA), but cross-reactivity occurs; PCR on blood and tissue.

Therapy: Treatment of uncomplicated *B. quintana* bacteremia is with a macrolide (erythromycin, azithromycin) or doxycyclin. In case of endocarditis 4–6 months of therapy is recommended in combination with a third-generation cephalosporin or gentamicin for the first 2–3 weeks. Heart valve replacement may be needed.

Prevention: Lice infestation (pediculosis) can be controlled by treating clothes and bedding with insecticides or boiling (bedding at shelters is a major source of lice infestation). The body does not need to be deloused as the lice live and lay their eggs in clothes or bedding. Oral ivermectin has been effective in delousing homeless people.

Epidemiology: Trench fever is named after infected soldiers in the trenches during World War I. Little data exist on the incidence and distribution of *B. quintana* infections. Infections have been reported from every continent. Trench fever is a sign of social turmoil and personal hardship. For instance, an epidemic of trench fever erupted in a refugee camp in Burundi. In Europe and North America, *B. quintana* infections are associated with poverty, alcoholism, and homelessness, known as urban trench fever. Crowded and unhygienic living conditions facilitate exposure of *B. quintana* infected individuals to lice that subsequently pass on the infection to others. Trench fever is a re-emerging disease due to the increase in homeless people and HIV-infected individuals.

Map sources: The *Bartonella quintana* map was made by geolocating reported cases (1990–2010) in the medical literature.

Key references

Foucault C, et al. (2006) *Bartonella quintana* characteristics and clinical management. *Emerg Infect Dis* **12**(2):217–223.

Maguina C, et al. (2009) Bartonellosis. *Clin Dermatol* **27**:271–280.

Ohl ME, et al. (2000) *Bartonella quintana* and urban trench fever. *Clin Infect Dis* **31**:131–135.

Atlas of Human Infectious Diseases, First Edition. Heiman F.L. Wertheim, Peter Horby and John P. Woodall.
© 2012 Blackwell Publishing Ltd. Published 2012 by Blackwell Publishing Ltd.

Botulism

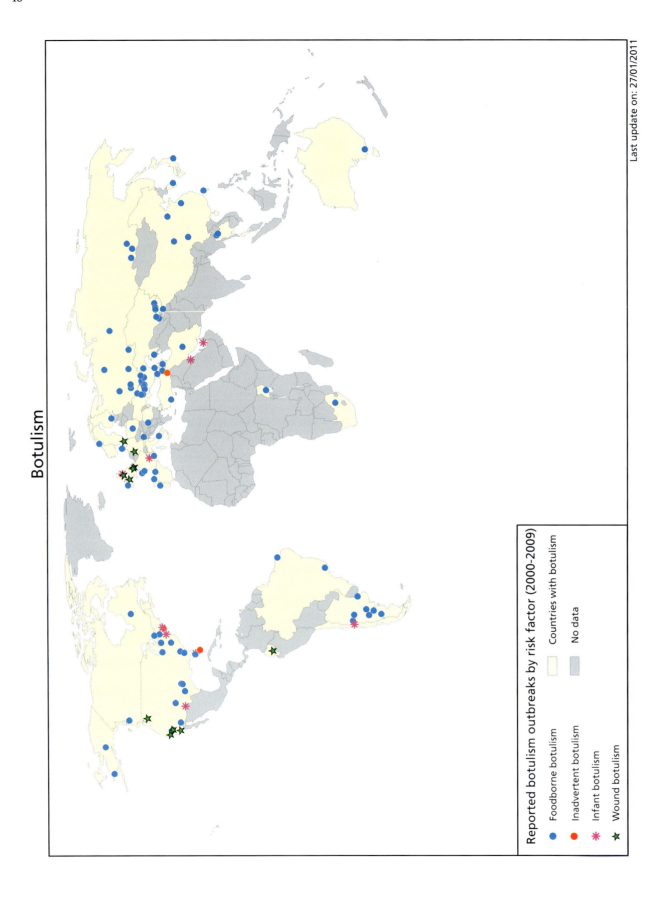

Reported botulism outbreaks by risk factor (2000-2009)

	Countries with botulism
	No data

- ● Foodborne botulism
- ● Inadvertent botulism
- ✳ Infant botulism
- ★ Wound botulism

Last update on: 27/01/2011

Disease: **Botulism**

Classification: ICD-9 005.1; ICD-10 A05.1

Syndromes and synonyms: None.

Agent: Botulinum toxin, produced by the anerobic spore-forming bacterium *Clostridium botulinum* types A, B, E and rarely F. Type E and F neurotoxins have been recovered from infants with botulism due to *C. butyricum* and *C. barati*. *C. botulinum* is considered a biological warfare agent.

Reservoir: *C. botulinum* spores are found in soil, dust, honey, marine sediments, and in intestines of fish and land animals.

Vector: None.

Transmission: By ingestion of contaminated food (honey in infant botulism), injection of contaminated drugs, or contamination of wounds by soil, dust or gravel. There is no human-to-human transmission.

Incubation period: Usually 12–36 hours; sometimes several days; up to 2 weeks for wound botulism.

Clinical findings: Descending flaccid skeletal muscle paralysis beginning at the shoulders in the absence of fever; fatigue, weakness, vertigo, blurred vision, dry mouth, difficulty in speaking and swallowing, progressing to an inability to breathe without assistance. Vomiting, diarrhea or constipation may occur. The CFR in the USA after treatment is 5–10%; recovery may take months. Infants present with constipation, anorexia, weakness, an altered cry, difficulty sucking, and swallowing. Muscle weakness progresses in a symmetric descending fashion over hours to a few days. The prognosis is excellent when treated timely.

Diagnostic tests: Detection of toxin in serum, stool or wound by mouse inoculation or ELISA; culture of the bacterium from stool or wound; electromyography.

Therapy: Food-borne botulism: intensive supportive care and polyvalent botulinum antitoxin iv. Wound botulism: wound debridement, antibiotics (penicillin) and polyvalent botulinum antitoxin iv. Equine botulinum antitoxin can prevent progression of illness and shorten symptoms in food-borne and wound botulism if administered early. Avoid aminoglycoside antibiotics as these may potentiate the toxin and result in a complete neuromuscular blockade and resultant paralysis.

Prevention: Food for canning or bottling should be thoroughly cooked; consumption of inadequately smoked or salted food and uneviscerated fish should be avoided. Also avoid honey and dusty excavation sites with infants. A pentavalent botulinum toxoid (PBT) vaccine is available from the CDC.

Epidemiology: Rare, but good disease burden data are lacking. Underdiagnosis is common. There are four main types of botulism: intestinal/infant, food-borne, wound and inadvertent. Infant botulism is the most common form of botulism in the USA and is caused by growth of spores germinating the immature gut of infants and releasing the toxin, or rarely in adults with abnormal intestinal tracts. Honey is a common source, but in 85% of infants, the source is unknown. Infant cases occur from 6 days to 12 months of age and affect equally both sexes. Food-borne botulism is the result of eating fermented, salted, or smoked fish, seafood or meat that has not been cured for long enough to eliminate contamination. It is also due to incorrect home canning or bottling of vegetables or fruit. Botulism usually occurs in outbreaks in those exposed to the same food. The largest numer of reported cases per country over the decade 2000–2009 in ProMED mail have occurred in Thailand (83 cases from deer meat, 163 from bamboo shoots), Poland (276 from preserved food), and Georgia (217 from home-preserved – vegetables). Food-borne botulism outbreaks occur in indigenous tribes in Alaska and Canada by consuming improperly preserved fish products (seal, salmon, salmon eggs). Wound botulism results from failure to remove contaminated soil completely from wounds and sealing them, permitting anaerobic growth of the bacteria. Inadvertent botulism is a recent phenomenon resulting from the use of diluted Botulinum toxin to treat patients for several disorders and for cosmetic reasons.

Map sources: Reported human botulism outbreaks in ProMED-mail between 2000 and 2009, available at: www.promedmail.org.

Key references

Brook I (2006) Botulism: the challenge of diagnosis and treatment. *Rev Neurol Dis* **3**(4):182–189.
Brook I (2007) Infant botulism. *J Perinat* **27**:175–180.
Smith LA (2009) Botulism and vaccines for its prevention. *Vaccine* **27**(4):33–39.
Sobel J (2005) Botulism. *Clin Infect Dis* **41**(8):1167–1173.

Atlas of Human Infectious Diseases, First Edition. Heiman F.L. Wertheim, Peter Horby and John P. Woodall.
© 2012 Blackwell Publishing Ltd. Published 2012 by Blackwell Publishing Ltd.

Brucellosis

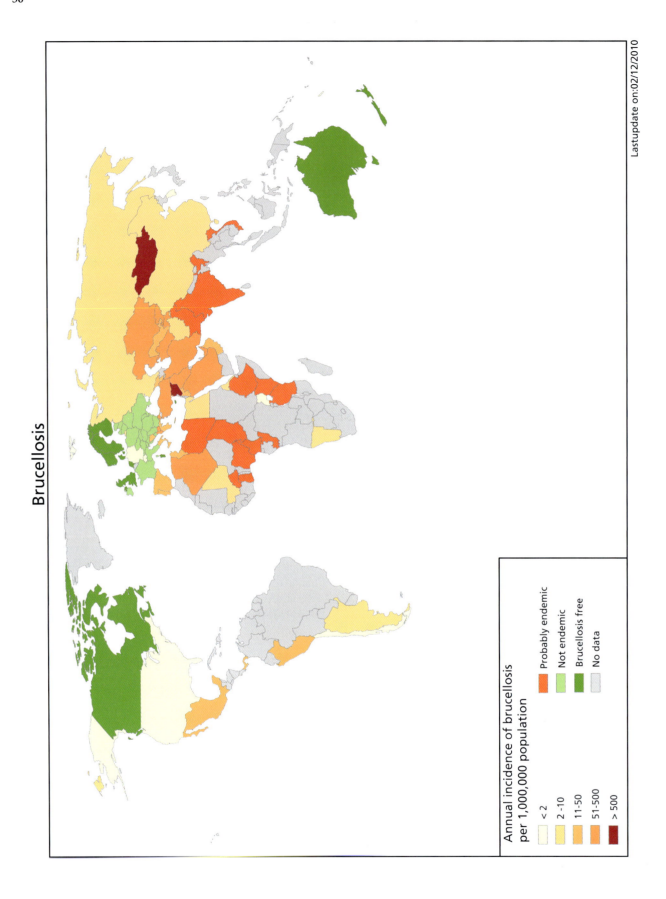

Annual incidence of brucellosis
per 1,000,000 population

< 2

2 -10

11-50

51-500

> 500

Probably endemic

Not endemic

Brucellosis free

No data

Disease: **Brucellosis**

Classification: ICD-9 023; ICD-10 A23.1

Syndromes and synonyms: Undulant fever, malta fever, Mediterranean fever.

Agent: *Brucella melitensis*, *B. abortus*, *B. suis*, and *B. canis*, intracellular Gram-negative bacilli.

Reservoir: Cattle, swine, goats, sheep, and various wildlife species. *B. canis* in dogs and coyottes.

Transmission: Enteric by ingestion of unpasteurized milk or milk products (soft cheese, yoghurt) from infected animals; direct inoculation of mucosa or skin with infected animal tissue (usually occupational in farmers or butchers); inhalation in housing of infected animals. Brucellosis is an occupational disease in shepherds, abattoir workers, veterinarians, dairy industry workers, and microbiology laboratory staff. No person-to-person transmission apart from isolated case reports of sexual transmission.

Cycle: *Brucella* spp. is introduced into animals via inhalation, broken skin, or mucosa and invades local lymph nodes where it propagates and enters the bloodstream and disseminates to mainly the reticulo-endothelial system (bone marrow, spleen, liver, lymph nodes), kidneys and placenta in pregnant animals. From infected organs, like mammary glands, kidneys, and placenta, viable bacteria are shedded into the environment by milk, urine, and uterine discharge, leading to new infections in exposed animals and humans.

Incubation period: Usually 14–21 days, up to several months.

Clinical findings: Acute irregular fever, chills, sweating, arthralgia, headache, and depression. Evidence of localized suppurative infections may be found in liver, spleen, genitourinary tract, and osteo-articular (joints and sacrum). Symptoms may last for months and vary from mild to severe and even fatal (CFR: <2%).

Diagnostic tests: Blood or bone marrow culture and other infected bodily tissues (urine, CSF); serology; PCR.

Therapy: Doxycycline for 6 weeks, in combination with either rifampicin for 6 weeks, or streptomycin for 2–3 weeks, or gentamicin for 1–2 weeks.

Prevention: Pasteurize milk; do not eat unpasteurized dairy products, especially in endemic areas; brucellosis control in domestic animals; hygienic measures in farms and slaughter houses; screening of livestock. Laboratory infections occur where biosafety measures are not adequate.

Epidemiology: Brucellosis is a common zoonosis with approximately 500,000 new cases per year world wide. The disease occurs mostly in areas where it is common to consume unpasteurized dairy products (soft cheese) and where poor veterinary health systems exist. The main *Brucella* infecting species vary by region. Incidence is highest in males with occupational exposure. The highest incidences are recorded in Mediterranean countries, Middle East, Central America, and Central Asia. Five of 10 countries with highest incidences are in the Middle East, with Syria leading. Many of the high-incidence countries were formerly part of the Soviet Union. Since their independence the veterinary health system has deteriorated, leading to an increase in brucellosis cases. In the USA it is mainly reported in Hispanics eating imported infected food. The disease is not considered highly endemic in South America. Data from Brazil is lacking, despite high cattle densities in this country (see Livestock map). Many western European countries have brucellosis-free status. Mediterannean European countries implemented eradication campaigns, but still a high prevalence exists, especially in the Balkan peninsula. In eastern Europe the disease is limited to veterinarians.

Map sources: The Brucellosis map is a modified version from Pappas et al. (2006).

Key references

Akhvlediani T, et al. (2010) The changing pattern of human brucellosis: clinical manifestations, epidemiology, and treatment outcomes over three decades in Georgia. *BMC Infect Dis* **10**:346.

Pappas G, et al. (2006) The new global map of human brucellosis. *Lancet Infect Dis* **6**:91–99.

Atlas of Human Infectious Diseases, First Edition. Heiman F.L. Wertheim, Peter Horby and John P. Woodall.
© 2012 Blackwell Publishing Ltd. Published 2012 by Blackwell Publishing Ltd.

Buruli Ulcer

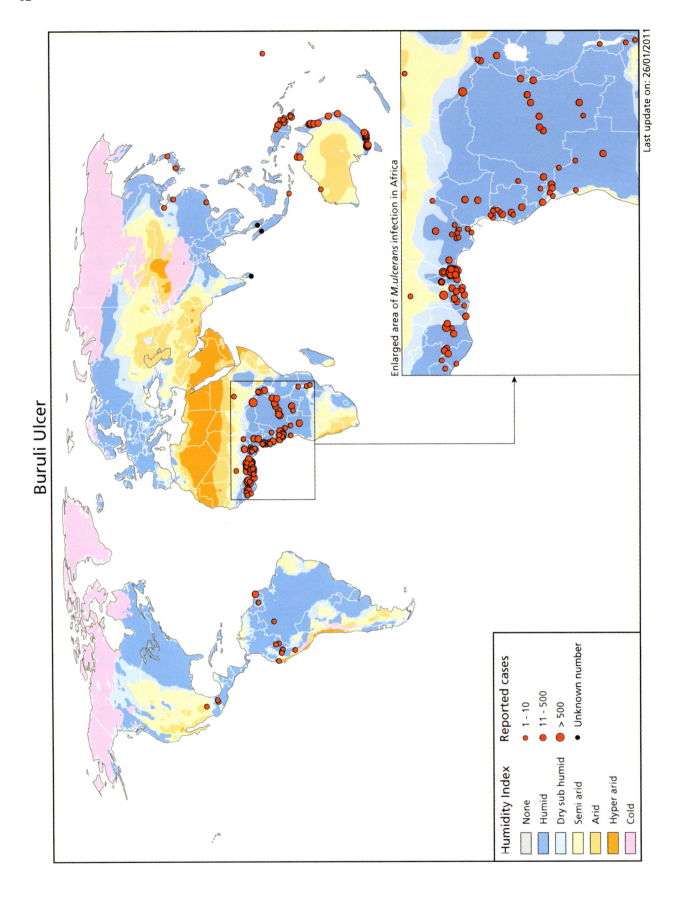

Enlarged area of *M.ulcerans* infection in Africa

Last update on: 26/01/2011

Humidity Index

- None
- Humid
- Dry sub humid
- Semi arid
- Arid
- Hyper arid
- Cold

Reported cases

- 1 - 10
- 11 - 500
- > 500
- Unknown number

Disease: Buruli Ulcer

Classification: ICD-9 031.1; ICD-10 A31.1

Syndromes and synonyms: Bairnsdale ulcer (southern Australia), Daintree ulcer (northern Australia) Kumusi ulcer (Papua New Guinea), Searl ulcer.

Agent: *Mycobacterium ulcerans*, an acid-fast, slow-growing bacillus. There are at least four geographically distinct strains: African, American, Asian, and Australian. They all produce mycolactone, which destroys tissue and suppresses the immune system. Variations in the structure of mycolactone may correlate with disease severity in different regions.

Reservoir: This is unknown at present. *M. ulcerans* has been found in biofilms on vegetation in swamps and other permanent wetlands, aquatic insects, snails, and fish. In Australia, some land animals, particularly native possums, have been found to carry *M. ulcerans* in their gastrointestinal tracts.

Vector: Aquatic insects; in southern Australia mosquitoes; not yet fully understood.

Transmission: Contamination of a break in the skin by bacilli in the environment, or by the bite of an infected aquatic insect or mosquito. Person to person transmission is rare.

Cycle: The disease ecology is not completely understood. Humans are likely dead end hosts.

Incubation period: From 2–3 months to several years. Most infections do not progress to disease.

Clinical findings: Chronic, painless skin nodule that progresses to a severe, deforming ulcer. One-third of early nodules heal spontaneously. Most nodules appear on limbs, but also face and breast; skin lesions may also appear as plaques or indurated edematous lesions; osteomyelitis. Typical characteristic is the presence of deeply undermined ulcers. Sequelae include contracture, deformity, and permanent disability.

Diagnostic tests: Ziehl–Neelsen stain on smears or biopsies, culture (takes 6–12 weeks), PCR, histopathology.

Therapy: In early and limited disease: 4 weeks of streptomycin and rifampicin followed by 4 weeks of rifampicin and clarithromycin. For more extensive disease: rifampicin plus streptomycin for 8 weeks; extensive lesions may require reconstructive surgery and physiotherapy. Lesions < 5cm can be excised under local anesthetic.

Prevention: Wear clothes that cover extremities; cover skin lesions; insect repellent; cover water supply.

Epidemiology: Buruli ulcer is named after Buruli county in Uganda, where the disease was common in the 1960s. The disease is reported in 30 countries with tropical climates, but it may occur in some temperate regions. West Africa is the most affected region. Typical Buruli endemic regions are areas with slow-flowing or stagnant water. Flooding due to deforestation or the construction of dams, and irrigation systems such as rice fields, can lead to outbreaks. Outbreaks have also been associated with mining activities in Africa, due to creation of pits with stagnant water. In southern Australia several coastal towns have reported local outbreaks. It is unclear what triggered these outbreaks. World wide, mainly children are susceptible to Buruli ulcer disease.

Map sources: The Buruli ulcer map was made by geolocating confirmed cases reported in the medical literature up to 2010. As Buruli ulcer is associated with water, the humidity index is also shown.

Key references

Johnson PDR, et al. (2005) Buruli ulcer (*M. ulcerans* infection): New insights, new hope for disease control. *PLoS Med* **2**(4):e108.

Fyfe JAM, et al. (2010) A major role for mammals in the ecology of *Mycobacterium ulcerans*. *PLoS Negl Trop Dis* **4**(8):e791.

Nienhuis WA, et al. (2010) Antimicrobial treatment for early, limited *Mycobacterium ulcerans* infection: a randomised controlled trial. *Lancet* **375**(9715):664–672.

Portaels F, et al. (2008) First cultivation and characterization of *Mycobacterium ulcerans* from the environment. *PLoS Negl Trop Dis* **2**(3):e178.

Atlas of Human Infectious Diseases, First Edition. Heiman F.L. Wertheim, Peter Horby and John P. Woodall.
© 2012 Blackwell Publishing Ltd. Published 2012 by Blackwell Publishing Ltd.

Cholera

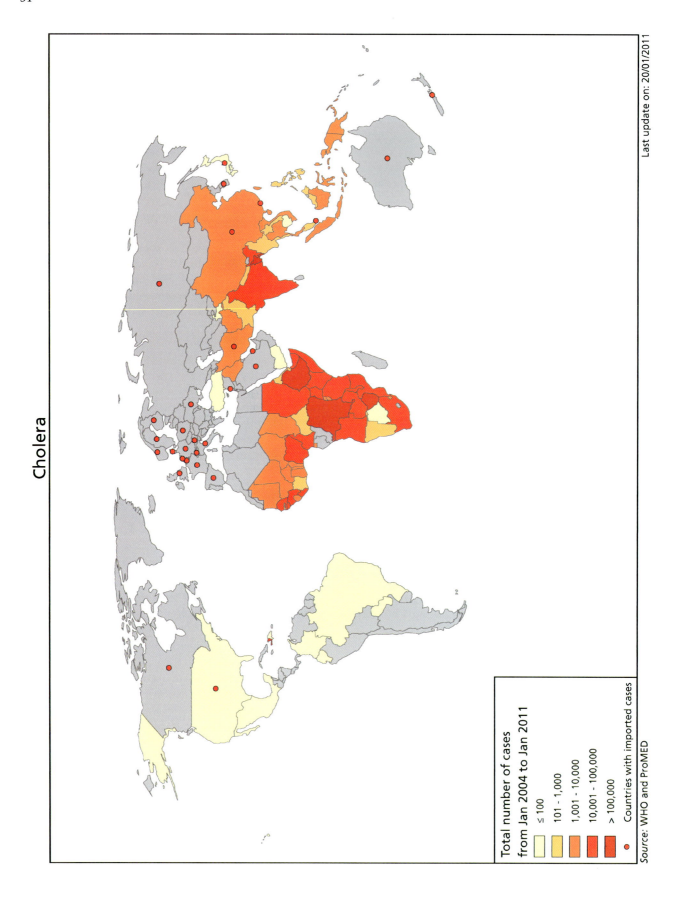

Total number of cases
from Jan 2004 to Jan 2011

≤ 100
101 - 1,000
1,001 - 10,000
10,001 - 100,000
> 100,000
Countries with imported cases

Source: WHO and ProMED

Last update on: 20/01/2011

Disease: **Cholera**

Classification: ICD-9 001; ICD-10 A00

Syndromes and synonyms: Summer diarrhea, acute diarrhea.

Agent: Enterotoxin-producing *Vibrio cholerae* 01 and 0139 Bengal. Serogroup 01 has two biotypes, classical and El Tor, each with three serotypes: Inaba, Ogawa, and the rarer Hikojima.

Reservoir: Principally humans; also warm-water marine and estuarine copepods, other zooplankton. Crabs, shrimps, and shellfish carry the vibrio on their carapaces and shells.

Vector: Main transmission is fecal–oral, but houseflies act as supplementary vectors by contaminating food after feeding on exposed human feces.

Transmission: Consuming fecally contaminated food or water, raw or undercooked contaminated shellfish. Person-to-person transmission through indirect fecal–oral transmission occurs. The role of bacteriophages needs further elucidation.

Cycle: Two interacting cycles can be distinguished: (1) a persistent cycle in the aquatic reservoir, and (2) in the human host, leading to amplification through fecal–oral spread.

Incubation period: A few hours to 5 days; usually 2–3 days.

Clinical findings: Among those infected, about 20% develop acute watery diarrhea, of which 10–20% develop severe watery diarrhea with vomiting, leading to severe dehydration which may be lethal if not treated. The CFR is typically below 5%, but in crowded refugee camps it can run as high as 50%.

Diagnostic tests: Dipstick test, dark-field or phase microscopy on fecal or rectal swab smear; bacterial culture.

Therapy: Oral rehydration therapy (ORT) using reduced osmolarity ORS; intravenous rehydration in severe cases. Antibiotics are only useful to prevent spread, as they do not affect the already released toxin.

Prevention: Hygiene, access to clean water and sanitation. An oral cholera vaccine is available which is safe and provides sustained protection of > 50% that lasts for 2 years in endemic populations. The vaccine does not protect against infections with O139 strains. Chemoprophylaxis for contacts may consist of tetracycline or doxycycline. Breast-feeding protects infants. Quarantine is ineffective. Infection results in limited protection against homologous strains, but there is no cross-protection. Cholera must be reported to national health authorities as small local outbreaks may become large epidemics.

Epidemiology: Cholera is a common cause of epidemic diarrhea throughout the developing world. There are an estimated 3 to 5 million cholera cases and 100,000 to 130,000 deaths due to cholera each year. The disease is endemic on the Indian subcontinent, Southeast Asia and Sub-Saharan Africa. It has a seasonal pattern with one or two peaks corresponding to the warm season. Areas with overcrowding and poor sanitation such as slums, refugee camps, and regions with political conflicts are at high risk for cholera outbreaks. Natural disasters (e.g. flooding) can be followed by cholera outbreaks due to disruption of the sanitation system (see Natural Disasters map). In 2010, a severe cholera epidemic was introduced into Haiti by human activity from a distant geographic source. Cholera was absent from Haiti for at least 100 years. Cases have also been detected in Florida and the Dominican Republic.

Current-circulating *V. cholerae* strains are of the O1 and O139 serotype. Cholera caused by O1 strains of the El Tor biotype occurs world wide. The O1 classical biotype is confined to Bangladesh. In India, some recently isolated strains display characteristics of both the classical and El Tor biotype. Since 1992, the O139 serotype has caused cholera in Bangladesh and India. Other serotypes of toxin-producing *Vibrio cholerae* (e.g. O141 and O75) have caused severe diarrhea in patients who consumed seafood from the Gulf Coast of the USA.

Map sources: The Cholera map was made with data obtained from WHO and the medical literature from 2004 to 2010. The Haiti cholera outbreak was reported at the end of 2010.

Key references

Chin CS, et al. (2011) The origin of the Haitian cholera outbreak strain. *N Engl J Med* **364**(1):33–42.

Emch M, et al. (2008) Seasonality of cholera from 1974 to 2005: a review of global patterns. *Int J Health Geogr* **7**:31.

Nelson EJ, et al. (2009) Cholera transmission: the host, pathogen and bacteriophage dynamic. *Nat Rev Microbiol* **7**(10):693–702.

Reidl J, et al. (2002) Vibrio cholerae and cholera: out of the water and into the host. *FEMS Microbiol Rev* **26**(2):125–139.

Atlas of Human Infectious Diseases, First Edition. Heiman F.L. Wertheim, Peter Horby and John P. Woodall.
© 2012 Blackwell Publishing Ltd. Published 2012 by Blackwell Publishing Ltd.

Diphtheria

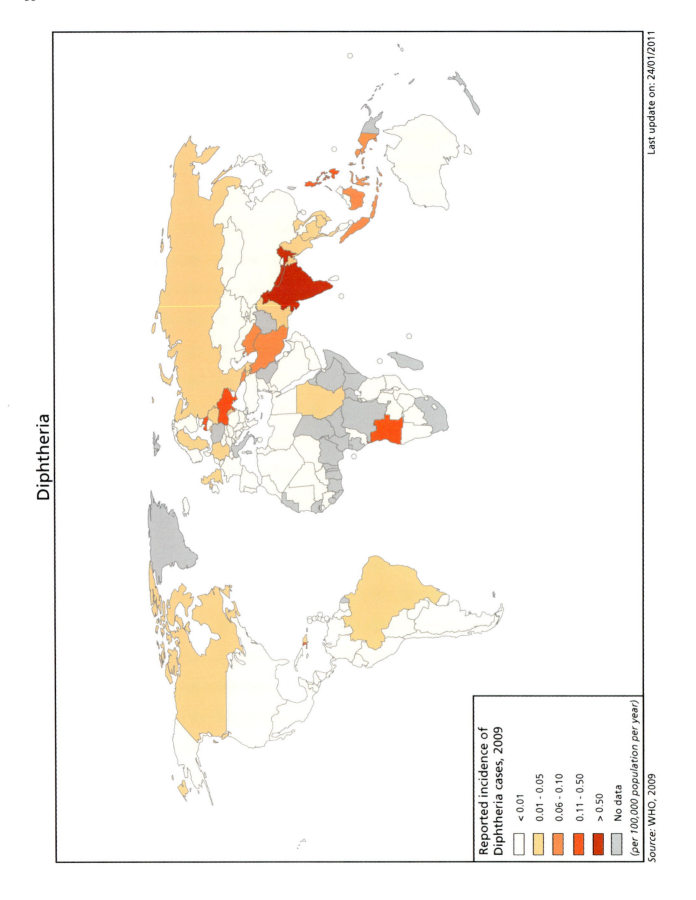

Reported incidence of
Diphtheria cases, 2009

	< 0.01
	0.01 - 0.05
	0.06 - 0.10
	0.11 - 0.50
	> 0.50
	No data

(per 100,000 population per year)

Source: WHO, 2009

Last update on: 24/01/2011

Disease: **Diphtheria**

Classification: ICD-9 032; ICD-10 A36

Syndromes and synonyms: Veldt sore (cutaneous diphtheria).

Agent: *Corynebacterium diphtheriae* is a Gram-positive, aerobic rod that is classified into three potentially toxigenic biotypes, *intermedius, mitis,* and *gravis.* Toxin producing strains of *C. diphtheriae* carry a bacteriophage-derived *tox* gene. Toxin-producing strains of *C. ulcerans* may also cause respiratory diphtheria.

Reservoir: Humans. Cattle and other livestock may harbor *C. ulcerans.*

Transmission: Respiratory droplets from people with respiratory diphtheria, or from asymptomatic throat or nasal carriers. Direct contact with discharge from the skin of cutaneous diphtheria cases. People recovering from diphtheria may carry the organism in the nasopharynx for weeks. Rarely from contaminated items. In the past, outbreaks have been linked to consumption of contaminated raw milk.

Incubation period: Usually 2–5 days (range 1–10 days).

Clinical findings: Respiratory diphtheria is classically associated with fever, inflammation of the pharynx or larynx, pseudomembrane formation, lymphadenopathy and edema of the soft tissues of the neck. However, most cases are mild and may resemble streptococcal pharyngitis and the pseudomembrane may be absent. The exotoxin of *C. diphtheriae* can cause polyneuritis and myocarditis. Nasal diphtheria is usually mild and chronic with nasal discharge and ulceration. Cutaneous diphtheria is characterized by chronic, sharply demarcated ulcers with an adherent gray pseudomembrane. It is usually associated with skin infections caused by *Staphylococcus aureus* and group A streptococci.

Diagnostic tests: Isolation of *C. diphtheriae* and *C. ulcerans* by culture and toxigenicity testing of strains at reference labs.

Therapy: Therapy is aimed at neutralizing the potent exotoxin, eradicating the organism, and providing supportive care. Immediate treatment with diphtheria antitoxin and iv antibiotics (penicillin or macrolide).

Prevention: Immunization with diphtheria toxoid, usually formulated in a multivalent vaccine (see DTP3 map). Recommended schedule is a primary course of three doses in the first 4 months of life and one or two boosters between 18 months and 5 years. Treatment of cases and carriers with antibiotics to eradicate the organism and prevent further transmission.

Epidemiology: In the early 20th century diphtheria was the leading cause of death in children aged 4–10 years in Europe, and many countries experienced large diphtheria outbreaks during World War II. Childhood vaccination has now virtually eliminated diphtheria as a public health problem in most developed countries, and diphtheria cases reported to WHO have fallen by almost 93% between 1980 and 2008. The WHO has estimated that around 5,000 deaths from diphtheria occurred in 2004, with 4,000 of these in children under 5 years of age. However, a steady decline in the global number of reported diphtheria cases from 1980 was interrupted by a large recrudescence in the early to mid-1990s in the former Soviet Union. Since 1990, diphtheria outbreaks have also occurred in Africa, the Middle East, Asia, and South America. Without periodic immunological boosting through vaccination or natural exposure to toxigenic strains of *C. diphtheriae,* adults may become susceptible to infection. Epidemics may then occur, exacerbated by poor living conditions or the emergence of new toxigenic variants. This has led to the introduction of booster doses of toxoid in adolescents in some non-endemic countries.

Map sources: The Diphtheria map was made with data obtained from WHO, available at: http://www.who.int/immunization_monitoring/en/.

Key references

Galazka A (2000) The changing epidemiology of diphtheria in the vaccine era. *JID* **181**(Suppl 1):S2–9.

World Health Organization (2009) *State of the World's Vaccines and Immunization*, 3rd edn. Geneva, WHO, UNICEF, World Bank Report.

World Health Organization (2009) *WHO Vaccine-Preventable Diseases: Monitoring System*. 2009 Global Summary: Immunization, Vaccines, and Biologicals.

Atlas of Human Infectious Diseases, First Edition. Heiman F.L. Wertheim, Peter Horby and John P. Woodall.
© 2012 Blackwell Publishing Ltd. Published 2012 by Blackwell Publishing Ltd.

Donovanosis

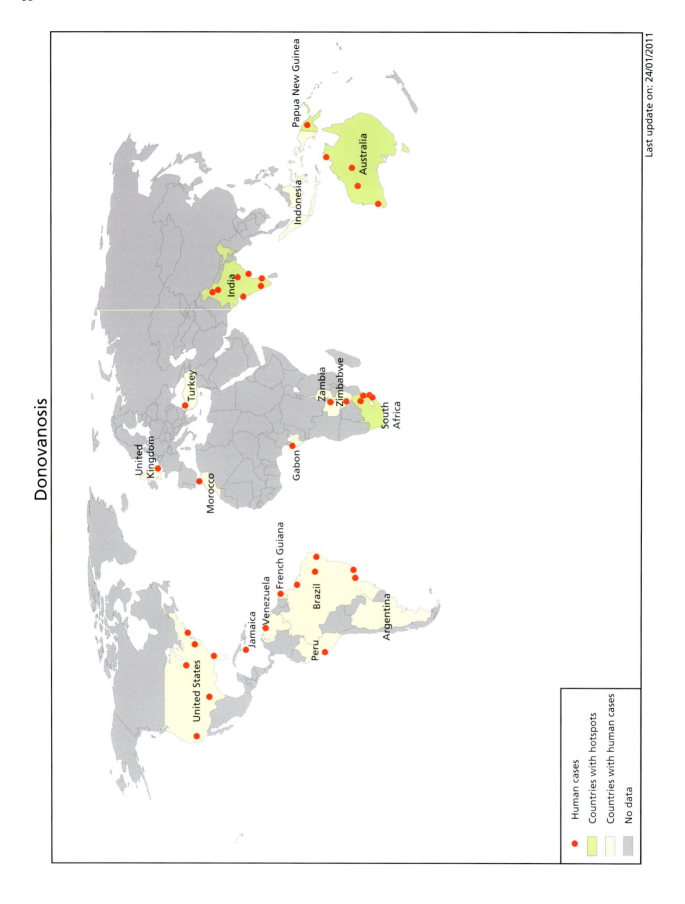

Last update on: 24/01/2011

Human cases

Countries with hotspots

Countries with human cases

No data

Disease: **Donovanosis**

Classification: ICD-9 99.2; ICD-10 A58

Syndromes and synonyms: Granuloma inguinale, granuloma venereum.

Agent: *Klebsiella granulomatis*, formerly *Calymmatobacterium granulomatis*, a Gram-negative facultative aerobic coccobacillus.

Reservoir: Human.

Vector: None.

Transmission: By sexual contact. In children with no history of abuse, the route of transmission is unclear. Several reported pediatric cases have been in contact with infected adults, but without evidence of sexual contact.

Incubation period: Approximately 50 days, but varies.

Clinical findings: A progressive chronic illness of the skin and mucous membranes in the genital and perigenital regions with painless granulomatous ulcers and regional lymphadenopathy. Nodular skin lesions can appear as lymphadenopathy, known as 'pseudobulbar.' The painless lesions are often found in warm moist body regions and bleed easily. Lesions can be progressive and cause local tissue destruction. Systemic spread is rare but bones and internal organs may eventually be infected.

Diagnostic tests: Detection of Donovan bodies in cytodiagnostic or histopathologic examination (may be absent when pretreated with antibiotics); histology is similar to that of rhinoscleroma; PCR.

Therapy: Doxycycline; erythromycin for pregnant women; alternatives are ceftriaxone, norfloxacin and trovofloxacin; in cases of no response: gentamicin; surgery in advanced cases.

Prevention: Early diagnosis and treatment; safe sexual practices (condom use). Proper bodily hygiene.

Epidemiology: It is endemic in tropical and subtropical climates, such as Papua New Guinea, South Africa, parts of India and Indonesia, and among the aborigines of Australia. Some cases have been reported in the countries of Central and South America and the Caribbean. The disease may be related more to socioeconomic conditions than to racial or geographical factors. In some settings it is a common cause of chronic genital ulcers in HIV patients. In the USA, it is more common in African-Americans, of people in lower socioeconomic status, and those with poor hygiene. It has been hypothesized that the natural habitat of *K. granulomatis* is the intestine and that the skin is affected by direct contact during anal coitus, or indirectly through contamination of the genitals by fecal material. There is no gender difference in incidence; most cases occur in adults between the ages of 20 and 40 years. There are no reports of congenital infections, but cases have been reported in newborn and nursing babies; the course of the disease is more aggressive during gestation. Donovanosis increases the risk of subsequent HIV infection.

Map sources: The Donovanosis map was made by geolocating reported cases in the medical literature from 1990 to 2009. Countries considered hotspots (relative high number of cases) by experts are visualized.

Key references
O'Farrell N (2002) Donovanosis. *Sex Transm Inf* **78**(6):452–457.
Velho P, et al. (2008) Donovanosis. *Braz J Infect Dis* **12**(6):521–525.

Atlas of Human Infectious Diseases, First Edition. Heiman F.L. Wertheim, Peter Horby and John P. Woodall.
© 2012 Blackwell Publishing Ltd. Published 2012 by Blackwell Publishing Ltd.

Ehrlichioses

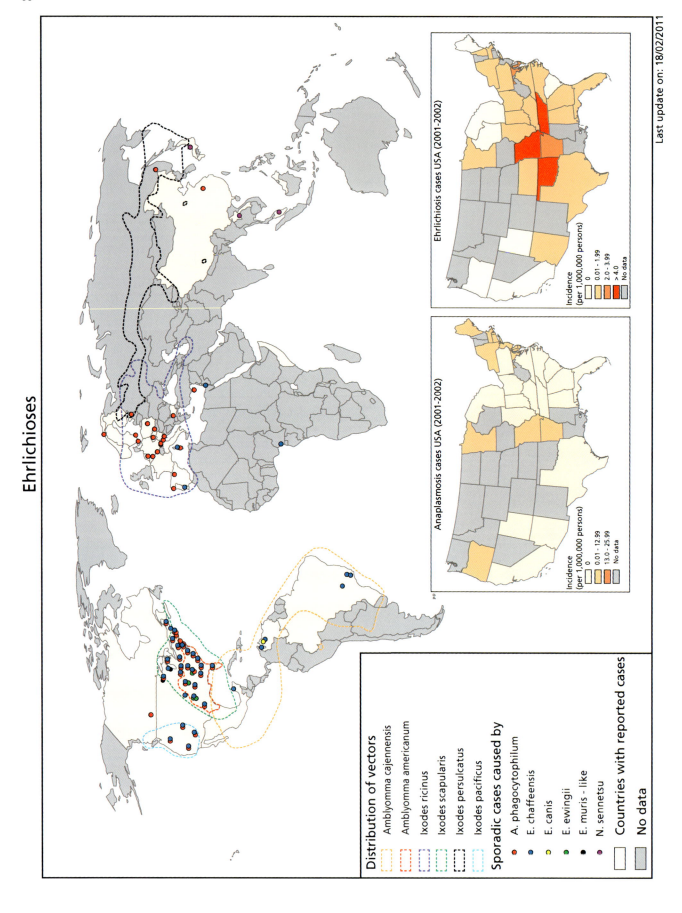

Ehrlichiosis cases USA (2001-2002)

Incidence
(per 1,000,000 persons)

- 0
- 0.01 - 1.99
- 2.0 - 3.99
- > 4.0
- No data

Anaplasmosis cases USA (2001-2002)

Incidence
(per 1,000,000 persons)

- 0
- 0.01 - 12.99
- 13.0 - 25.99
- No data

Distribution of vectors

- Amblyomma cajennensis
- Amblyomma americanum
- Ixodes ricinus
- Ixodes scapularis
- Ixodes persulcatus
- Ixodes pacificus

Sporadic cases caused by

- A. phagocytophilum
- E. chaffeensis
- E. canis
- E. ewingii
- E. muris - like
- N. sennetsu

Countries with reported cases

No data

Last update on: 18/02/2011

Disease: Ehrlichioses

Classification: ICD-9 083.8; ICD-10 A77.4

Syndromes and synonyms: Human monocytic ehrlichioses (HME), human granulocytic anaplasmosis (HGA), Sennetsu fever.

Agent: Obligate intracellular, pleomorphic bacteria of the family *Anaplasmataceae*, which invade host leukocytes. *Ehrlichia chaffeensis* infects mononuclear phagocytes; *E. ewingii* and *Anaplasma phagocytophilum* infects neutrophils. *E. canis* may cause human disease in Venezuela. In 2009 an *E. muris*-like organism was discovered in USA. *Neorickettsia sennetsu* causes Sennetsu fever.

Reservoir: Deer and dogs (*E. chaffeensis*, *E. ewingii*). The white-tailed deer is a complete host for maintaining the transmission cycle of *E. chaffeensis*. Deer, ruminants, and field rodents (*A. phagocytophilum*); unknown for *N. sennetsu*; other members of the genus parasitize the trematode worms of aquatic vertebrates and invertebrates.

Vector: Ticks of the genera *Amblyomma* and *Ixodes*.

Transmission: By tick bites, except for *N. sennetsu*, which is probably transmitted through ingestion of uncooked, parasitized aquatic hosts. No person-to-person spread except by blood transfusion.

Cycle: Tick to mammalian host to tick for *Ehrlichia* and *Anaplasma*; trematode to aquatic host to trematode for *Neorickettsia*. Human is a dead-end host for all. During the eclipse phase of both HME and HGA infection, the blood remains potentially infectious by blood transfusion.

Incubation period: 7–10 days for HME, 7–14 days for HGA, 14 days for Sennetsu fever.

Clinical findings: HME, HGA: fever, headache, anorexia, myalgia, nausea, and vomiting; occasionally a rash. Leucopenia and thrombopenia are common and thrombopenia may be life-threatening. HME cases may progress to meningoencephalitis. Sennetsu fever: sudden onset fever, chills, malaise, headache, muscle and joint pain, sore throat; generalized lymphadenopathy. Reinfection can occur. CFR is 2.7% for HME, <1% for HGA, and absent for *E. ewingii* infection.

Diagnostic tests: Serology (IFA on acute and convalescent serum); cross-reactivity occurs. Microscopy of blood or bone marrow smears is insensitive; PCR on acute phase whole blood; isolation by cell culture in reference labs.

Therapy: Doxycycline for all patients. Rifampicin may be useful for HGA in younger children and pregnant patients.

Prevention: Standard antitick precautions; avoidance of raw aquatic food from *N. sennetsu* endemic regions.

Epidemiology: Ehrlichiosis occurs worldwide, principally following the distribution of the transmitting tick vectors and reservoir species. Less is known of the epidemiology and ecology of *E. chaffeensis* as compared to *A. phagocytophilum*. Most HME cases are reported in the south-central and -eastern USA, where *A. americanum* reaches high population densities. Approximately 70% of HME cases occur from May to July in the USA, corresponding to the peak feeding activity period of the ticks. HME is most commonly diagnosed in adults, with a male-to-female ratio of >2:1. Most HME cases are single and not clustered. Recreational or occupational activities in rural tick-infested habitats are at risk. Majority of the cases have a history of a tick bite. Ehrlichiosis is often not recognized in Africa, where the primary diagnostic focus is malaria and typhoid fever. Sennetsu fever occurs in Asian regions where the eating of raw fish is common, such as in Japan. *N. sennetsu* has been detected in the climbing perch in Laos, a fish common throughout the Mekong River, Basin. Climbing perch is widely distributed and eaten in Asia.

Map sources: The Ehrlichioses map was made with the following data and updates from medical literature:

- Average annual incidence of ehrlichiosis and anaplasmosis reported to CDC (2001–2002), available at: www.cdc.gov
- Vector distributions from *Fauna of Ixodid Ticks of the World*, at: www.kolonin.org.

Key references

Ganguly S, et al. (2008) Tick-borne ehrlichiosis infection in human beings. *J Vector Borne Dis* **45**:273–280.

Ndip LM, et al. (2009) Molecular and clinical evidence of *Ehrlichia chaffeensis* infection in Cameroonian patients with undifferentiated febrile illness. *Ann Trop Med Parasitol* **103**(8):719–725.

Newton P, et al. (2009) Sennetsu neorickettsiosis: a probable fish-borne cause of fever rediscovered in Laos. *Am J Trop Med Hyg* **81**(2):190–194.

Paddock CD, et al. (2003) *Ehrlichia chaffeensis*: a prototypical emerging pathogen. *Clin Microbiol Rev* **16**(1):37–64.

Atlas of Human Infectious Diseases, First Edition. Heiman F.L. Wertheim, Peter Horby and John P. Woodall.
© 2012 Blackwell Publishing Ltd. Published 2012 by Blackwell Publishing Ltd.

Endemic Treponematosis

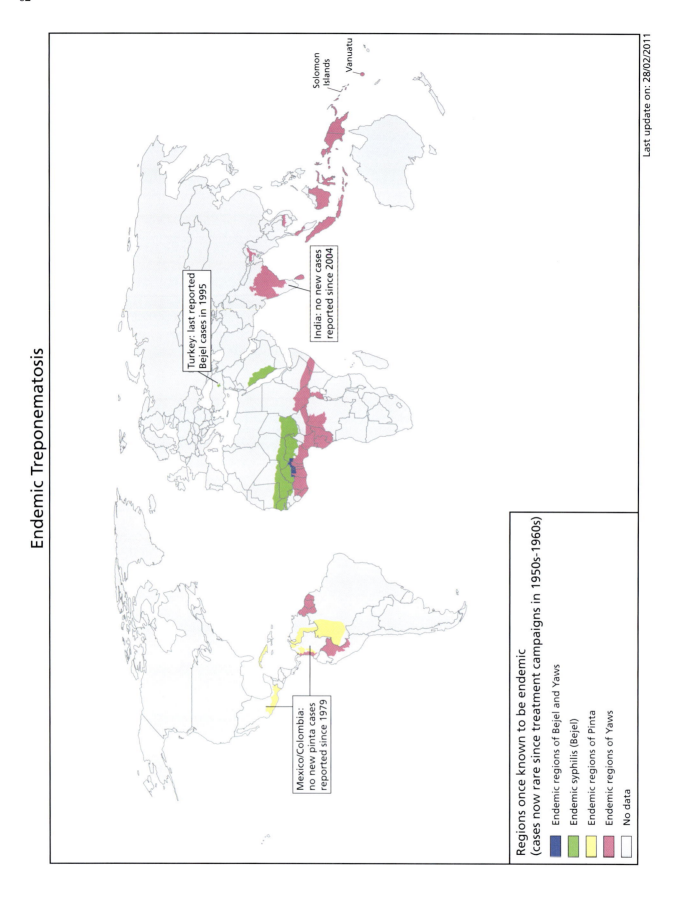

Vanuatu

Solomon
Islands

Turkey: last reported
Bejel cases in 1995

India: no new cases
reported since 2004

Mexico/Colombia:
no new pinta cases
reported since 1979

Regions once known to be endemic
(cases now rare since treatment campaigns in 1950s-1960s)

Endemic regions of Bejel and Yaws

Endemic syphilis (Bejel)

Endemic regions of Pinta

Endemic regions of Yaws

No data

Last update on: 28/02/2011

Disease: Endemic Treponematosis

Classification: ICD-9 102.0 (yaws), 103.0 (pinta), 104.0 (endemic syphilis); ICD-10 A65 (endemic syphilis), A66 (yaws), A67 (pinta).

Syndromes and synonyms: Endemic syphilis (bejel, non-venereal) syphilis, pinta (carate), yaws (frambesia), non-venereal treponematosis.

Agent: *Treponema pallidum* ssp. *endemicum* (bejel), *T. pallidum* ssp. *pertenue* (yaws), and *T. carateum* (pinta), spirochetes that are morphologically and serologically similar to *T. pallidum* ssp. *pallidum*, the agent of syphilis.

Reservoir: Mainly humans; yaws is also found in non-human primates (baboons, chimpanzees, and gorillas).

Vector: Possibly mechanic transmission by non-biting flies (*Hippelates pallipes*) in the transmission of yaws.

Transmission: Direct transmission via skin to skin or oral contact (also via sharing drinking and eating utensils). Sharing of drinking vessels plays an important role in transmission of endemic syphilis in arid regions. There is little or no mother-to-child transmission during pregnancy.

Incubation period: Endemic syphilis and yaws: 2 weeks to 3 months; pinta: 18 weeks.

Clinical findings: Similar to syphilis, the clinical manifestations can be classified into early and late stages. Early-stage lesions are generally infectious and may last up to 5 years, with periods of latency. The disease has a relapsing clinical course with mainly skin manifestations, which is the only finding in pinta. In yaws and endemic syphilis there is also involvement of the mucous membranes and the bones. Cardiovascular and neurological lesions are extremely rare.

Diagnostic tests: Serology; there is no serological test that can distinguish between *T. pallidum* and the non-venereal *T. pallidum* subspecies. Definitively diagnosis by PCR and sequencing.

Therapy: Single im injection with benzathine penicillin G.

Prevention: Prevent intimate contact with cases and contamination of environment from lesions. Lesions or discharge from the lesions are infectious. Treat close contacts. There has been a drastic decline in global disease prevalence since mass treatment campaigns with penicillin under the technical guidance of WHO and with material support from UNICEF in the 1950s and 1960s.

Epidemiology: Endemic treponematoses is now rarely reported since the eradication campaign. Complete eradication may have been achieved if surveillance was continued and rural healthcare services improved. Disease foci still exist, but reports are lacking. Several nations fail to report to avoid the stigma of 'being backward.' The WHO has estimated that 2.5 million people are still infected with endemic treponemes, and about 460,000 are actively infectious. The disease primarily afflicts children in tropical and subtropical areas. The distribution of endemic treponematoses is patchy and associated with poverty and poor access to social and healthcare services; it thus affects mainly rural communities in developing countries (see Human Development map). Endemic syphilis generally affects individuals in hot, arid climates, and yaws affects those in hot and humid areas. Pinta is found only in Central and South America, but has not been reported for over 40 years. No endemic syphilis cases have been reported since the 1980s. Yaws is also rare and currently is only reported from foci in West Africa and Indonesia. Also, no new yaws cases have been reported in India since 2004. It has been suggested that the presence of non-venereal treponematoses indicates that the country or region has a poor-quality healthcare system.

Map sources: The Endemic Treponematosis map was made by combining data from Farnsworth et al. (2006) and WHO.

Key references

Antal GM, et al. (2002) The endemic treponematoses. *Microbes Infect* **4**(1):8394.

Asiedu K, et al. (2008) Yaws eradication: past efforts and future perspectives. *WHO Bulletin* **86**(7):499.

Farnsworth N, et al. (2006) Endemic treponematosis: review and update. *Clin Dermatol*.

Harper KN, et al. (2008) On the origin of the treponematoses: a phylogenetic approach. *PLoS Negl Trop Dis* **2**(1):e148.

Atlas of Human Infectious Diseases, First Edition. Heiman F.L. Wertheim, Peter Horby and John P. Woodall.
© 2012 Blackwell Publishing Ltd. Published 2012 by Blackwell Publishing Ltd.

Haemophilus influenzae Type b (Hib)

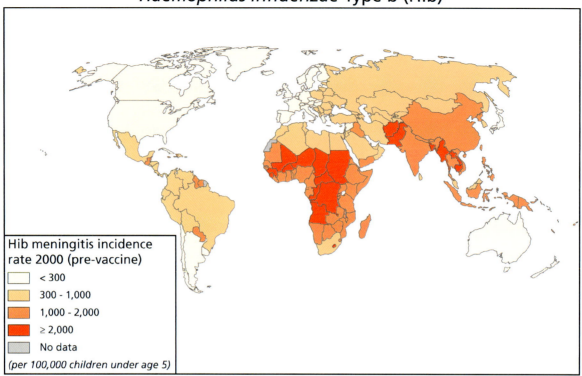

Hib meningitis incidence rate 2000 (pre-vaccine)
- < 300
- 300 - 1,000
- 1,000 - 2,000
- ≥ 2,000
- No data

(per 100,000 children under age 5)

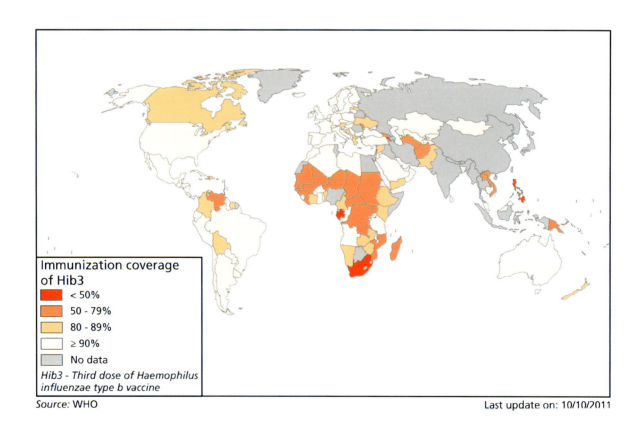

Immunization coverage of Hib3
- < 50%
- 50 - 79%
- 80 - 89%
- ≥ 90%
- No data

Hib3 - Third dose of Haemophilus influenzae type b vaccine

Source: WHO

Last update on: 10/10/2011

Disease: *Haemophilus influenzae* Type b

Classification: ICD-9 320.0; ICD-10 G00.0

Syndromes and synonyms: None.

Agent: *Haemophilus influenzae,* a Gram-negative bacterium that can be uncapsulated or capsulated. Capsulated strains are classified into serotypes a–f. *H. influenzae* type b (Hib) is the most pathogenic serotype.

Reservoir: Humans.

Transmission: Hib is transmitted from person to person via airborne droplets or direct contact with respiratory secretions.

Incubation period: Approximately 2–4 days.

Clinical findings: Hib is a common invasive bacterial infection that primarily causes pneumonia, meningitis, and bacteremia. Pneumonia due to Hib is clinically indistinguishable from other causes of bacterial pneumonia. Hib meningitis may present acutely or subacutely with fever, vomiting, lethargy, irritability, and a bulging fontanelle in infants or a stiff neck in older children. Bacteremia may be present with meningitis or pneumonia but may also occur without an obvious focus of infection. Hib may also cause epiglottitis, which presents with fever, sore throat, and difficulty swallowing, talking and breathing. Infections of soft tissue, bones, and joints with *H. influenzae* may occur.

Diagnostic tests: Gram stain and culture of CSF, blood, or synovial fluid. Capsular polysaccharide antigen detection by latex agglutination or other techniques. PCR from normally sterile site.

Therapy: Third generation cephalosporins (e.g. ceftriaxone or cefotaxime). Other beta-lactam antibiotics may be used in case the organism is susceptible, like amoxicillin. Alternative agents are: fluoroquinolones, macrolides, and tetracyclines.

Prevention: Vaccination of children with three doses of Hib conjugate vaccine from the age of 2 months, with a booster dose aged 12–15 months. Since household contacts of confirmed cases of invasive Hib disease are at increased risk of disease, rifampicin prophylaxis is recommended for all household members if the household contains an infant or inadequately immunized children under the age of 3 years.

Epidemiology: In the absence of vaccination, Hib is commonly carried in the nose and throats of healthy individuals and almost all children are exposed to Hib by the age of 5. In developed countries (prior to immunization), Hib was the commonest cause of bacterial meningitis in young children, but in countries with high vaccination coverage Hib is now almost eliminated as a public health problem. In developing countries Hib meningitis is common but Hib pneumonia appears to be even more common, with pneumonia morbidity and mortality exceeding that of meningitis. In 2000 Hib is estimated to have caused around 8 million cases of severe invasive disease and 360,000 deaths in children under 5 years of age. Ten countries, all in Africa and Asia, accounted for an estimated 61% of all these Hib deaths. Hib pneumonia is estimated to be responsible for around 16% of pneumonia deaths in HIV-negative children, therefore Hib makes an important contribution to the high childhood mortality rates and low life expectancy of Sub-Saharan Africa. Global coverage with three doses of Hib vaccine was estimated at 28% in 2008, with overall coverage of around 90% in the Americas, 65% in Europe, 40% in Africa, and less than 5% in Asia and the Pacific. The introduction of Hib vaccination has however been accelerating and by the end of 2009, in 83% of WHO Member States (160/193), Hib is included in the national immunization schedule.

Map sources: Data for the *Haemophilus influenzae* map were obtained from WHO, available at: http://apps.who.int/immunization_monitoring/en/globalsummary/timeseries/tscoveragehib3.htm (vaccination coverage) and http://www.who.int/nuvi/hib/db_hib1.jpg (incidence).

Key references

Levine OS, et al. (2010) Global status of Haemophilus influenzae type b and pneumococcal conjugate vaccines: evidence, policies, and introductions. *Curr Opin Infect Dis* **23** (3):236–241.

Watt J.P, et al. (2009) Burden of disease caused by Haemophilus influenzae type b in children younger than 5 years: global estimates. *Lancet* **374**(9693):903–911.

WHO, UNICEF, World Bank (2009) *State of the World's Vaccines and Immunization*, 3rd edn. Geneva, World Health Organization, Report.

Leprosy

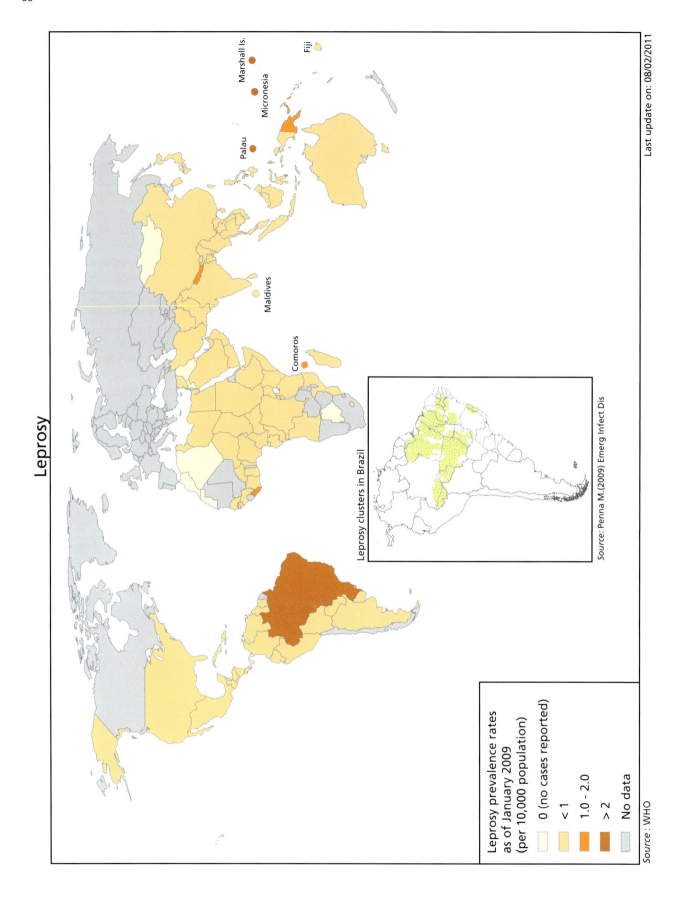

Last update on: 08/02/2011

Marshall Is.

Fiji

Micronesia

Palau

Maldives

Comoros

Leprosy clusters in Brazil

Source: Penna M.(2009) Emerg Infect Dis

Leprosy prevalence rates
as of January 2009
(per 10,000 population)

0 (no cases reported)

< 1

1.0 - 2.0

> 2

No data

Source : WHO

Disease: Leprosy

Classification: ICD-9 030; ICD-10 A30

Syndromes and synonyms: Hansen disease, multibacillary leprosy (ML), paucibacillary leprosy (PL), lepromatous leprosy, tuberculoid leprosy.

Agent: *Mycobacterium leprae*, a slow-growing, acid-fast, intracellular bacterium. It grows best at 27–30 °C, which explains the main target organs of *M. leprae*: skin, peripheral nerves, nasal mucosa, upper respiratory tract, and eyes.

Reservoir: Humans are the main reservoir. Subclinical infection is likely common in endemic areas, as *M. leprae* DNA can be found in nasal swabs in up to 5% of healthy individuals in Asian endemic regions. Subclinical infection generally does not develop into clinical disease. Natural infection occurs in armadillos and several primates.

Transmission: The precise mechanism is unclear: probably by aerosol spread of nasal secretions from a case to respiratory mucosa of close contacts. *M. leprae* cannot cross intact skin. The relative risk for leprosy disease in household contacts is 8 to 10 for multibacillary (lepromatous) leprosy and 2 to 4 for paucibacillary (tuberculoid) leprosy.

Incubation period: 3 to 5 years (range 9 months to >20 years); shorter for PL than for ML.

Clinical findings: The disease mainly affects the skin, peripheral nerves, mucosa of the upper respiratory tract and the eyes, shown by patches of pigmented or reddish skin with loss of sensation, peripheral nerve enlargement with loss of sensation, sometimes paralysis, muscle wasting and trophic ulcers. Patients are classified as having either PL or ML. PL is milder and characterized by <5 skin patches or lesions. ML is defined as ≥5 skin patches or lesions. Skin lesions are often symmetric. Involvement of the nasal mucosa results in nasal congestion and epistaxis. Reduced sensation of digits may lead to their loss due to trauma. Up to 10% of cases with early lesions may resolve spontaneously.

Diagnostic tests: According to the WHO leprosy case definition, at least one of the following: (1) hypopigmented or reddish skin lesion(s) with loss of sensation, (2) thickening of the peripheral nerves with loss of sensation, and (3) acid-fast bacilli in skin smear (often negative). Histology is the gold standard. *M. leprae* cannot be cultured *in vitro*.

Therapy: PL: dapsone and rifampicin for 6 months. ML: dapsone, rifampicin, amd clofazimine for 24 months. Relapses may occur in up to 2.5% of treated cases.

Prevention: Leprosy control is achieved by timely detection and treatment of new cases. BCG vaccination provides variable protection: from 34% to 80%. Chemoprophylaxis and quarantine are not recommended. *M. leprae* bacilli remain viable for 9 days in dried nasal secretions and about 6 weeks in moist soil.

Epidemiology: The disease is thought to have originated in the tropics and subtropics of Africa and Asia. WHO reported 213,036 leprosy cases at the beginning of 2009. Although the worldwide prevalence has declined in the last two decades, the incidence has remained the same. India had the most new cases in 2008 (134,000), followed by Brazil (39,000), and Indonesia (17,000). Males are affected more than females (2:1); young children are rarely infected. Epicurves for PL show a peak at age 15 followed by a trough at age 20. WHO considers that leprosy has been eliminated as a public health problem in any country when the prevalence is less than 1 case per 10,000 population. In 2007, the DRC and Mozambique achieved that status. Also India reported that their national prevalence is below 1/10,000. However, pockets of high endemicity still remain in some areas within those countries. Decreased prevalence without a reduction in incidence may lead to an increase of cases as countries may be less committed to control them once they meet elimination status. Foci in Brazil are found in the Amazonian jungle, but also in arid areas. Poverty and crowded dwellings are important risk factors. Leprosy in North America and Europe has declined to zero cases in line with improvement in living conditions.

Map sources: Data for the Leprosy map were obtained from WHO: www.who.int/lep/situation/en/. The leprosy clusters in Brazil were obtained from Penna et al. (2009).

Key references

Britton WJ, et al. (2004) Leprosy. *Lancet* **363**:1209–1219.

Penna MLF, et al. (2009) Spatial distribution of leprosy in the Amazon region of Brazil. *Emerg Infect Dis* **15**(4):650–652.

Scollard DM, et al. (2008) The continuing challenges of leprosy. *Clin Microbiol Rev* **19**(2):338–381.

World Health Organization (2009) Global leprosy situation, 2009. *Weekly Epidemiol Rec* **33**(84):333–340.

Atlas of Human Infectious Diseases, First Edition. Heiman F.L. Wertheim, Peter Horby and John P. Woodall.
© 2012 Blackwell Publishing Ltd. Published 2012 by Blackwell Publishing Ltd.

Leptospirosis

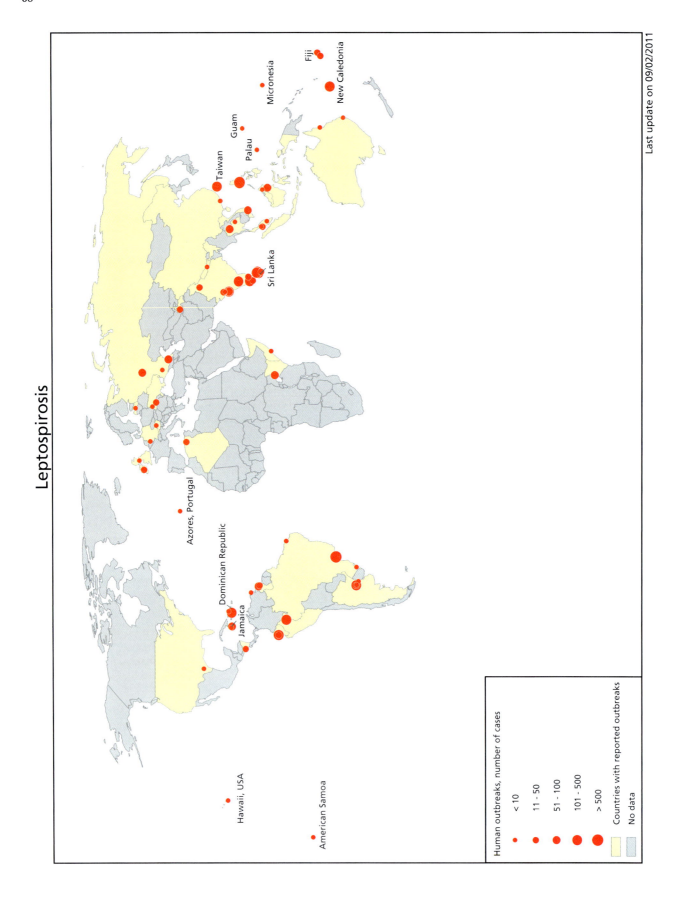

Micronesia

Fiji

New Caledonia

Guam

Taiwan

Palau

Sri Lanka

Azores, Portugal

Dominican Republic

Jamaica

Hawaii, USA

American Samoa

Human outbreaks, number of cases

< 10

11 - 50

51 - 100

101 - 500

> 500

Countries with reported outbreaks

No data

Last update on 09/02/2011

Disease: Leptospirosis

Classification: ICD-9 100; ICD-10 A27

Syndromes and synonyms: Weil disease, swamp fever, cane cutters disease, hemorrhagic jaundice, swineherd disease.

Agent: Multiple species of the spirochetal genus, including *Leptospira interrogans*, which is the species associated with most severe disease. There are currently 8 species found to be pathogenic for humans, associated with >250 serovars belonging to the pathogenic species. Antigenically related serovars are grouped into 24 serogroups. A single serovar may belong to different *Leptospira* species.

Reservoir: Rats and other rodents, dogs, cattle, and pigs are the most important zoonotic reservoirs of human infection.

Transmission: Direct contact of abraded skin or conjunctival mucosa to urine of infected animals or exposure to environmental sources where urine is deposited. Infection via ingestion is uncommon.

Cycle: *Leptospira* chronically colonize the proximal renal tubules of many animals and are excreted in the urine into the environment. Animals can shed *Leptospira* into the environment for prolonged periods without any signs of disease

Incubation period: 1–3 weeks.

Clinical findings: From asymptomatic to fatal. Acute febrile illness with chills, headache, severe myalgia (with mild rhabdomyolysis), conjunctivitis and gastrointestinal symptoms. Less common findings are hepatomegaly, rash, lymphadenopathy, jaundice, and aseptic meningo-encephalitis. Pulmonary symptoms may occur varying from cough, dyspnea, and hemoptysis, to adult respiratory distress syndrome. Weil disease is a severe form of leptospirosis and is characterized by jaundice, renal failure and hemorrhage with a CFR of 5–20%.

Diagnostic tests: Serology (acute and convalescent sera) using the microscopic agglutination test (MAT). Isolation of leptospira from blood or CSF during first 10 days of illness and urine during the 2nd and 3rd weeks; PCR may provide early diagnosis. Dark-field microscopy is not recommended.

Therapy: Supportive and antibiotics: oral doxycycline, ampicillin or amoxicillin for mild disease, parenteral penicillin G, ceftriaxone or cefotaxime for severe disease.

Prevention: Occupational hygiene by the use of protective clothing and avoiding contaminated surface waters (difficult in case of flooding in developing countries). Environmental control measures, like rodent and flood control, are difficult to implement. Chemoprophylaxis for adventure travelers, military personnel who visit endemic areas, and after an accidental lab exposure.

Epidemiology: Leptospirosis has a worldwide distribution, is more common in tropical regions where it is both an occupational disease and a disease of 'daily lives,' mainly during heavy rainfall. Most foci are found in Latin America and the Caribbean, India, Southeast Asia, Oceania, and eastern Europe. The agent favors warm, humid environments. The prevalence of different serovars depends on the reservoir in which animals are present, local environmental conditions, local occupation, and agricultural practices. Protective measures have decreased the occupational risk in high-risk jobs, like mining, sewer maintenance, farming, veterinary work, and the military. In the tropics, occupational exposures (rice and sugar cane farming, fishing) and other agricultural activities remain an important risk. Leptospirosis is an emerging disease in slums, especially during rainy seasons. Also large recreational events with water exposure can be an important source of big multinational outbreaks.

Map sources: The Leptospirosis map was made by geocoding reported human leptospirosis outbreaks in ProMED-mail and the medical literature between 2000 and 2010.

Key references

Adler B, et al. (2010) Leptospira and leptospirosis. *Vet Microbiol* **140**(3–4):287–296.

Bhart AR, et al. (2003) Leptospirosis: a zoonotic disease of global importance. *Lancet Infect Dis* **3**:757–771.

Pappas G, et al. (2008) The globalization of leptospirosis: worldwide incidence trends. *Int J Infect Dis* **12**:351–357.

Reis RB, et al. (2008) Impact of environment and social gradient on leptospira infection in urban slums. *PLoS Negl Trop Dis* **2**(4):e228.

Atlas of Human Infectious Diseases, First Edition. Heiman F.L. Wertheim, Peter Horby and John P. Woodall.
© 2012 Blackwell Publishing Ltd. Published 2012 by Blackwell Publishing Ltd.

Listeriosis

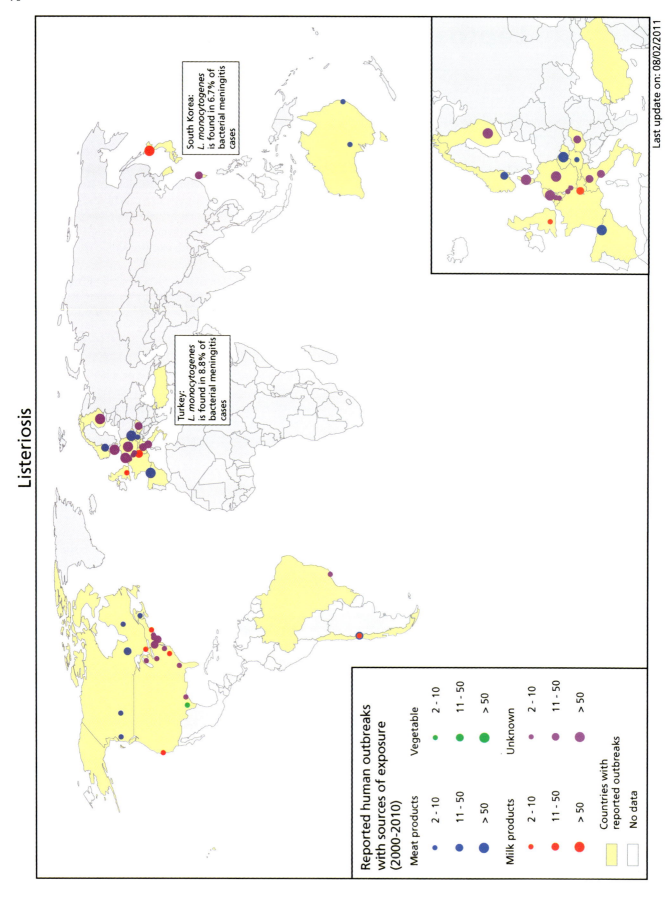

South Korea:
L. monocytogenes
is found in 6.7% of
bacterial meningitis
cases

Turkey:
L. monocytogenes
is found in 8.8% of
bacterial meningitis
cases

Last update on: 08/02/2011

Reported human outbreaks with sources of exposure (2000-2010)

Meat products
- 2 - 10
- 11 - 50
- > 50

Milk products
- 2 - 10
- 11 - 50
- > 50

Vegetable
- 2 - 10
- 11 - 50
- > 50

Unknown
- 2 - 10
- 11 - 50
- > 50

Countries with reported outbreaks

No data

Disease: **Listeriosis**

Classification: ICD-9 027.0; ICD-10 A 32.1

Syndromes and synonyms: Listeriasis, listerellosis.

Agent: *Listeria monocytogenes,* a Gram-positive rod-shaped intracellular bacterium. There are at least 13 serotypes, with serotypes 1/2a, 1/2b, and 4b causing most disease. *L. ivanovii* is a very rare enteric opportunistic human pathogen.

Reservoir: Soil, (decaying) vegetation, and ruminants. Humans and ruminants can carry listeria in their intestines.

Transmission: Food-borne and transplacental (mother to child). Ingestion of *L. monocytogenes* occurs commonly world wide. Development of the disease depends on the host immunity.

Cycle: Listeria bacteria in the environment or food are ingested by ruminants and humans, colonize the intestine and shed again into the environment with the feces. *L. monocytogenes* is able to cross the intestinal mucosa under specific conditions, resulting in systemic disease or hematogeneous spread to the central nervous system and, in the case of pregnancy, fetus.

Incubation period: 3 to 70 days, usually about 3 weeks. For gastroenteritis: hours to 10 days with a mean of 24 hours.

Clinical findings: Non-invasive GI listeriosis: fever, muscle aches, nausea and diarrhea. Invasive listeriosis: septicemia, meningoencephalitis, and perinatal listeriosis. Meningoencephalitis: headache, stiff neck (often absent), confusion, convulsions and coma (CFR: 20–30%). Infection during pregnancy can lead to miscarriage, stillbirth and infection of the newborn. Pregnant women most commonly have flu-like symptoms. Focal infections in any organ may occur. Focal cutaneous and eye infections can occur after direct inoculation with contaminated tissue, usually occupational. Listerial gastroenteritis is uncommon.

Diagnostic tests: *L. monocytogenes* can be detected from blood and CSF by microscopy/culture or PCR. MRI is indicated for suspected brainstem infection (rhombencephalitis). Serology is not useful for diagnosis.

Therapy: First choice is ampicillin or penicillin G. Gentamicin is added in case of immunosuppression, endocarditis, and meningitis. Alternative: trimethoprim-sulfamethoxazole.

Prevention: Pasteurization. Persons at high risk of infection should avoid high-risk foods (smoked fish, raw meat sausage, soft cheeses) and sufficiently heat foods (e.g. left-overs), chemoprophylaxis can be given to susceptible persons at risk after exposure to contaminated food. The organism can replicate at refrigerator temperatures.

Epidemiology: The disease is distributed worldwide, with the majority cases attributed to contaminated processed foods. Listeriosis is, after salmonellosis, the second most frequent cause of food-borne infection-related deaths in Europe. The disease incidence has decreased in the USA, while it increased in Europe for unknown reasons. The more regular use of immunosuppressive medications and the increasing size of the elderly population has increased the population at risk in both Europe and the USA. The majority of invasive listerial infections occurs in individuals with predisposing conditions: pregnancy, corticosteroid use, or other immunosuppressive conditions. One-third of reported cases occur in pregnant women. In non-pregnant patients corticosteroid use is the most important predisposing factor. Clinical data from Asia, Africa, and South America are lacking. *L.monocytogenes* has been found in food products from these regions. Food-borne outbreaks, many of which are manifested by febrile gastroenteritis, have been described with a variety of foods. The most common are processed/delicatessen meats, hot dogs, soft cheeses, smoked seafood, meat spreads, and pates. Infections from animal contact are uncommon and generally occur in veterinarians, abattoir workers, and farmers.

Map sources: The Listeria map was made by geocoding human listeria outbreaks (at least two related cases) reported in ProMED-mail and the medical literature between 2000 and 2010.

Key references

Allerberger F, et al. (2010) Listeriosis: a resurgent foodborne infection. *Clin Microbiol Infect* **16**(1):16–23.

Guillet C, et al. (2010) Human listeriosis caused by *Listeria ivanovii*. *Emerg Infect Dis* **16**(1):136–138.

Siegman-Igra Y, et al. (2003) Listeria monocytogenes infection in Israel and review of cases worldwide. *Emerg Infect Dis* **8**(3):305–310.

Atlas of Human Infectious Diseases, First Edition. Heiman F.L. Wertheim, Peter Horby and John P. Woodall.
© 2012 Blackwell Publishing Ltd. Published 2012 by Blackwell Publishing Ltd.

Lyme Disease

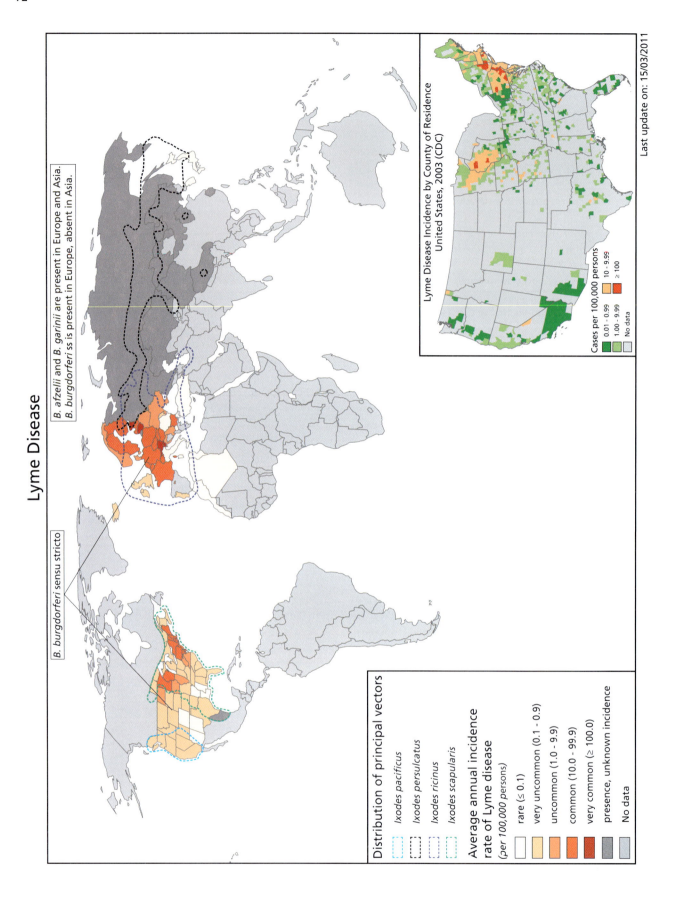

B. afzelii and B. garinii are present in Europe and Asia.
B. burgdorferi ss is present in Europe, absent in Asia.

B. burgdorferi sensu stricto

Distribution of principal vectors

Ixodes pacificus
Ixodes persulcatus
Ixodes ricinus
Ixodes scapularis

Average annual incidence rate of Lyme disease
(per 100,000 persons)

rare (≤ 0.1)
very uncommon (0.1 - 0.9)
uncommon (1.0 - 9.9)
common (10.0 - 99.9)
very common (≥ 100.0)
presence, unknown incidence
No data

Lyme Disease Incidence by County of Residence
United States, 2003 (CDC)

Cases per 100,000 persons

0.01 - 0.99   10 - 9.99
1.00 - 9.99   ≥ 100
No data

Last update on: 15/03/2011

Disease: Lyme Disease

Classification: ICD-9 088.81; ICD-10 A69.2

Syndromes and synonyms: Lyme borreliosis, erythema (chronicum) migrans (EM), tick-borne meningopolyneuritis, acrodermatitis chronica atrophicans.

Agent: The spirochete *Borrelia burgdorferi*. Initially identified as a single species, *B. burgdorferi* has been separated into at least 12 species. Almost all cases of Lyme disease are caused by *B. burgdorferi* sensu stricto, *B. garinii*, and *B. afzelii*, and very few by *B. spielmanii* and *B. lusitaniae*.

Reservoir: Small rodents (mice, voles, rats) and insectivores (shrews, hedgehogs) are the most common animal reservoirs of *Borrelia*, while larger animals (deer, livestock) serve as hosts for the tick vectors. Hares and birds may also serve as reservoirs. Ticks by trans-stadial transmission; trans-ovarial transmission in ticks is limited.

Vector: Hard ticks, principally *Ixodes scapularis* (formerly *I. dammini*) and *I. pacificus* in North America, *I. persulcatus* and *I. ricinus* in Eurasia. In Russia, the principal vectors are *I. persulcatus* in the west and *I. ricinus* in the east.

Transmission: By tick bite or blood transfusion. Most transmission to humans is by the nymphal tick stage.

Cycle: Tick-small mammals and birds-tick; large mammals are necessary to maintain tick populations. Humans and lizards are dead-end hosts.

Incubation period: 3–32 days, mean 7–10 days for EM. Since EM can remain absent, the interval between the tick bite and disease can be much longer.

Clinical findings: Lyme borreliosis is a multisystem disease that can affect the skin, heart, nervous system and, less commonly, the eyes, kidneys, and liver. Often there is an annular skin rash that develops at the bite site, known as EM. After several months, approximately 60% of patients with untreated infection will have intermittent arthritis. Up to 5% of untreated patients develop chronic neurological complaints months to years after infection. Re-infection can occur.

Diagnostic tests: Lyme disease is a clinical diagnosis and laboratory testing is supportive. ELISA or IFA, confirmed by IgM and IgG Western or striped blot test. PCR on blood, CSF, urine and tissues, but is not standardized.

Therapy: Early Lyme disease is generally treated for 10–14 days, late Lyme disease for 21–30 days. Oral antibiotics commonly used are: doxycycline or amoxicillin. Patients with neurological or cardiac forms of illness may need iv ceftriaxone or penicillin.

Prevention: Tick bite prevention by avoiding wooded and bushy areas with high grass and leaf litter, especially in summer months; insect repellents; minimize bare skin check for tick bites and remove them within 24 hours.

Epidemiology: Lyme disease is the most commonly reported vector-borne disease in both North America and Europe, where its incidence is increasing. Incidence is seasonal, corresponding to increased vector activity during summer. The three *Borrelia* species differ in geographic location, vectors, and clinical manifestations: *B. burgdorferi* ss is present both in North America and Europe, but is absent from Asia; *B. garinii* and *B. afzelii* occur in Europe and Asia. A recent study showed that *B. garinii* is the main genotype in China. Data of *B. burgdorferi* presence are lacking for South America, Sub-Saharan Africa, South and Southeast Asia. In the USA the disease is focal: most cases come from limited areas in the northeastern and upper midwestern regions. In the Baltic region, disease rates are several fold higher than in the USA. Incidences vary, ranging from 0.3/100,000 in the UK to 130/100,000 in Austria. Climate change, more housing in wooded areas, and expanding populations of deer, and small rodents may be responsible for the increase in Lyme disease cases. None of the mammal species identified as reservoir hosts and none of the transmitting ticks are present in Australia.

Map sources: The Lyme disease map was made with data obtained from the CDC for USA (www.cdc.gov/ncidod/dvbid/lyme/) and R. Smith et al. (2006) for Europe. Tick distributions were redrawn from Kolonin's website on *Fauna of Ixodid Ticks of the World*, available at: www.kolonin.org.

Key references

Goodman JL (eds), et al. (2005) *Tick-Borne Diseases of Humans*. ASM Press.

Gratz N (2004) *The Vector-Borne Human Infections of Europe: Their Distribution and Burden on Public Health*. WHO Regional Office for Europe, pp. 1–144.

Hao Q, et al. (2011) Distribution of *Borrelia burgdorferi* sensu lato in China. *J Clin Microbiol* **49**(2):647–650.

Smith R, et al. (2006) Lyme borreliosis: Europe-wide coordinated surveillance and action needed? *Euro Surveill* **11**(25).

Atlas of Human Infectious Diseases, First Edition. Heiman F.L. Wertheim, Peter Horby and John P. Woodall.
© 2012 Blackwell Publishing Ltd. Published 2012 by Blackwell Publishing Ltd.

Melioidosis

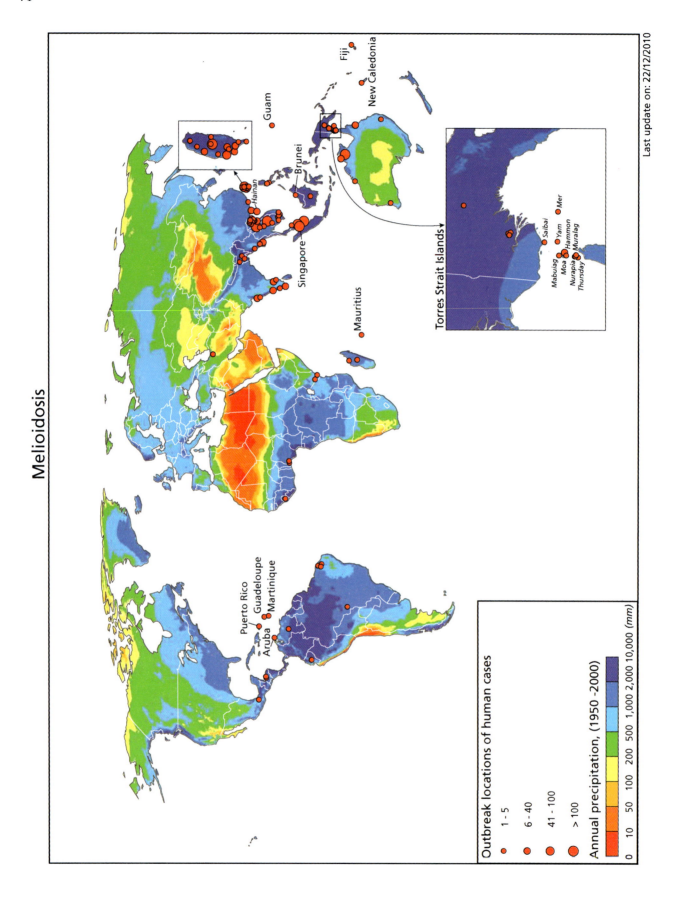

Outbreak locations of human cases

- 1 - 5
- 6 - 40
- 41 - 100
- > 100

Annual precipitation, (1950 -2000)

0 10 50 100 200 500 1,000 2,000 10,000 (mm)

Torres Strait Islands

Mabuiag Saibai Yam Mer
Moa Hammon
Nurapia Muralag
Thursday

Guam

Fiji

New Caledonia

Brunei

Hainan

Singapore

Mauritius

Puerto Rico
Guadeloupe
Martinique
Aruba

Disease: **Melioidosis**

Classification: ICD-9 025; ICD-10 A24.1-A24.4

Syndromes and synonyms: Whitmore disease.

Agent: *Burkholderia pseudomallei,* (formerly *Pseudomonas pseudomallei*), an aerobic, motile Gram-negative bacillus of the beta-proteobacteria group. It is oxidase positive, resistant to a wide range of antibiotics including gentamicin, polymyxin, and the second-generation cephalosporins. A similar disease of equines called *glanders*, now rare (extinct in the Americas), is caused by the related bacterium *B. mallei*. Both *B. mallei* and *B. pseudomallei* are listed as potential biological warfare agents.

Reservoir: *B. pseudomallei* is a soil and water saprophyte and can survive for long periods in moist soil and mammalian tissues. Infection has been found in a wide range of animals, but none is thought to be a reservoir host.

Transmission: Through breaks in skin, ingestion or aspiration of contaminated water, inhalation of contaminated dust. There are rare reports of transmission from human or animal cases to humans. Laboratory workers have been infected by aerosols.

Incubation period: 1–21 days for most acute cases but activation of latent infection has occurred from 25 to 63 years after exposure.

Clinical findings: Range from asymptomatic pulmonary consolidation to mild bronchitis, through acute pneumonic or rapidly fatal septicemic presentations to chronic suppurative infection. Pulmonary cavitation, osteomyelitis and empyema may also be seen. Easily confused clinically with typhoid fever and tuberculosis, and laboratories may not recognize the causative organism and report it as a contaminant.

Diagnostic tests: Isolation of agent from blood, urine, sputum, pus or skin lesions; direct immunofluorescence; serology. PCR may be of value on samples other than blood.

Therapy: Drain abscesses, iv ceftazidime, meropenem or imipenem followed by eradication treatment using cotrimoxazole, with or without doxycycline. Amoxicillin-clavulanic acid is an alternative for those with resistant strains or where co-trimoxazole is contraindicated. Also usually sensitive to piperacillin or ticarcillin with clavulanic acid. There is an up to 10% relapse rate.

Prevention: Avoid contamination of skin by potentially infected soil or water. There is no vaccine available.

Epidemiology: The true worldwide distribution and incidence is unknown. Antibody prevalence in humans and livestock in countries with sporadic cases suggest that most human infections are subclinical or benign, or misdiagnosed and underreported.

Cases are mainly sporadic and have been reported in humid areas of the tropics and subtropics world wide, mainly during the rainy season. Cases have been reported in dryer areas, like northeastern Brazil and north Iran. This is likely explained by the fact that these two areas have irrigated rice fields. In Southeast Asia, it is a disease of mainly rice farmers and others who are occupationally exposed to contaminated soil or water. In northeast Thailand, 20% of community-acquired septicemic cases are due to melioidosis, which accounts for 39% of fatal septicemias and 36% of fatal community-acquired pneumonias. Up to 80% of cases occur in those who are predisposed by underlying immunocompromising conditions such as diabetes, chronic renal disease, or alcoholism, age, chronic infection, or immunosuppressive therapy. Sporadic human infections with glanders (*B. mallei*), occur in equine veterinarians and pathologists, horse butchers, and laboratory workers.

Map sources: The Melioidosis map was made by geocoding confirmed cases reported in the medical literature up to 2010. Imported cases were excluded. The global precipitation data are obtained from WorldClim (www.worldclim.org).

References

Cheng AC (2010) Melioidosis: advances in diagnosis and treatment. *Curr Opin Infect Dis* **23**(6):554–559.

Cheng AC, et al. (2005) Melioidosis: epidemiology, pathophysiology, and management. *Clin Microbiol Rev* **18**(2):383–416.

Currie BJ (2008) Advances and remaining uncertainties in the epidemiology of Burkholderia pseudomallei and melioidosis. *Trans R Soc Trop Med Hyg* **102**(3):225–227.

Peacock SJ (2006) Melioidosis. *Curr Opin Infect Dis* **19**(5):421–428.

Atlas of Human Infectious Diseases, First Edition. Heiman F.L. Wertheim, Peter Horby and John P. Woodall.
© 2012 Blackwell Publishing Ltd. Published 2012 by Blackwell Publishing Ltd.

Meningococcal Meningitis

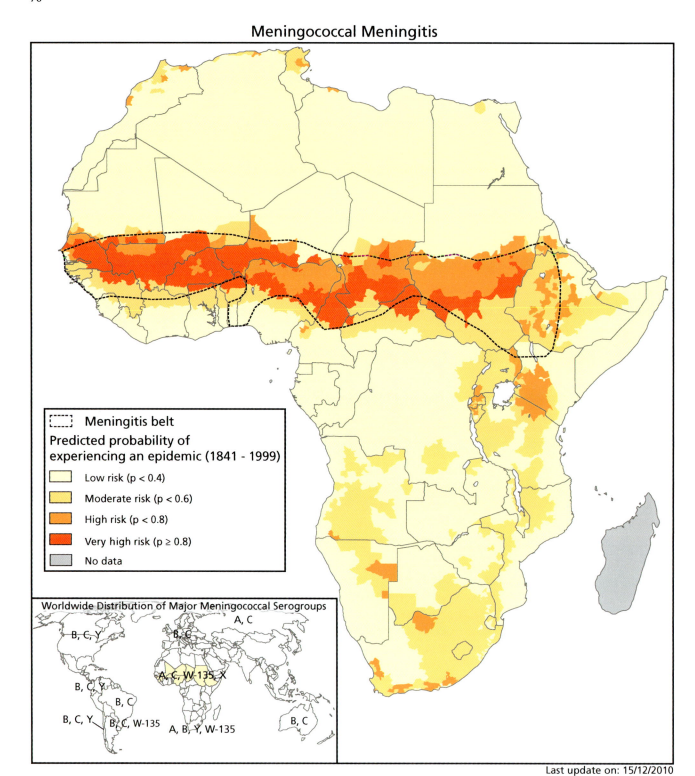

Meningitis belt

Predicted probability of
experiencing an epidemic (1841 - 1999)

Low risk (p < 0.4)

Moderate risk (p < 0.6)

High risk (p < 0.8)

Very high risk (p ≥ 0.8)

No data

Worldwide Distribution of Major Meningococcal Serogroups

A, C

B, C, Y

B, C

B, C, Y

B, C

A, C, W-135, X

B, C, Y

B, C, W-135

A, B, Y, W-135

B, C

Last update on: 15/12/2010

Disease: Meningococcal Meningitis

Classification: ICD-9 036.0; ICD-10 A39.0

Syndromes and synonyms: None

Agent: *Neisseria meningitidis*, a Gram-negative aerobic diplococcus. Pathogenic *N. meningitidis* produce a polysaccharide capsule, used for serogrouping. Five serogroups are responsible for most cases: A, B, C, W135, and Y.

Reservoir: Humans. Asymptomatic carriage of *N. meningitidis* in the oropharynx is common, although carriage rates vary widely by geographic and epidemiological setting. The carrier state is immunizing and development of meningococcal disease is associated with recent acquisition.

Route of transmission: *N. meningitidis* is transmitted from person to person by respiratory droplets.

Incubation period: 2–10 days, commonly 3–4 days

Clinical findings: Classically meningococcal meningitis presents with fever, headache, neck stiffness, photophobia, nausea, and vomiting. In infants and young children the clinical picture may be non-specific. If the patient also has meningococcal bacteremia, a hemorrhagic skin rash may be seen.

Diagnostic tests: Gram stain and microscopy of cerebrospinal fluid, and culture. Latex agglutination tests for detection of group-specific capsular polysaccharide. PCR.

Therapy: Early iv or im antibiotic therapy: iv benzylpenicillin, third-generation cephalosporin or chloramphenicol.

Prevention: Polysaccharide vaccines against A, C, Y, and W135 are available. These vaccines are safe and effective in adults and older children but are poorly immunogenic in children under the age of 2 and the duration of protection is limited to 3–5 years. The development of a group C conjugated meningococcal vaccine that is effective in children under the age of 2 years has been an important advance, and conjugate vaccines are now available for A, C, Y, and W135. The development of a group B vaccine remains a challenge. Chemoprophylaxis of close contacts eradicates carriage and reduces the incidence of secondary cases. Vaccination of household contacts may also prevent further cases.

Epidemiology: World wide, but the epidemiology of the meningococcal meningitis is regionally heterogeneous and dynamic. Group A causes the highest incidence and is responsible for large epidemics every 5–10 years in a belt that stretches across the semi-arid regions of Sub-Saharan Africa: the 'meningitis belt.' These epidemics occur in the dry season and are associated with periods of low absolute humidity and dusty conditions. The map opposite shows the probability of meningococcal meningitis epidemics in Africa based on reported epidemics occurring between 1841 and 1999 and predicted from differences in physical environmental conditions between the regions where epidemics have ever and never occurred. The map provides a reasonable description of 'at-risk' areas and matches well with the WHO defined 'meningitis belt.' However, other factors will also influence the epidemiology, e.g. demographic and social patterns, and immunological susceptibility. While epidemic meningococcal disease does occur in Asia (China – serogroups A, C; India – serogroup A; Philippines – serogroup A) endemic disease activity appears to be low, for reasons that are unclear. Group A epidemics used to occur in western countries but disappeared after World War II and now groups B and C predominate, tending to cause sporadic cases or small clusters in temperate climates and in South America. A significant proportion of disease due to serogroup Y has been reported from Canada, the USA, Columbia, and South Africa. Group W135 had been rare until outbreaks were detected in association with the annual Islamic pilgrimage to Mecca in Saudi Arabia (The Hajj) in 2000. It has now emerged as a cause of epidemics in the meningitis belt, South Africa and Argentina.

Map sources: The Meningococcal Meningitis map was made with data from the International Research Institute for Climate and Society (http://portal.iri.columbia.edu/portal/server.pt), Harisson et al. (2009), and Savory et al. (2006).

Key references

Harrison LH, et al. (2009) Global epidemiology of meningococcal disease. *Vaccine* **27S**:B51–B63.

Molesworth AM, et al. (2003) Environmental risk and meningitis epidemics in Africa. *Emerg Infect Dis* **9**(10): 1287–1293.

Savory EC, et al. (2006) Evaluation of the meningitis epidemics risk model in Africa. *Epidemiol Infect* **134**(5):1047–1051.

Stephens DS, et al. (2007) Epidemic meningitis, meningococcaemia, and Neisseria meningitidis. *Lancet* **369**:2196–2210.

Atlas of Human Infectious Diseases, First Edition. Heiman F.L. Wertheim, Peter Horby and John P. Woodall.
© 2012 Blackwell Publishing Ltd. Published 2012 by Blackwell Publishing Ltd.

Noma

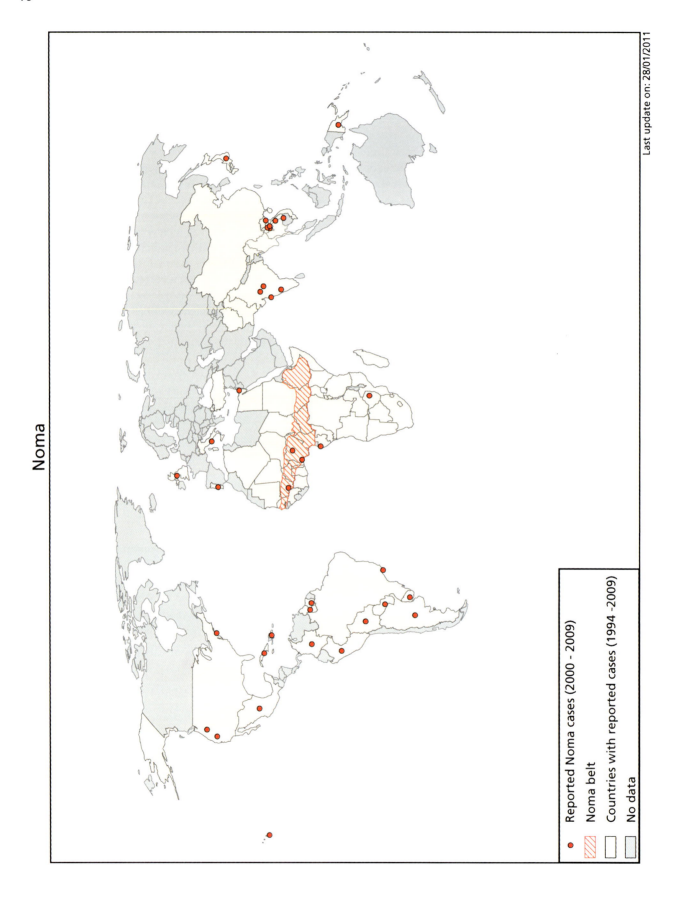

Last update on: 28/01/2011

- • Reported Noma cases (2000 - 2009)
- Noma belt
- Countries with reported cases (1994 -2009)
- No data

Disease: **Noma**

Classification: ICD-9 528.1; ICD-10 A69.0

Syndromes and synonyms: Cancrum oris, gangrenous stomatitis

Agent: Oral commensal bacteria such as *Fusobacterium necrophorum, F. nucleatum* and a spirochete (formerly identified as *Borrelia vincenti*) are the suspected etiological agents.

Reservoir: Human buccal flora.

Transmission: Noma is an opportunistic infection with endogenous buccal flora.

Incubation period: Days to weeks.

Clinical findings: Noma is an opportunistic infection that evolves rapidly from a gingival inflammation to severe, mutilating orofacial gangrene, which is painless and usually unilateral. It begins as a small vesicle or ulcer on the gingiva that rapidly becomes necrotic and spreads to produce extensive destruction of the buccal and labial mucosa and tissues of the face, including the bone, which may result in severe disfigurement and even death. Noma can also cause tissue damage to the genitals (noma pudenda)

Diagnostic tests: None. Diagnosis is made by clinical examination.

Therapy: Penicillin and metronidazole; rehydration; nutritional rehabilitation; treatment of predisposing diseases (e.g. malaria, measles, tuberculosis); wound disinfection; reconstructive surgery.

Prevention: Noma can be prevented through health education, poverty reduction, improved nutrition, promotion of breastfeeding, proper prenatal care and immunisations against childhood diseases.

Epidemiology: The incidence of Noma and the prevalence of survivors of Noma are not well known. In 1998, WHO estimated that 770,000 people had been affected in the past and survived the affection, and that 140,000 new cases were reported each year, of which 100,000 were between 1 and 7 years old and living in Sub-Saharan Africa. An estimation of the global incidence based on epidemiological field work in north-west Nigeria indicates 30,000 to 40,000 new cases per year. It occurs predominantly in debilitated and malnourished children, especially in underdeveloped countries. Peak incidence is at age 1–4 years, the period of growth retardation in deprived children. The etiology is multifactorial: malnutrition, concurrent infections with malaria or measles, bad oral hygiene, severe diarrhea and severe necrotic ulcerative gingivitis are risk factors. In developed countries sporadic cases occur in immune-compromised patients, neonates, HIV-positive and diabetic patients.

Map sources: The Noma map is modified from Enwonwu et al. (2006) and updated with cases reported in the medical literature (2000–2009). The Noma belt was drawn based on expert opinion that stated that African countries directly under Sahara (Senegal to Ethiopia) are 'the noma belt of the world'.

Key references

Enwonwu CO, et al. (2006) Noma (cancrum oris). *Lancet* **368**:147–156.

Fieger A, et al. (2003) An estimation of the incidence of noma in north-west Nigeria. *Trop Med Int Health* **5**:402–407.

Pertussis

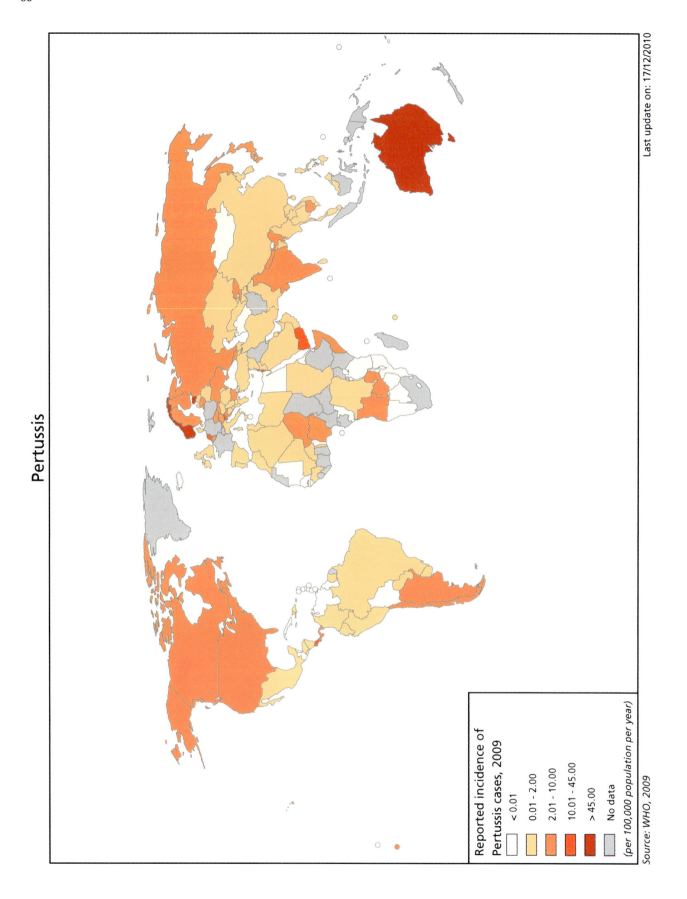

Reported incidence of
Pertussis cases, 2009

- < 0.01
- 0.01 - 2.00
- 2.01 - 10.00
- 10.01 - 45.00
- > 45.00
- No data

(per 100,000 population per year)

Source: WHO, 2009

Last update on: 17/12/2010

Disease: Pertussis

Classification: ICD-9 033.0, 033.9; ICD-10 A37.0, A37.9

Syndromes and synonyms: Whooping cough

Agent *: Bordetella pertussis* a Gram-negative, fastidious bacterium (*Bordetella parapertussis* causes a milder illness called parapertussis).

Reservoir: Humans.

Transmission: Direct person-to-person transmission via respiratory droplets.

Incubation period: Average 7–10 days (range 5–21 days).

Clinical findings: Classical pertussis has a prodromal stage of 1–2 weeks with coryza and a mild, persistent cough that progresses to paroxysms of violent coughing interspersed with an inspiratory whoop. Vomiting may follow coughing bouts. This stage can last 4–6 weeks. Adolescents and adults often do not have paroxysms and whooping, presenting more commonly with a prolonged cough. Asymptomatic infection may also occur. Infants under 6 months may present with apnea, and deaths occur mostly in this age group. Serious complications include pneumonia, seizures, cerebral hypoxia, and encephalopathy.

Diagnostic tests: Culture is the gold standard but is insensitive. PCR is more sensitive than culture. Serology may be helpful in patients presenting 3 weeks or more after cough onset, when both culture and PCR are likely to be negative.

Therapy: Antibiotic treatment with a macrolide antibiotic is mainly indicated to reduce communicability in those presenting within 3 weeks of onset. Hospitalization may be needed in severe causes for supportive care.

Prevention: Two or more doses of a pertussis-containing vaccine are necessary for protection. Global coverage with three doses of a pertussis-containing vaccine are shown elsewhere (see DTP3 map). Infants under the age of 3–5 months are, depending on the vaccination schedule, too young to have received two doses and are also vulnerable to complications of pertussis. This group therefore suffers the greatest burden of pertussis mortality. Post-exposure prophylaxis with a macrolide antibiotic may be recommended for contacts in households where there is a susceptible member (e.g. an infant).

Epidemiology: Pertussis immunization has been successful in reducing the burden of pertussis disease and deaths, with around 150,000 cases reported in 2008 compared to almost 2 million cases in 1980. However, these figures must be interpreted with great caution since reporting is mostly based on clinical diagnosis, which is not easy in neonates, older children, and adults. The WHO estimated that nearly 18 million cases and 254,000 deaths occurred in 2004, of which 90% were in developing countries. Although pertussis disease has clearly been reduced by immunization, it is not clear to what extent immunization has reduced circulation of *B. pertussis*. The continued risk of pertussis in unimmunized infants and the persistence of epidemic cycles indicate that *B. pertussis* transmission continues despite vaccination programs. Several developed countries with high coverage in children have experienced outbreaks of pertussis in adolescents and adults. Immunity following natural pertussis infection or vaccination is not permanent, therefore high coverage with pertussis vaccines in children has shifted susceptibility and peak incidence to adolescents and young adults; these age groups are then transmitting infection to young infants. Since pertussis in adults usually manifests as only a prolonged cough it is difficult to identify cases and protect infants.

Map sources: The Pertussis map was made with pertussis incidence and immunization data obtained from WHO, available at: http://apps.who.int/immunization_monitoring/en/.

Key references

Cherry JD (2005) The epidemiology of pertussis: a comparison of the epidemiology of the disease pertussis with the epidemiology of Bordetella pertussis infection. *Pediatrics* **15**:1422–1427.

Wood N et al. (2008) Pertussis: review of epidemiology, diagnosis, management and prevention. *Pediatric Resp Rev* **9**:201–212.

World Health Organization (2009) *State of the World's Vaccines and Immunization*, 3rd edn. WHO, UNICEF, World Bank Geneva.

Atlas of Human Infectious Diseases, First Edition. Heiman F.L. Wertheim, Peter Horby and John P. Woodall.
© 2012 Blackwell Publishing Ltd. Published 2012 by Blackwell Publishing Ltd.

Plague

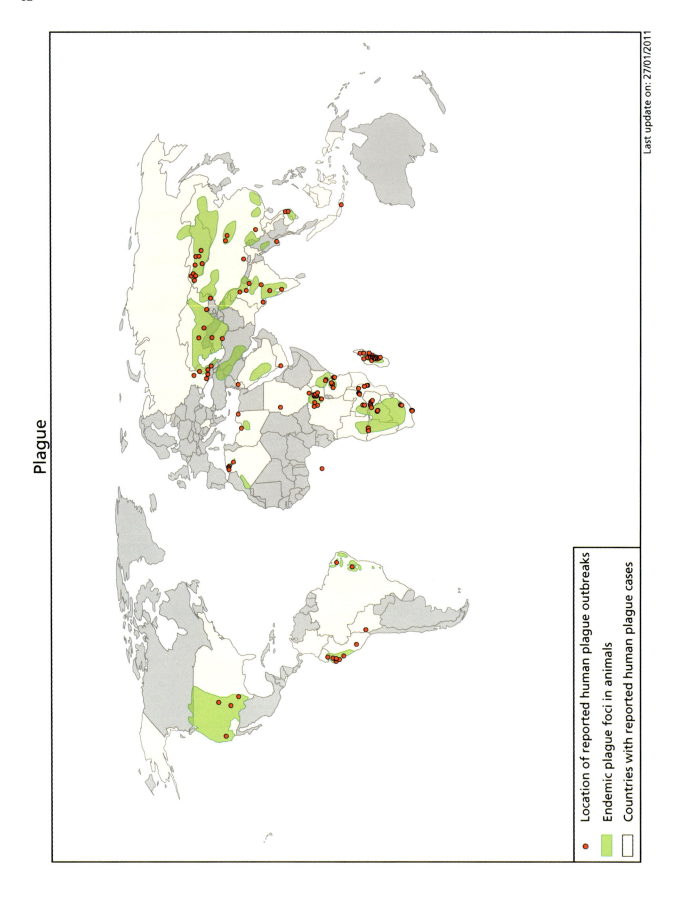

Location of reported human plague outbreaks

Endemic plague foci in animals

Countries with reported human plague cases

Last update on: 27/01/2011

Disease: **Plague**

Classification: ICD-9 020; ICD-10 A20

Syndromes and synonyms: Pestis, pest, bubonic plague, pneumonic plague, black plague, black death.

Agent: *Yersinia pestis*, a Gram-negative bacillus. *Y. pestis* is considered a potential biological warfare agent.

Reservoir: Rodents, principally rats and sylvatic ground squirrels: marmots, susliks, and prairie dogs. Rabbits, camels, carnivores, and domestic cats may also be infected. Cats can also develop pneumonic plague. The desert regions of Central Asia contain endemic plague foci where the great gerbil is the main host.

Vector: Fleas, especially the rat flea (*Xenopsylla cheopis*) and possibly human flea (*Pulex irritans*).

Transmission: By flea bite for the bubonic form, by the respiratory route for the pneumonic form; handling carcasses or eating meat of infected animals. Person-to-person transmission occurs through the bite of fleas (bubonic form) or respiratory droplets (pneumonic form).

Cycle: There are different cycles, including a sylvatic rodent–flea cycle, a commensal rodent–flea cycle, and a cycle of pneumonic transmission in humans. *Y. pestis* can survive in the environment, mainly in rodent burrows in a sylvatic cycle. In case an infected flea feeds on a commensal rodent (rat), a rodent–flee–rodent cycle starts. When the rodents dies, their fleas move to alternative hosts, possibly humans. If humans develop pneumonic plague, the infection can be transmitted from person to person via respiratory droplets.

Incubation period: 1–4 days for pneumonic, 2–7 days for bubonic plague.

Clinical findings: Sudden onset of fever, chills, headaches, body aches, sore throat, vomiting and nausea. Bubonic plague is most common, producing swollen, painful and eventually suppurating lymph nodes (buboes) which are usually inguinal. In the septicemic form, *Y. pestis* spreads through the bloodstream usually affecting the lungs, ending in fatal endotoxic shock and DIC. The CFR of the bubonic form is 40–70%; of pneumonic and septicemic plague in the absence of prompt treatment, nearly 100%.

Diagnostic tests: Microscopy of stained smear from a bubo, sputum or CSF shows characteristic 'safety-pin' shape; serology (IFA; ELISA); rapid dipstick test. Culture takes about 4 days.

Therapy: Streptomycin, tetracyclines, and sulfonamides are standard; alternatives are gentamicin and fluoroquinolones. Chloramphenicol in cases of plague meningitis. Treatment should be started within 18 hours of onset. Buboes may need to be drained.

Prevention: A killed vaccine is available for laboratory workers, but is not recommended for use in epidemics. In buildings or rodent burrows, flea control with insecticide should be followed by rat destruction (killing rats liberates fleas); rat control in ports and ships. Chemoprophylaxis of pneumonic plague contacts. Pneumonic cases should be isolated.

Epidemiology: There are an estimated 1,000–3,000 human cases per year, but there is considerable underreporting and underdiagnosis. The last plague pandemic of 1894 started in Hong Kong establishing many endemic foci world wide. New foci continue to arise, as was seen in Algiers, in 2003. Warm springs and wet summers have increased the plague prevalence in the great gerbil in Kazakhstan. Similar climatic conditions may have resulted in past plague pandemics. Infection control and antibiotics can decrease plague morbidity and mortality but plague cannot be eradicated as it is widespread in wild rodents. There has been a large shift in case load from Asia to Africa, with more than 90% of cases occurring in Africa. The most common form is bubonic plague, but outbreaks of pneumonic plague still occur. Plague is possibly more common in Africa as poor rural communities in Africa live in close proximity to rodents, which are widely hunted and eaten in plague-endemic areas.

Map sources: The Plague map is modified from the CDC map 'Distribution of Plague 1998', available at: www.cdc.gov/ncidod/dvbid/plague/world98.htm. The map is updated with recent literature and expert opinion. Africa plague distribution data was obtained from S.B. Neerinckx et al. (2008).

Key references

Gratz N. (1999) *Plague Manual Epidemiology, Distribution, Surveillance and Control*. WHO Report, Geneva.

Neerinckx SB, et al. (2008) Geographic distribution and ecological niche of plague in sub-Saharan Africa. *Int J Health Geog* **7**:54.

Stenseth NC, et al. (2008) Plague: past, present and future. *PLoS Med* **5**(1):e3.

World Health Organization (2005) Plague. *Weekly Epidemiol Rec* **80**:138–140.

Atlas of Human Infectious Diseases, First Edition. Heiman F.L. Wertheim, Peter Horby and John P. Woodall.
© 2012 Blackwell Publishing Ltd. Published 2012 by Blackwell Publishing Ltd.

Pneumococcal Disease

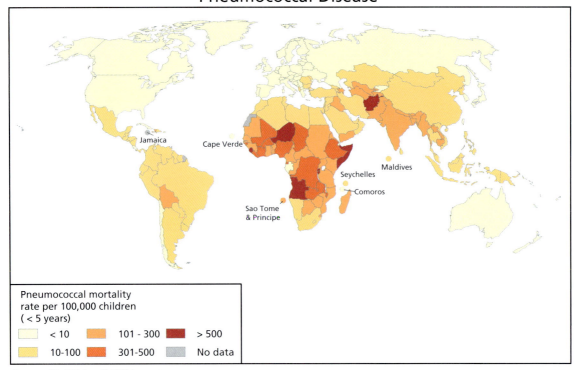

Pneumococcal mortality
rate per 100,000 children
(< 5 years)

< 10	101 - 300	> 500
10-100	301-500	No data

Source: KL O'Brien (2009) Lancet

Pneumococcal Vaccine

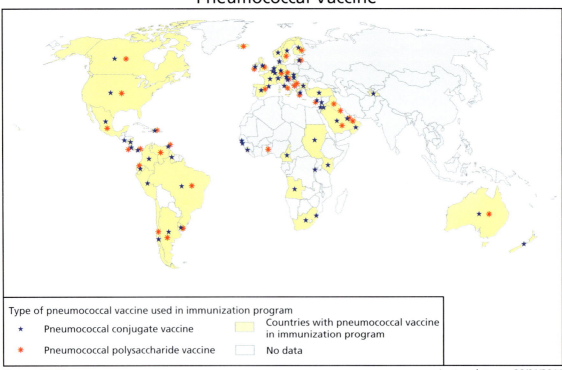

Type of pneumococcal vaccine used in immunization program

★ Pneumococcal conjugate vaccine

✳ Pneumococcal polysaccharide vaccine

Countries with pneumococcal vaccine
in immunization program

No data

Source: WHO   Last update on: 28/01/2011

Disease: Pneumococcal Disease

Classification: ICD-9 041.2; ICD-10 A40.3

Syndromes and synonyms: None.

Agent: *Streptococcus pneumoniae* (pneumococcus), an encapsulated Gram-positive bacterium, with >90 serotypes based on capsular polysaccharide antigens. Approximately 23 serotypes are responsible for 90% if the infections in the developed world.

Reservoir: Healthy humans can carry *S. pneumoniae* in their upper respiratory tract.

Transmission: Direct person-to-person transmission between close contacts by droplet spread or direct oral contact; through objects contaminated with respiratory secretions.

Incubation period: 1 to 3 days.

Clinical findings: Depends on the type of infection and severity. *S. pneumoniae* is an important cause of severe pneumonia, meningitis, and sepsis. It also is a common cause of otitis media and sinusitis. It can cause deep-seated infections involving any organ in a disseminated disease.

Diagnostic tests: Recovery of *S. pneumoniae* from sputum, blood, CSF or other normally sterile fluids by culture or PCR. *S. pneumoniae* antigen test in urine.

Therapy: Depends on disease severity and type of disease. In areas with high penicillin resistance, ceftriaxone can be used for severe disease. In case of ceftriaxone resistance, vancomycin is used. For meningitis, dexamethasone is added to antibiotic treatment.

Prevention: Vaccination with vaccines based on capsular polysaccharides. Both conjugated and non-jugated vaccines are available. Conjugated vaccines targeting either 7, 9, 10, or 13 capsule types are recommended for children under 5 years of age and risk groups. The 23-valent non-conjugated vaccine can only be used in individuals older than 2 years and at high risk of disease. National surveillance of pneumococcal disease and infecting serotypes is required to detect vaccine escapees, requiring vaccine modification. Individuals are not protected against pneumococcal capsule types not in the vaccine. Through the GAVI Alliance, low-income countries can access pneumococcal vaccines with a small contribution. Rwanda was the first GAVI-eligible country that introduced the vaccine in 2009.

Epidemiology: *S. pneumoniae* is an important cause of severe pneumonia, meningitis, and sepsis in children and adults. Risk factors for severe disease are: older age (>65 years), diabetes, chronic disease (heart, lung, kidney, liver), alcoholism, cancer, HIV, non-functioning or absent spleen, and sickle cell disease. A global burden of disease study estimated that in 2000 about 14.5 million episodes of serious pneumococcal disease occurred world wide, leading to about 826,000 deaths in children <5 years. The most common presentation of severe disease is pneumonia. The majority of deaths (95%) occurred in Africa and Asia. Since 2000 the pneumococcal vaccine has been introduced, mostly in developed countries, while developing countries need them most. In 2008, 24 high-income and two middle-income countries had pneumococcal vaccination in their program, accounting for less than 0.2% of childhood pneumococcal deaths in 2000. Many deaths in low-income countries are due to poor healthcare infrastructure and inadequate treatment options. Penicillin and chloramphenicol are still widely used to treat meningitis despite high resistance levels against these agents in some areas. Vaccination and access to proper treatment are needed in Africa and Asia. Interventions should be targeted on countries with large populations and moderate incidence, and countries with high incidence and mortality.

Map sources: The Pneumococcal Disease map is reproduced from K.L. O'Brien et al. (2009). The Vaccination schedule data was obtained from WHO (www.who.int).

Key reference
O'Brien KL, et al. (2009) Burden of disease caused by *Streptococcus pneumoniae* in children younger than 5 years: global estimates. *Lancet* **374**:893–902.

Atlas of Human Infectious Diseases, First Edition. Heiman F.L. Wertheim, Peter Horby and John P. Woodall.
© 2012 Blackwell Publishing Ltd. Published 2012 by Blackwell Publishing Ltd.

Q Fever

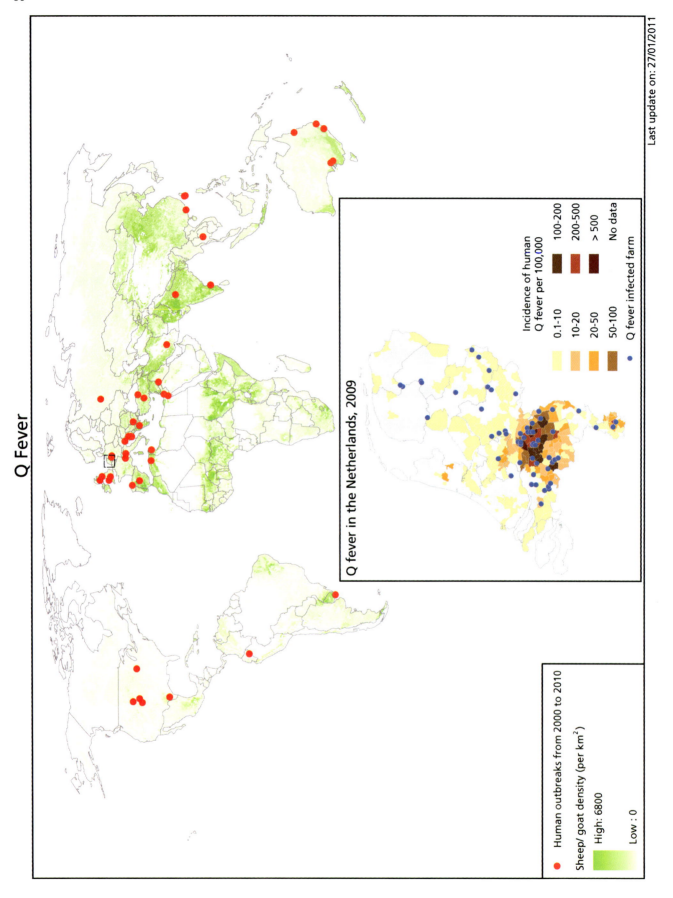

Q fever in the Netherlands, 2009

Incidence of human
Q fever per 100,000

0.1-10	100-200
10-20	200-500
20-50	> 500
50-100	No data

● Q fever infected farm

● Human outbreaks from 2000 to 2010

Sheep/ goat density (per km²)

High: 6800

Low : 0

Last update on: 27/01/2011

Disease: Q Fever

Classification: ICD-9 083.0; ICD-10 A78.

Syndromes and synonyms: Coxiellosis, Query fever.

Agent: A zoonosis caused by *Coxiella burnetii*, an intracellular Gram-negative bacterium, and is closely related to *Legionella* spp., *Francisella tularensis*, and *Rickettsia* spp. *C. burnetii* is classified as a potential biological warfare agent.

Reservoir: Domestic and free living ungulates (cattle, sheep, and goats). Also found in other livestock, birds, pets (cats and dogs), and ticks. Infected animals are generally asymptomatic, but infection may lead to late abortion.

Vector: Rarely by tick bite.

Cycle: Animals inhale *C. burnetii* aerosols or ingest contaminated straw or hay. *C. burnetii* bacteria invade local lymph nodes, where they complete their life cycle within phagosomes. From the lymph nodes the agent spreads to other organs via the bloodstream. This bacteremic phase lasts for one week. From infected organs, like mammary glands, placenta, and kidneys, it can be excreted into the environment and lead to infection in exposed animals and humans.

Transmission: Inhalation of contaminated aerosols generated from infected animal body fluids (placenta, urine, milk, feces) or dust contaminated with dried animal excretions. Less common routes are enterally when consuming contaminated food products and possibly through skin inoculation. Person-to-person transmission is rare.

Incubation period: About 2–3 weeks for acute Q fever. One to 20 years for chronic Q fever.

Clinical findings: Half of the infected patients are asymptomatic and those with symptoms usually have mild disease. The most common presentations of acute Q fever are pneumonia, hepatitis, and isolated fever. Other symptoms are neurological (headache, confusion, peripheral neuropathy), sore throat, chills, sweats, rash, and non-productive cough. Proportion of people presenting with pneumonia or hepatitis varies by region and immune status. CFR: 1–2%. Chronic Q fever occurs 1 to 20 years after acute infection and most often presents as endocarditis in patients with pre-existing heart disease (valve abnormality).

Diagnostic tests: IgG and IgM antibody detection to phase I and II antigens by IFA, CFT, or ELISA; immunohistology; PCR; ultrasound for endocarditis.

Therapy: Doxycycline for acute Q fever. Chronic Q fever endocarditis: a combination of doxycycline and hydroxychloroquine for approximately 18 months.

Prevention: *C. burnetii* is resistant to many disinfectants and extreme environmental conditions. The organism can survive in aerosols for 2 weeks and in soil up to 5 months. Prevention is targeted to those working with livestock, mainly sheep and goats; appropriate disposal of birth products; routine testing of risk animals; restricted movement of animals in infected regions; culling of infected animals; a human and veterinary vaccine is available in several countries; pasteurize milk.

Epidemiology: Q fever has been described world wide, with the exception of New Zealand. Though small outbreaks are reported from tropical countries, serological studies do show that the prevalence of disease is higher there than in temperate regions. Most human outbreaks involve either goats or sheep. The largest global outbreak ever reported occurred in the Netherlands between 2007 and 2010, mainly in the southeast where there is a high density of dairy goat farms. The outbreak led to a high incidence of infections in people exposed to aerosols living in the vicinity of infected farms but had no occupational exposure. People living within 2 km of a farm had a much higher risk than those living >5km away. The hospitalization rate was relatively high, 20% versus around 5% which is normally reported.

Map sources: The Q-fever map was made by geocoding reported Q-fever outbreaks in ProMED-mail and the medical literature between 2000 and 2010. The Netherlands outbreak map is modified from W. van der Hoek et al. (2010). The sheep and goat density data was obtained from FAO.

Key references

Angelakis E, et al. (2010) Q fever. *Vet Microbiol* **140**:297–309.
Raoult D, et al. (2005) Natural history and pathophysiology of Q fever. *Lancet Infect Dis* **5**:219–226.
Van der Hoek W, et al. (2010) *Euro Surveill* **15**(12):19520.
Woldehiwet Z. (2004) Q fever (coxiellosis): epidemiology and pathogenesis. *Vet Sci* **77**:93–100.

Atlas of Human Infectious Diseases, First Edition. Heiman F.L. Wertheim, Peter Horby and John P. Woodall.
© 2012 Blackwell Publishing Ltd. Published 2012 by Blackwell Publishing Ltd.

Rat Bite Fever

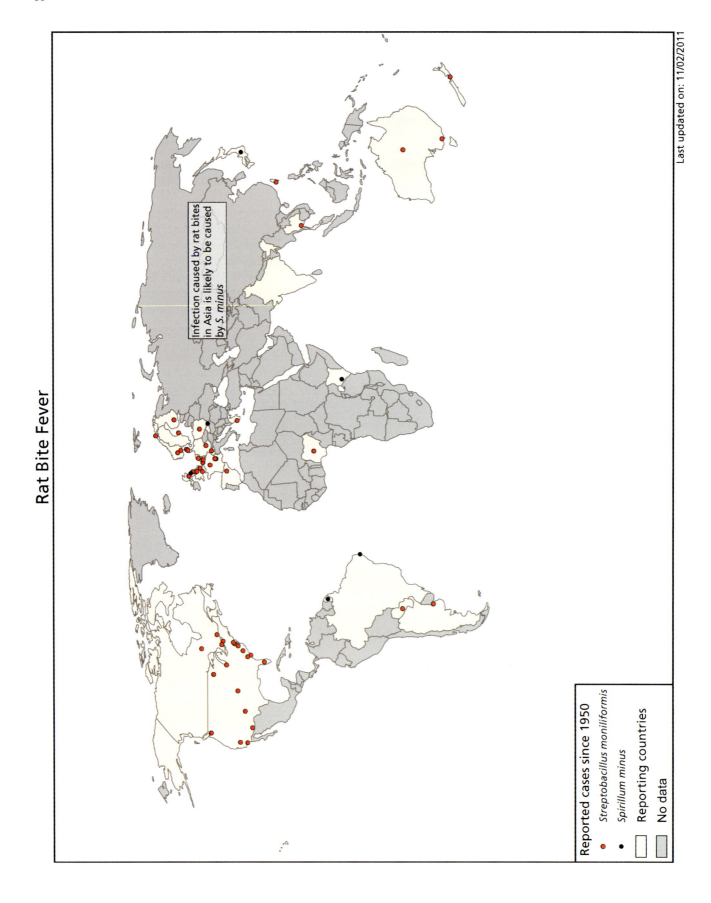

Infection caused by rat bites in Asia is likely to be caused by *S. minus*

Reported cases since 1950
- ● Streptobacillus moniliformis
- ● Spirillum minus
- ☐ Reporting countries
- ▨ No data

Last updated on: 11/02/2011

Disease: **Rat Bite Fever**

Classification: ICD-9 026; ICD-10 A25

Syndromes and synonyms: Streptobacillosis, streptobacillary fever, Haverhill fever, epidemic arthritic erythema, spirillosis, spirillary fever, sodoku.

Agents: Streptobacillosis: *Streptobacillus moniliformis* (formerly *Actinobacillus muris, Haverhillia multiformis*), a Gram-negative, non-motile pleiomorphic rod-like bacterium. Spirillosis: *Spirillum minus (minor)*, a Gram-negative motile spiral bacterium.

Reservoir: Rats are the main host species involved in human rat bite fever for both agents. The main location for *S. moniliformis* in rats is the pharynx. *S. minus* is mainly present in the blood and tongue of rats and salivary glands of mice. Other rodent species such as mouse, squirrel, and gerbil – and non-rodent species – have occasionally been identified as possible sources of infection. The rat population is estimated to be 10 billion, which is one-third of the total global mammalian population.

Cycle: Rodent to rodent with spill over to humans in case of adequate exposure.

Transmission: Via a bite or a scratch by an infected host animal. Human infection via *S. moniliformis* ingestion (milk, water, food) is known as Haverhill fever. Some streptobacillosis cases may occur by close contact with the oral flora of pet rats through kissing and sharing food. There is no person-to-person transmission.

Incubation period: 3–10 days for streptobacillosis, 1–3 weeks for spirillosis.

Clinical findings: The most common clinical presentation for streptobacillosis is a triad of (1) relapsing fever, (2) severe, migratory polyarthralgias, and (3) a peripheral, hemorrhagic maculopapular rash. The most prominent symptom is severe myalgia with prostration. Polyarthralgias occur in two-thirds of reported cases. In spirillosis, the bite site becomes indurated and may ulcerate with regional lymphadenopathy; arthritic symptoms are rare. If untreated, the disease may progress to bacterial endocarditis, pericarditis, parotitis, tenosynovitis, and focal abscesses of soft tissues or the brain.

CFR in untreated cases may be as much as 13%. There is a significant risk of streptobacillary endocarditis with associated CFR of 50%.

Diagnostic tests: Microscopy, isolation of the agent from lesion, blood or pus by inoculation into mouse footpad or guinea pigs, or culture; serum agglutination test; PCR.

Therapy: Penicillin for both forms of rat bite fever. Penicillin resistance in *S. moniliformis* is rare. Tetracycline in penicillin-allergic patients.

Prevention: Rodent control; those with occupational exposure to rodents (e.g. sewage workers) should wear personal protective clothing; avoid close contact with reservoir animals, including pets; prophylaxis with penicillin or doxycycline following rat bite.

Epidemiology: Rat bite fever is a rare and underreported disease with a worldwide distribution. *S. minus* infection is reported less frequently than *S. moniliformis* and occurs mainly in Asia, particularly Japan. World wide, millions of people are bitten by animals each year and rats are responsible for about 1% of these bites. It is estimated that 2% of rat bites lead to an infection (all causes). It is unknown what the proportion of rat bite fever is of these infections. The relation between humans and animals is changing which may alter the epidemiology of rat bite fever. Rats have become a pet in several countries, while it used to be considered a pest. Children handling pet rats may be a special risk group. More than half of the reported cases of rat bite fever occur in children.

Map sources: The Rat Bite Fever map was made by geocoding reported case in the medical literature between 1950 and 2010.

Key references

Gaastra W, et al. (2009) Rat bite fever. *Vet Microbiol* **133**:211–228.

Elliott SP. (2007) Rat bite fever and Streptobacillus moniliformis. *Clin Microbiol Rev* **20**:13–22.

Wullenweber M. (1995) Streptobacillus moniliformis – a zoonotic pathogen. Taxonomic considerations, host species, diagnosis, therapy, geographical distribution. *Lab Anim* **29**:1–15.

Atlas of Human Infectious Diseases, First Edition. Heiman F.L. Wertheim, Peter Horby and John P. Woodall.
© 2012 Blackwell Publishing Ltd. Published 2012 by Blackwell Publishing Ltd.

Relapsing Fever

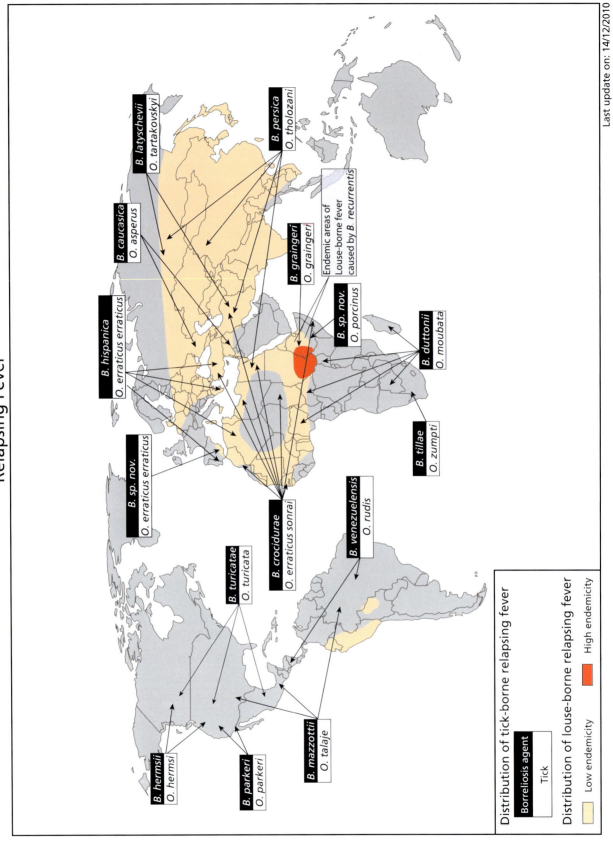

Last update on: 14/12/2010

B. latyschevii
O. tartakovskyi

B. persica
O. tholozani

B. caucasica
O. asperus

Endemic areas of
Louse-borne fever
caused by B. recurrentis

B. graingeri
O. graingeri

B. hispanica
O. erraticus erraticus

B. sp. nov.
O. porcinus

B. duttonii
O. moubata

B. sp. nov.
O. erraticus erraticus

B. tillae
O. zumpti

B. crocidurae
O. erraticus sonrai

B. venezuelensis
O. rudis

B. turicatae
O. turicata

B. hermsii
O. hermsi

B. parkeri
O. parkeri

B. mazzottii
O. talaje

Distribution of tick-borne relapsing fever

Borreliosis agent

Tick

Distribution of louse-borne relapsing fever

Low endemicity   High endemicity

Disease: Relapsing Fever

Classification: ICD-9 087; ICD-10 A68.0 – A68.1

Syndromes and synonyms: Epidemic or louse-borne relapsing fever (LBRF), endemic or tick-borne relapsing fever (TBRF).

Agent: For LBRF, *Borrelia recurrentis*, a Gram-negative spirochete. For TBRF, at least 15 *Borrelia* species, each specific to a particular species of tick vector. Since the 1980s, the number of new *Borrelia* species associated with relapsing fever has increased, in part due to improved diagnostics.

Reservoir: For LBRF, humans; for TBRF, wild rodents, bats and ticks (by trans-stadial and transovarian transmission). *B. duttonii* has thus far not been detected in wild animals, only in humans and tick vector *O. moubata*. Livestock may also become infected.

Vector: TBRF is primarily transmitted by *Ornithodoros* ticks. LBRF is transmitted by the human body louse *(Pediculus humanus)*; neither the head louse nor the pubic louse has been shown to transmit the disease.

Transmission: LBRF is not transmitted by the bite itself but by feces or louse gut fluid entering broken skin by scratching. TBRF: by bite or coxal fluid of infected ticks. Transmission may also occur through blood transfusion or transplacental.

Cycle: Lice become infective 4–5 days after an infectious blood meal and remain so for life (20–30 days). Infected ticks remain infective for life (in excess of 10 years).

Incubation period: LBRF: 5–15 days (usually 8); TBRF: 2–18 days (usually 7).

Clinical findings: Characterized by high fever of 2–7 days alternating with afebrile periods of 4–14 days, relapsing up to 13 times. Initial symptoms include generalized body aches, myalgias, arthralgias, headache, chills, sweats, and a transitory rash. Later symptoms may include nausea, vomiting, dry cough, photophobia, neck pain, conjunctivitis, jaundice, hepatosplenomegaly, confusion; rarely hematuria and epistaxis. Long-term sequelae of TBRF include cardiac, neurological, and renal abnormalities, ophthalmia and abortion.

LBRF is generally more severe than TBRF, but associated with fewer relapses.

Diagnostic tests: Detection of spirochetemia in blood smears with dark-field or conventional microscopy; blood culture in special media or mouse inoculation; quantitative buffy coat (QBC) fluorescence; PCR.

Therapy: Tetracyclines, chloramphenicol, or penicillins for 7 days have all been shown to be effective for treating TBRF. LBRF can be treated with a single dose of antibiotics. When initiating antibiotic therapy, watch closely for a Jarisch–Herxheimer reaction.

Prevention: Standard louse control and personal tick protection. Chemoprophylaxis may be used for bite victims.

Epidemiology: The louse-borne agent is responsible for epidemics, with a CFR of 30–70%; tick-borne agents cause endemic disease, with a CFR of 2–10%. LBRF has disappeared from Europe; tick-borne relapsing fever is found world wide, except in Australia and New Zealand, and is rare in Europe and North America. Human TBRF is frequent in endemic areas where people live in close proximity to burrows of reservoir animals. Otherwise, the disease is sporadic. LBRF is now found sporadically in epidemics in Africa, and is associated with refugee camps, natural disasters, and famine. LBRF used to be common world wide with large epidemics during the two world wars. It may re-establish anywhere in louse-infested human populations.

Map sources: The Relapsing Fever map was made with data from: S. Rebaudet et al. (2006), CIESIN (http://www.ciesin.org/docs/001-613/map30.gif), and P. Parola et al. (2001).

Key references

Gratz N (2006) *The Vector- and Rodent-Borne Diseases of Europe and North America: Their Distribution and Public Health Burden.* Cambridge University Press.

Parola P, et al. (2001) Ticks and tickborne bacterial diseases in humans: an emerging infectious threat. *Clin Infect Dis* **32**(6):897–928.

Rebaudet S, et al. (2006) Epidemiology of relapsing fever borreliosis in Europe. *FEMS Immunol Med Microbiol* **48**(1):11–15.

Rickettsioses, Tick-borne, New World

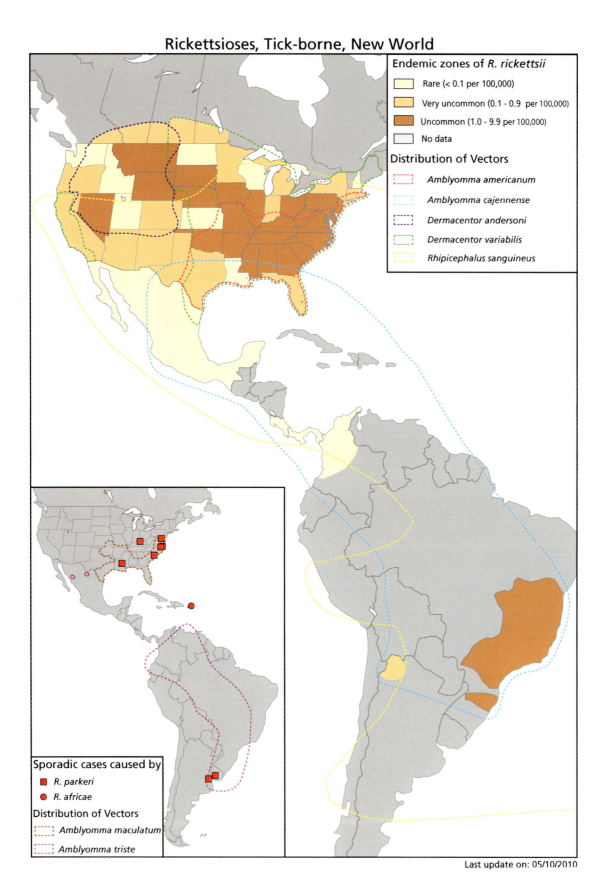

Endemic zones of *R. rickettsii*

- Rare (< 0.1 per 100,000)
- Very uncommon (0.1 - 0.9 per 100,000)
- Uncommon (1.0 - 9.9 per 100,000)
- No data

Distribution of Vectors

- *Amblyomma americanum*
- *Amblyomma cajennense*
- *Dermacentor andersoni*
- *Dermacentor variabilis*
- *Rhipicephalus sanguineus*

Sporadic cases caused by

- R. parkeri
- R. africae

Distribution of Vectors

- *Amblyomma maculatum*
- *Amblyomma triste*

Last update on: 05/10/2010

Disease: **Rickettsioses, Tick-borne, New World**

Classification: ICD-9 082.0; ICD-10 A77.0

Syndromes and synonyms: Rocky Mountain spotted fever (RMSF), North American tick typhus, New World spotted fever, Tick-borne or tick typhus, Tobia fever (Colombia), Sao Paulo fever or 'febre maculosa' (Brazil), and fiebre manchada (Mexico).

Agent: *Rickettsia rickettsii, R. parkeri* and *R. africae*, Gram-negative intracellular bacilli. *R. rickettsii* is the agent of RMSF, *R. parkeri* causes a RMSF-like illness. *R. africae* causes African tick bite fever and is rarely found in the new world. New agents are still being discovered regularly.

Reservoir: Hard ticks (*Ixodidae*). Depending on the tick species, they can acquire infection via feeding on animals with rickettsemia, or via venereal, transovarial, and trans-stadial passage. Animals preferred for feeding varies by tick species and their life stage. Rodent hosts include ground squirrels, mice, and voles.

Vector: The Ixodid ticks are both vector and reservoir. *Amblyomma americanum, Dermacentor andersoni* and *D. variabilis* (American dog tick) in Canada and the USA, *Rhipicephalus sanguineus* in Mexico and Central America, and *A. cajennense* from the southern states of the USA southwards as far as Argentina. *D. variabilis* is the primary vector for RMSF in the USA. *A. maculatum* is the main vector of *R. parkeri* in North America and *A. triste* in South America.

Transmission: By tick bite or crushing an infected tick or its feces into a break in the skin or mucous membrane. Also by blood transfusion and, in the laboratory, aerosol.

Cycle: Tick–vertebrate–tick with humans as accidental host. Animals preferred for feeding depends on tick species and their life stage.

Incubation period: 2–14 days (usually 5–7).

Clinical findings: RMSF and *R. parkeri* rickettsiosis are characterized by fever, myalgia, malaise, headache, and a maculopapular eruption that can involve the palms or soles. *R. parkeri* rickettsiosis is milder than RMSF, and often does not require hospitalization. RMSF cases may progress and develop stupor, delirium, ataxia, or coma; RMSF CFR is about 7%. Untreated RMSF is often progressive with a CFR of 20%, which is not the case for untreated *R. parkeri* rickettsiosis. Most (>90%) *R. parkeri* cases have an eschar, which is rare in RMSF. GI symptoms are common in RMSF and rare in *R. parkeri* disease.

Diagnostic tests: PCR on blood or skin biopsy, or IFA on the latter. Serology is unspecific due to cross-reactivity. Until recently, *R. parkeri* cases were misdiagnosed as RMSF.

Therapy: Doxycycline is the treatment of choice. Generally, treatment is continued for at least 3 days after the patient is afebrile.

Prevention: Search for ticks on the whole body daily and remove them without crushing. Use tick repellent on skin and an acaricide on clothing. There is no effective vaccine.

Epidemiology: The distribution of RMSF and *R. parkeri* rickettsiosis is limited by the tick vector distribution. Average annual RMSF incidence of the disease in the USA was 2.2 cases per million between 1997 and 2002, and approximately 250–1,200 cases are reported each year. Many cases of RMSF may actually have been caused by other rickettsial agents, as was seen with *R. parkeri*. Many rickettsiae of unknown pathogenicity are present in ticks and new disease causing agents are still being discovered. RMSF in the USA follows a seasonal pattern with most cases in warmer months, when ticks are most active. RMSF cases are usually found in rural areas, and less commonly in urban areas. Residing in wooded regions or areas with high grass and exposure to dogs increases the risk of RMSF. RMSF is sporadic and rarely occurs in clusters.

Map sources: The Spotted Fever, New World map was made with data from: CDC (www.cdc.gov/ticks/geographic_distribution.html), CIESIN (www.ciesin.org/docs/001-613/001-613.html), G.V. Kolonin (2009), recent literature and expert opinion.

Key references

Dantas-Torres F (2007) Rocky Mountain spotted fever. *Lancet Infect Dis* **7**(11):724–732.

Kolonin GV (2009) *Fauna of Ixodid Ticks of the World (Acari, Ixodidae)*. Moscow. Website: www.kolonin.org.

Paddock CD, et al. (2008) *Rickettsia parkeri* rickettsiosis and its clinical distinction from Rocky Mountain spotted fever. *Clin Infect Dis* **47**:1188–1196.

Parola P, et al. (2005) Tick-borne rickettsioses around the world: emerging diseases challenging old concepts. *Clin Microbiol Rev* **18**(4):719–756.

Atlas of Human Infectious Diseases, First Edition. Heiman F.L. Wertheim, Peter Horby and John P. Woodall.
© 2012 Blackwell Publishing Ltd. Published 2012 by Blackwell Publishing Ltd.

Rickettsioses, Tick-borne, Old World

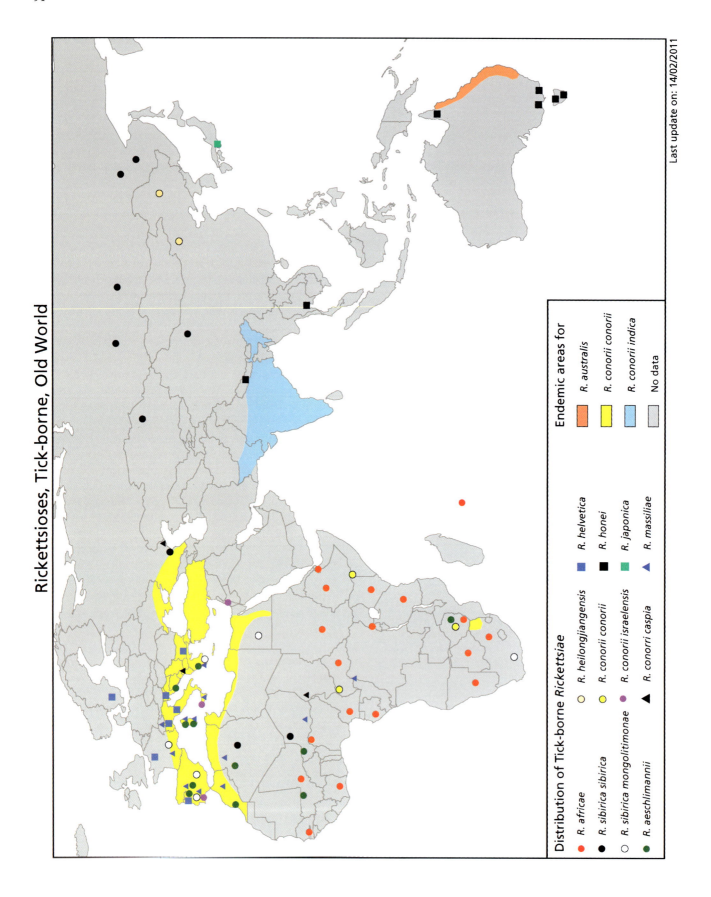

Last update on: 14/02/2011

Distribution of Tick-borne *Rickettsiae*

○ *R. africae*	○ *R. heilongjiangensis*	■ *R. helvetica*
● *R. sibirica sibirica*	○ *R. conorii conorii*	■ *R. honei*
○ *R. sibirica mongolitimonae*	● *R. conorii israelensis*	■ *R. japonica*
● *R. aeschlimannii*	▲ *R. conorii caspia*	◄ *R. massiliae*

Endemic areas for

■ *R. australis*	
■ *R. conorii conorii*	
■ *R. conorii indica*	
■ No data	

Disease: Rickettsioses, Tick-borne, Old World

Classification: ICD-9 082; ICD-10 A77

Synonyms: Mediterranean spotted fever (MSF), Israeli spotted fever (ISF), Siberian or North Asian tick typhus (STT/NATT), Queensland tick typhus (QTT), Japanese or Oriental spotted fever (JSF/OSF), Astrakhan fever (AF), African tick bite fever (ATBF), Flinders Island spotted fever (FISF), Indian tick typhus (ITT), Boutonneuse fever.

Agent: *Rickettsia aeschlimannii, R. africae* (ATBF), *R. australis* (QTT), *R. conorii caspia* (AF), *R. conorii conorii* (MSF), *R. conorii indica* (ITT), *R. conorii israelensis* (ISF), *R. helvetica, R. honei* (FISF), *R. japonica* (JSF/OSF), *R. massiliae, R. sibirica* (STT/NATT), Gram-negative intracellular bacilli. New agents are still being discovered regularly.

Reservoir: Hard ticks (Ixodidae). Depending on the tick species, they can acquire infection via feeding on animals with rickettsemia, or via venereal, transovarial, and transstadial passage. Animals preferred for feeding varies by tick species and their life stage. Hosts include dogs, rodents, and other animals.

Vector: Hard ticks (Ixodidae). The brown dog tick (*Rhipicephalus sanguineus*), the principal vector of MSF, ISF, ITT, and AF, is most active during spring and summer, has a low human affinity, and prefers dogs in a peridomestic environment. The southern African bont tick (*Amblyomma hebraeum*) and *A. africanum* are the principal vectors of *R. africae* in southern Africa. *A. hebraeum* is an aggressive, human-biting tick and has high rates of rickettsia infection, and ATBF cases therefore often occur in clusters. See key references for further reading on ticks and tick-borne rickettsioses.

Transmission: By tick bite or crushing an infected tick or its feces into a break in the skin or mucous membrane. Also by blood transfusion and, in the laboratory, aerosol.

Cycle: There is a natural cycle between ticks and animals with humans as accidental host.

Incubation period: Varies by agent but is generally 7 days with a range from 1 to 15 days.

Clinical findings: Boutonneuse fever (group name for *R.conorii* infections: MSF, ISF, ITT), QTT and STT/NATT: mild febrile illness that may last up to 2 weeks, eschar at bite site with regional lymphadenopathy (in ISF, eschars are rare), generalized maculopapular erythematous rash on palms on soles after 4–5 days. The disease can be severe with a CFR up to 3%. ATBF is milder than other rickettsioses, fever and rash are less common, multiple eschars may be present with regional lymphadenopathy.

Diagnostic tests: PCR on blood or skin biopsy, or IFA on the latter. Serology is unspecific due to cross-reactivity.

Therapy: Doxycycline is the treatment of choice. Generally, treatment is continued for at least 3 days after the patient is afebrile.

Prevention: Search for ticks on the whole body daily and remove them without crushing. Use tick repellent on skin and an acaricide on clothing.

Epidemiology: Ecological characteristics of the ticks influence the epidemiology of tick-borne rickettsioses. In 1910, the first case of Mediterranean spotted fever (MSF) *R. conorii* was considered to be the only agent of tick-borne spotted fever group rickettsioses in Europe and Africa. Similarly, *R. sibirica* was thought to be the only agent in Russia and China and *R. australis* in Australia. The reason for this was that diagnosis was made by serologic testing, which cross-reacts with other rickettsial species. Due to improved diagnostics, particularly molecular, the understanding of rickettsioses has increased, and new agents are being found regularly. Multiple distinct tick-borne spotted fever group rickettsioses are recognized. The name of the agent informs us where the agent was initially found, but most agents have a more widespread distribution.

Map sources: The Tick-Borne Rickettioses map (Old World) was made with data obtained from P. Parola et al. (2005), www.kolonin.org, and updated with recent publications and expert opinion.

Key references

Parola P, et al. (2001) Ticks and tickborne bacterial diseases in humans: an emerging infectious threat. *Clin Infect Dis* **32**:897–928.

Parola P, et al. (2005) Tick-borne rickettsioses around the world: emerging diseases challenging old concepts. *Clin Microbiol Rev* **18**(4):719–756.

Atlas of Human Infectious Diseases, First Edition. Heiman F.L. Wertheim, Peter Horby and John P. Woodall.
© 2012 Blackwell Publishing Ltd. Published 2012 by Blackwell Publishing Ltd.

Scrub Typhus

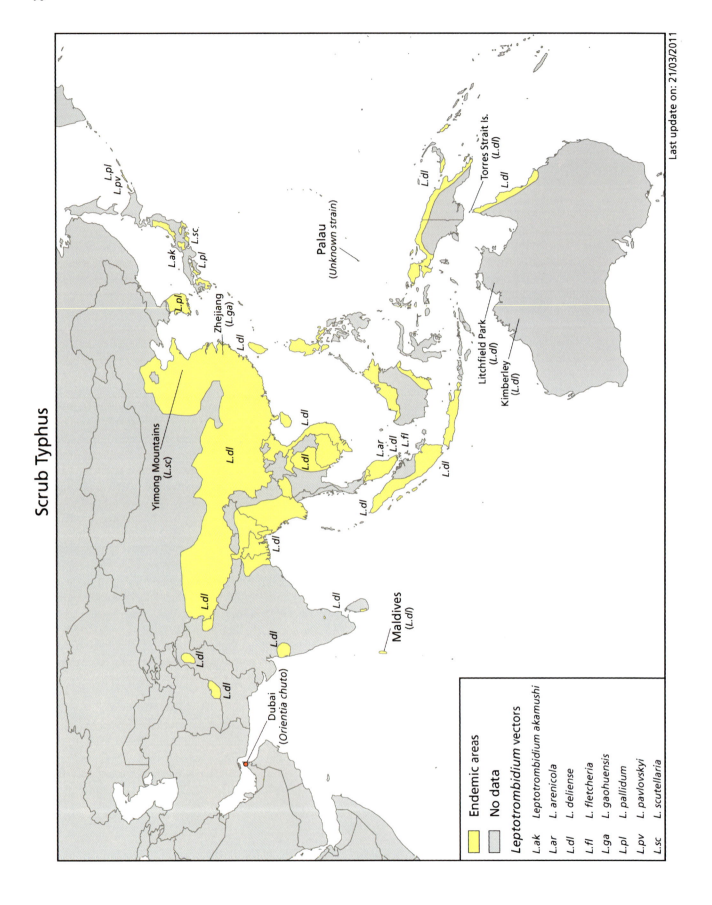

Last update on: 21/03/2011

L.pl
L.pv

L.ak

L.sc

L.pl

L.pl

Zhejiang
(L.ga)

L.dl

Yimong Mountains
(L.sc)

L.dl

L.dl

L.dl

L.ar
L.dl
L.fl

L.dl

L.dl

L.dl

L.dl

L.dl

L.dl

L.dl

L.dl

L.dl

L.dl

L.dl

Palau
(Unknown strain)

Torres Strait Is.
(L.dl)

L.dl

Litchfield Park
(L.dl)

Kimberley
(L.dl)

Maldives
(L.dl)

Dubai
(Orientia chuto)

	Endemic areas
	No data

Leptotrombidium **vectors**

L.ak	Leptotrombidium akamushi
L.ar	L. arenicola
L.dl	L. deliense
L.fl	L. fletcheria
L.ga	L. gaohuensis
L.pl	L. pallidum
L.pv	L. pavlovskyi
L.sc	L. scutellaria

Disease: Scrub Typhus

Classification: ICD-9 081.2; ICD-10 A75.3

Syndromes and synonyms: Tsutsugamushi disease, mite-borne typhus fever, chigger-borne rickettsioses, coastal fever (Australia).

Agent: *Orientia tsutsugamushi*, obligate intracellular bacterium, before 1995 known as *Rickettsia tsutsugamushi*. In 2010, a new species that can cause scrub typhus was discovered in Dubai, *O. chuto*.

Reservoir: Larval stage mites, so-called chiggers from the genus *Leptotrombidium*. A number of small rodents, particularly wild rats, are the natural hosts for scrub typhus without apparent disease.

Vector: Larval mites. Nymphs and adults do not feed on vetebrate hosts. The vector has adapted to various ecologies, including mountainous and tropical regions.

Transmission: Bite of infected larval mites (chiggers). There is no direct person-to-person transmission.

Cycle: The mites are infected by feeding on reservoir animals (small rodents), and maintain the infection throughout their life stages. The infection is passed on by transovarial transmission. *O. tsutsugamushi* are present in the salivary glands of the larvae and injected into the host during feeding.

Incubation period: 10–12 days, range: 6–21 days.

Clinical findings: Typical skin ulcer, eschar, may develop at the site of the mite's bite. Several days later fever, headache, myalgia, and lymphadenopathy may develop. Dry cough with signs of pneumonitis, jaundice, and meningoencepahlitis may occur. Scrub typhus severity and clinical presentation is probably strain dependent.

Diagnostic tests: Serology (IF, EIA); PCR; culture in mice or cell lines.

Therapy: Tetracycline, doxyxyline. Alternative: chloramphenicol.

Prevention: Avoid areas with mites; mite bite prevention by impregnating clothes with miticides; mite elimination in high-risk areas; no effective vaccine is available.

Epidemiology: It is estimated that over one million cases of scrub typhus occur each year. Infections most often occur in rural areas where diagnostic facilities are limited. Scrub typhus is thought to occur within the so-called 'Scrub typhus triangle,' bounded by Siberia (north), Kamchatka Peninsula (east), Pakistan (west), and Australia (south). *O. tsutsugamushi* infection primarily occurs in tropical climate in Asia, but is also found in temperate zones and semi-arid climates, including in scrub, gardens, forests, beach areas, and mountain deserts. In 2010 the western limit of the *Orientia* genus extended westwards to Dubai when a patient was diagnosed with a new *Orientia* species (*O. chuto*). In southern China, human infections typically occur in the summer and in northern areas the disease occurs mainly during autumn and winter. The migration of infested or infected rodents can lead to the establishment of new foci of disease.

Map sources: The Scrub Typhus map is modified from D.J. Kelly et al. (2). Data on vector distribution was obtained from the WHO report (1989) (see key references below).

Key references

Izzard L, et al. (2010) Isolation of a novel *Orientia* species (*O. chuto* sp. nov.) from a patient infected in Dubai. *J Clin Microbiol* **48**(12):4404–4409.

Kelly DJ, et al. (2009) Scrub typhus: the geographic distribution of phenotypic and genotypic variants of *Orientia tsutsugamushi*. *Clin Infect Dis* **48**:S203–S230.

World Health Organization (1989) *Areas of endemic chigger-borne rickettsiosis and distribution of the Leptotrombidium vectors. Geographical distribution of arthropod-borne diseases and their principal vectors.* Unpublished document WHO/VBC/89.967. Geneva.

Zhang et al. (2010) Scrub typhus in previously unrecorgnized areas of endemicity in China. *J Clin Microbiol* **48**:1241–1244.

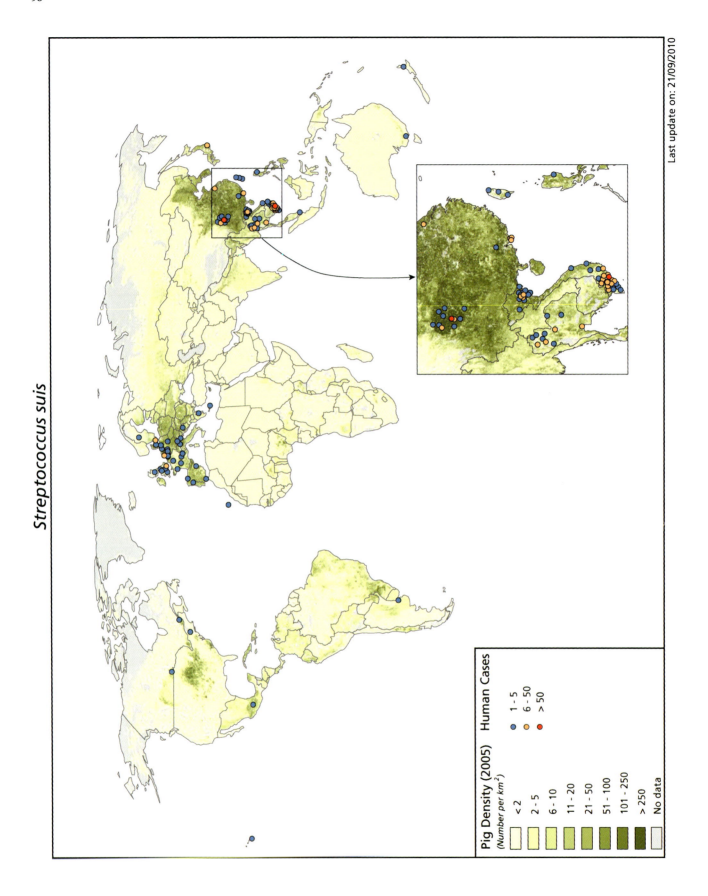

Streptococcus suis

Pig Density (2005)
(Number per km²)

- <2
- 2 - 5
- 6 - 10
- 11 - 20
- 21 - 50
- 51 - 100
- 101 - 250
- > 250
- No data

Human Cases

- 1 - 5
- 6 - 50
- > 50

Last update on: 21/09/2010

Disease: *Streptococcus suis*

Classification: ICD-9 A41.09; ICD-10 A40.8

Syndromes and synonyms: None.

Agent: *Streptococcus suis*, a Gram-positive alpha-hemolytic bacterium, with 35 serotypes based on capsular polysaccharide antigens. The predominant one causing human disease is serotype 2.

Reservoir: Pigs; occasionally found in wild boar, horses, dogs, cats, and birds. Asymptomatic pigs typically carry the bacteria in their tonsils.

Transmission: Through wounds on the skin, including minor abrasions. Infection via ingestion of contaminated improperly cooked pork products. No human-to-human transmission.

Cycle: Pig-to-pig, with occasional spill-over to humans.

Incubation period: From a few hours up to 3 days.

Clinical findings: Fever and signs of meningitis (headache, vomiting, neck stiffness, intolerance of light, and decreased level of consciousness). Hearing loss, generally permanent, in around 50% of those infected. Arthritis, pneumonia, and fatal toxic shock syndrome are possible complications.

Diagnostic tests: Recovery of bacteria from the cerebrospinal fluid, blood or fluid from arthritic joints; culture; PCR. *Streptococcus suis* is often misidentified as another streptococcus species and therefore underdiagnosed.

Therapy: For meningitis or septicemia, prompt treatment with appropriate antibiotics (penicillin, ceftriaxon) will lead to recovery. Specific organ involvement like the heart, requires specialist treatment. Early treatment with dexamethason can reduce the risk of hearing loss.

Prevention: During outbreaks: strict control on animal movements and slaughtering; health education of everyone who butchers, prepares, and cooks pork, including in their homes; wearing gloves to handle raw or uncooked pork, careful washing of hands and utensils. Adequate cooking essential; WHO recommends cooking pork to reach an internal temperature of 70 °C, or until the juices are clear rather than pink.

Epidemiology: Rarely reported in the Americas and Europe, sporadic in parts of Southeast Asia, especially Thailand, China, and Vietnam. Most important risk factor is contact with pigs or uncooked pig products, typically by farmers, veterinary personnel, abattoir workers, and butchers. Furthermore, in several Asian countries it is common to consume uncooked pork products, like blood, which is a risk for acquiring the disease. Individuals who are immunosuppressed, including those who have been splenectomized, are also at increased risk. Since *S. suis* is often misidentified, *S. suis* may be more common in certain parts of the world with high pig densities.

Map sources: The *Streptococcus suis* map was made by geocoding all reported human cases in the medical literature up to 2010. The pig density data is obtained from FAO, available at: www.fao.org/ag/againfo/resources/en/glw/home.html.

Key references

Gottschalk M, et al. (2007) Streptococcus suis infections in humans: the Chinese experience and the situation in North America. *Anim Health Res Rev* **8**(1):29–45.

Lun ZR, et al. (2007) Streptococcus suis, an emerging zoonotic pathogen. *Lancet Infect Dis* **7**(3):201–209.

Mai NT, et al. (2008) *Streptococcus suis* meningitis in adults in Vietnam. *Clin Infect Dis* **46**:659–667.

Wertheim H, et al. (2009) *Streptococcus suis*: an emerging pathogen. *Clin Infect Dis* **48**:617–625.

Atlas of Human Infectious Diseases, First Edition. Heiman F.L. Wertheim, Peter Horby and John P. Woodall.
© 2012 Blackwell Publishing Ltd. Published 2012 by Blackwell Publishing Ltd.

Tetanus

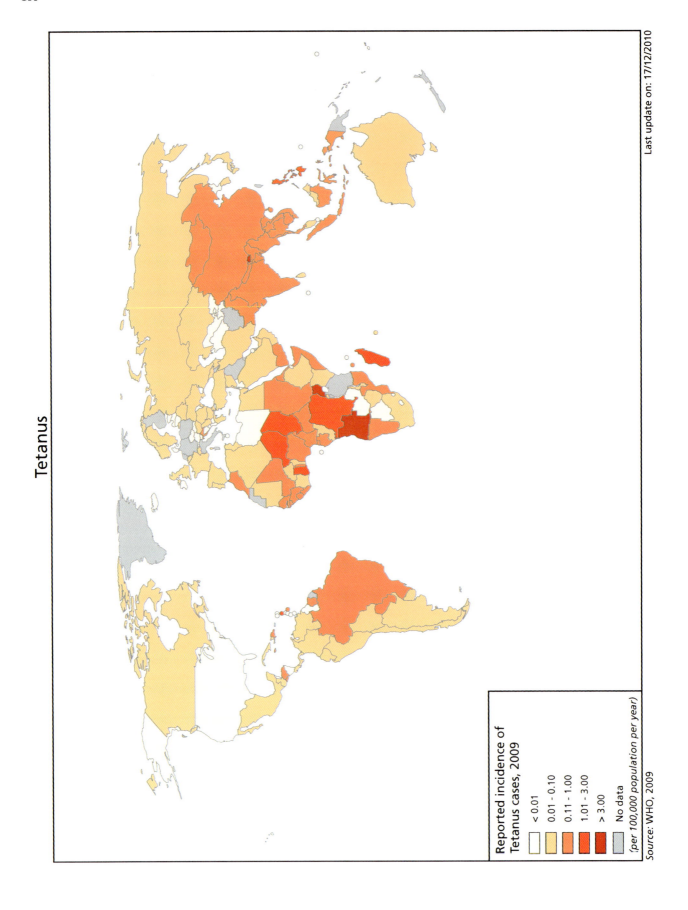

Reported incidence of
Tetanus cases, 2009

< 0.01
0.01 - 0.10
0.11 - 1.00
1.01 - 3.00
> 3.00
No data

(per 100,000 population per year)

Source: WHO, 2009

Last update on: 17/12/2010

Disease: Tetanus

Classification: ICD-9 037, 771.3; ICD-10 A33–35

Syndromes and synonyms: Lockjaw.

Agent: *Clostridium tetani,* a Gram-positive, spore-forming anaerobic bacterium. The spores can remain viable in the environment for years. *C. tetani* produces a highly potent exotoxin, tetanospasmin, which is responsible for the clinical features of tetanus.

Reservoir: Intestinal tract of animals and humans, and soil.

Route of transmission: Contamination of wounds with soil, dust or animal feces that contain *C. tetani* spores. Puncture wounds are most commonly associated with tetanus but it can result from even minor abrasions. Through injection of contaminated street drugs. Neonatal tetanus results from infection of the umbilical cord, either through the use of unclean instruments to cut the cord or through dressing the stump with contaminated materials.

Cycle: Tetanus spores enter the body through wounds and under anaerobic conditions, the spores germinate and produce toxin. The toxins are disseminated via the blood and lymphatic system and bind to nerve endings, preventing the release of inhibitory neurotransmitters. This results in unopposed skeletal muscle contraction.

Incubation period: Most cases occur within 14 days (range: 1 day to months). Shorter incubation periods are associated with more heavily contaminated wounds and an inoculation site closer to the central nervous system. Neonatal tetanus has a shorter incubation period, with an average of around 6 days.

Clinical findings: The principal clinical feature of tetanus is painful skeletal muscle spasms and rigidity. Three clinical forms are recognized. The commonest is generalized tetanus, which usually begins with spasms of the facial muscles and spreads in a descending pattern. On presentation patients commonly have 'lockjaw' (trismus), neck stiffness, difficulty swallowing, and abdominal rigidity. Generalized spasms may result in an arched posture (opisthotonus). Other symptoms include elevated temperature, blood pressure, and sweating. Localized tetanus presents as localized spasms of muscles around the entry wound. Cephalic tetanus is rare and results from infection in the head and neck, and affects cranial nerves.

Diagnostic tests: The diagnosis is based on characteristic clinical features. The bacterium is usually not cultured from wounds and a positive culture does not confirm the diagnosis.

Therapy: Clean wounds, perform debridement and remove foreign objects. A one-off dose of im or iv human tetanus immunoglobulin removes unbound toxin but does not affect bound toxin. Metronidazole in large doses for 7–14 days to eradicate *C. tetani* infection. Since the effect of bound toxin may last for 4–6 weeks, prolonged supportive care is required. Tetanus does not induce immunity. Vaccination with tetanus toxoid is therefore indicated during treatment.

Prevention: Immunization with tetanus toxoid (inactivated tetanus toxin). Immunization of pregnant women protects infants from neonatal tetanus.

Epidemiology: Tetanus is globally distributed but is more common in highly populated agricultural areas, and in warm and wet regions. In the late 1980s tetanus was estimated to cause around 1 million deaths per year, mostly in newborn infants. The current distribution of cases represents the coverage of tetanus immunization in children and adults. In countries with good vaccine coverage in children, adult cases may still be common, as natural immunity plays no role in the epidemiology of tetanus. The DTP3 Vaccination Coverage map shows coverage with the third dose of a tetanus-containing vaccine in childhood. The elimination of neonatal tetanus was set as a goal in 1989 and by mid-2010 neonatal tetanus had been eliminated in 79% (153/193) of WHO Member States. However, since *C. tetani* will always remain present in nature, tetanus will always remain a threat, and high levels of immunization must be maintained indefinitely.

Map sources: Data for the Tetanus map was obtained from WHO http://apps.who.int/immunization_monitoring/en/.

Key references

Thwaites CL, et al. (2003) Preventing and treating tetanus. *Br Med J* **326**(7381):117–118.

Roper MH, et al. (2007) Maternal and neonatal tetanus. *Lancet* **370**(9603):1947–1959.

World Health Organization (2009) *State of the World's Vaccines and Immunization,* 3rd edn. Geneva. WHO, UNICEF, World Bank.

Trachoma

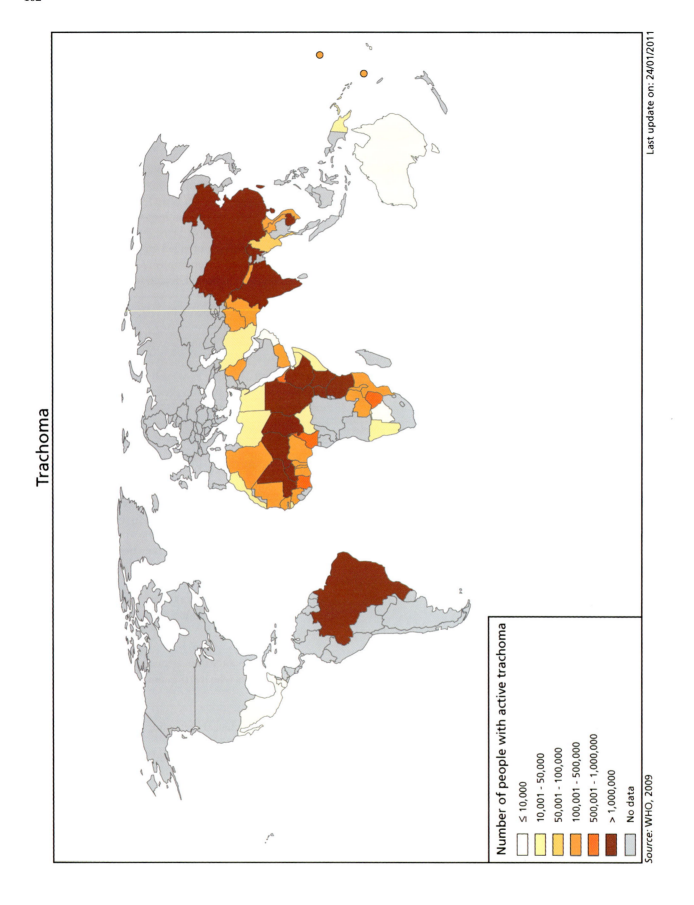

Number of people with active trachoma

≤ 10,000
10,001 - 50,000
50,001 - 100,000
100,001 - 500,000
500,001 - 1,000,000
> 1,000,000
No data

Source: WHO, 2009

Last update on: 24/01/2011

Disease: **Trachoma**

Classification: ICD-9 076.1; ICD-10 A71

Syndromes and synonyms: Chronic follicular conjunctivitis.

Agent: Repeated re-infection with *Chlamydia trachomatis* serovars A, B, Ba, and C, an obligate intracellular bacterium. The genital serovars D to K can infect the conjunctiva, but generally do not lead to blindness as they cause self-limited infections that typically do not recur.

Reservoir: Humans.

Vector: Flies contribute to the spread of ocular serovars of *C. trachomatis.*

Transmission: Repeated direct contact with infected secretions from infected individual (mainly from eye or nose); also by hands and fomites (shared clothes, towels or bedlinen). Flies also play a role in the transmission. High risk of infection in close contacts of infected individuals.

Incubation Period: 5 to 12 days for conjunctivitis; years to decades for trichiasis and eventually corneal damage and blindness. Repeated re-infection over many years is required for deposition of sufficient conjunctival scar to lead to the blinding complications; host genetic factors are probably also important.

Clinical findings: Self-limiting conjunctivitis, including watery or mucopurulent discharge. Typical findings are lymphoid follicles and papillary hypertrophy. Repeated infections lead to scarring of the conjunctiva and trichiasis. Trichiasis damages the corneal surface, resulting in keratitis, vascularization of the cornea, and impaired defence against secondary bacterial and fungal infection. Corneal damage produces corneal scar, leading to blindness.

Diagnostic tests: Clinical diagnosis of active disease by presence of follicles and papillae on the conjunctival epithelium of the upper eyelid. Trichiasis and corneal opacity are also diagnosed clinically. Presence or absence of infecting agent (by any method, including PCR) has poor correlation with presence or absence of disease or its severity; serology has no diagnostic value.

Therapy: Individuals with trichiasis require eyelid surgery. Active disease requires antibiotics: azithromycin or tetracycline eye ointment are recommended. Treatment of individual cases has little impact, because of rapid reinfection. Community management using the SAFE strategy (Surgery for trichiasis, Antibiotics to clear infection, Facial cleanliness and Environmental improvement [water and sanitation] to reduce transmission) is the recommended means for control in endemic areas; this strategy includes both treatment and prevention.

Prevention: Community management by SAFE strategy (see above). The WHO Alliance for the Global Elimination of Trachoma (GET 2020) seeks to eliminate trachoma as a public health problem by 2020.

Epidemiology: Trachoma is the leading infectious cause of blindness world wide and is generally a disease of poor rural communities. These communities are often in hot and dry regions. It is estimated that there are about 41 million people with active trachoma and 8 million with trichiasis. Highest prevalences are found in Sub-Saharan Africa. There is a high burden in Ethiopia and Sudan, where active trachoma in some communities can be found in >50% of 1–9-year-old children and trichiasis in >19% of adults. In Asia and Central and South America, the distribution is more focal. Overall the incidence of trachoma is declining and the disease has disappeared from Europe and North America due to improved living conditions.

Map sources: Data for the Active Trachoma map (all ages) is obtained from WHO, available at: www.who.int/blindness/ data_maps/en/. More detailed maps are available from the International Center of Eye Health, available at: https:// www.iceh.org.uk/display/WEB/Global + distribution + of + trachoma + maps.

Key references

Burton MJ, et al. (2010) The global burden of trachoma: a review. *PLoS Negl Trop Dis* **3**(10):e46.

Hu VH, et al. (2010) Epidemiology and control of trachoma: systematic review. *Trop Med Int Health* **15**(6):673–691.

Polack S, et al. (2005) Mapping the global distribution of trachoma. *WHO Bull* **83**:913–919.

Wright HR, et al. (2007) Trachoma. *Lancet* **371**:1945–1954.

104

Tuberculosis

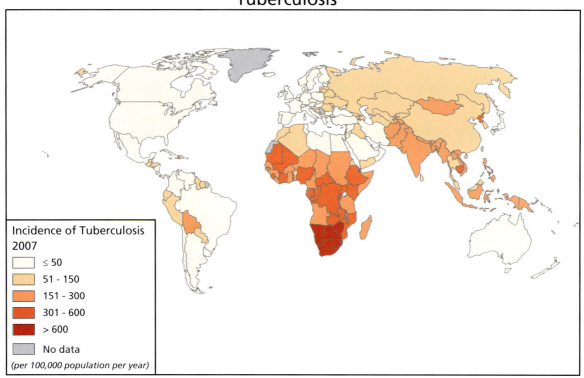

Incidence of Tuberculosis 2007
- ≤ 50
- 51 - 150
- 151 - 300
- 301 - 600
- > 600
- No data

(per 100,000 population per year)

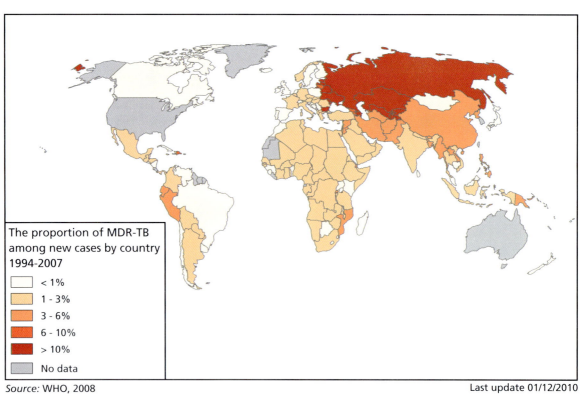

The proportion of MDR-TB among new cases by country 1994-2007
- < 1%
- 1 - 3%
- 3 - 6%
- 6 - 10%
- > 10%
- No data

Source: WHO, 2008

Last update 01/12/2010

Disease: **Tuberculosis**

Classification: ICD-9 010-018; ICD-10 A15–A19

Syndromes and synonyms: Consumption, white plague, TB.

Agent: *Mycobacterium tuberculosis* complex, including *M. tuberculosis, M. africanum, M. canetti,* and *M. bovis,* slow growing acid-fast rods. *M. bovis* is not discussed further.

Reservoir: Mainly humans; rarely non-human primates and other mammals.

Transmission: Person-to-person via inhalation of infectious aerosols from cases with pulmonary TB, particularly after prolonged exposure over time. Extrapulmonary tuberculosis is generally not communicable. HIV-infected individuals are more likely to develop TB.

Incubation period: 2–10 weeks to primary lesion or tuberculin-positive skin test; around 10% progresses to active disease annually, but it may remain latent for decades to lifelong,. This percentage is higher in children and in HIV-infected or otherwise immune-suppressed individuals.

Clinical findings: TB is a chronic disease with a gradual onset. Pulmonary lesions occur in 70% of cases, extrapulmonary (meningitis, skeletal, any other organ, disseminated) in 30%. Extrapulmonary TB is more common in children <5 years. Early symptoms of pulmonary TB are weight loss, fever, and night sweats, progressing to cough, chest pain, and hemoptysis. Findings of extrapulmonary TB depends on infected organ(s), and may present together with pulmonary TB.

Diagnostic tests: Direct: acid fast smear/culture and PCR of sputum and other body fluids, depending on clinical presentation; serological: tuberculin skin test (Mantoux); interferon gamma release assays (IGRAs). Culture in liquid media is gold standard and allows for antibiotic susceptibility testing but takes weeks to months; PCR allows for early detection, and recent assays include detection of resistance-associated mutations.

Therapy: WHO recommended regimen (Directly Observed Treatment Short-course or DOTS) is 2 months of rifampicin, isoniazid, pyrazinamide, and ethambutol, followed by 4 months of rifampicin plus isoniazid. If resistance to rifampicin or isoniazid is suspected, treatment must continue with second-line drugs for at least 18 months. Drug-resistant tuberculosis (MDR and XDR-TB) require special regimens.

MDR-TB is defined as resistance to two main first-line TB drugs: isoniazid and rifampicin. XDR-TB (Extensive Drug Resistant TB) is defined as MDR-TB with resistance to fluoroquinolones and one second-line injectable drug.

Prevention: Primary: BCG vaccination of children protects against disseminated disease. Secondary: intensive search for and treatment of source cases; contact investigation and treatment of positive cases with chemoprophylaxis. WHO has established a 'Stop TB Partnership' program to control TB world wide.

Epidemiology: TB is a major cause of death and disability world wide, especially in developing countries. Morbidity and mortality rates increase with age, and are higher in males. In regions of high incidence, morbidity peaks in adults of working age. Morbidity is higher in urban populations, among the poor, and in closed institutions such as prisons and military barracks. There were an estimated 9.27 million incident cases of TB in the world in 2007 (14% HIV positive), an almost 50% increase from 1990, and an estimated one-third of the world's population is either latently or actively infected with TB. Most of the cases in 2007 were in Asia (55%) and Africa (31%).

MDR-TB is a serious problem in Russia, former Russian republics, India and China. In 2007 there were an estimated 0.5 million MDR-TB cases. By 2008, 55 countries reported at least one XDR-TB case.

Map sources: The Tuberculosis map was made with incidence and resistance data from WHO, available at www.who.int/tb/country/global_tb_database/en/ and WHO report No. 4 (2008).

Key references

Dye C, et al. (2008) Measuring tuberculosis burden, trends, and the impact of control programmes. *Lancet Infect Dis* **8**:233–423.

World Health Organization (2008) *Anti-Tuberculous Drug Resistance in the World.* WHO Report No. 4, Geneva.

Wright A, et al. (2009) Epidemiology of antituberculosis drug resistance 2002–07. *Lancet* **373**:1861–1873.

Atlas of Human Infectious Diseases, First Edition. Heiman F.L. Wertheim, Peter Horby and John P. Woodall.
© 2012 Blackwell Publishing Ltd. Published 2012 by Blackwell Publishing Ltd.

Tularemia

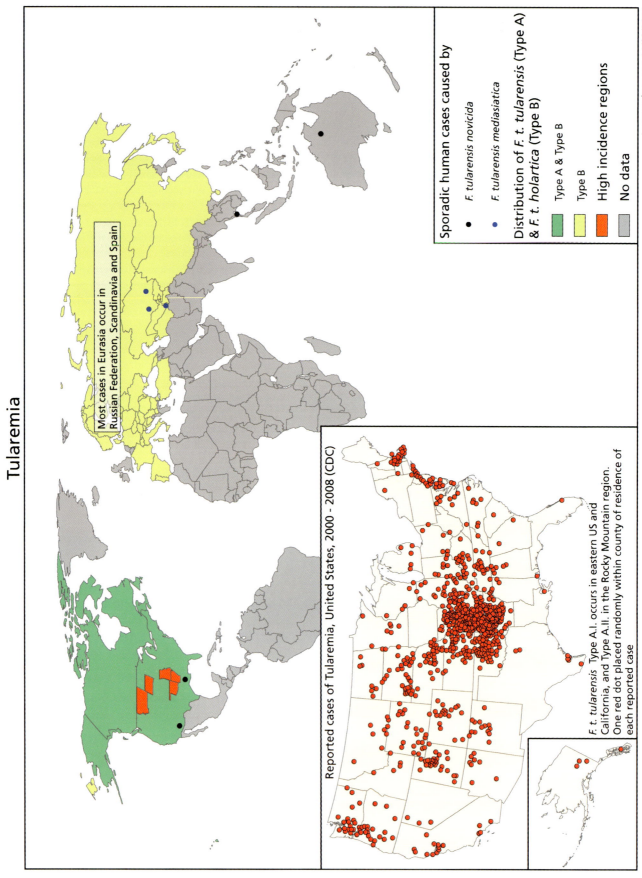

Most cases in Eurasia occur in Russian Federation, Scandinavia and Spain

Sporadic human cases caused by
- ● *F. tularensis novicida*
- ● *F. tularensis mediasiatica*

Distribution of *F. t. tularensis* (Type A)
& *F. t. holartica* (Type B)
- ■ Type A & Type B
- ■ Type B
- ■ High incidence regions
- ■ No data

Last update on: 14/02/2011

Reported cases of Tularemia, United States, 2000 - 2008 (CDC)

F. t. tularensis Type A.I. occurs in eastern US and California, and Type A.II. in the Rocky Mountain region. One red dot placed randomly within county of residence of each reported case

Disease: **Tularemia**

Classification: ICD-9 021; ICD-10 A21

Syndromes and synonyms: Rabbit fever, deerfly fever, hare fever, lemming fever, Ohara fever, Francis disease.

Agent: *Francisella tularensis tularensis* (Type A), *F. tularensis holarctica* (Type B), *F. tularensis mediasiatica*, Gram-negative non-motile intracellular coccobacilli that infect macrophages. Type A is highly virulent and divided into two clades: A.I and A.II. *F. tularensis* is considered a potential biological warfare agent. *F. novicida* is rarely virulent.

Reservoir: Lagomorphs and rodents (ground squirrels) for *F. tularensis* (Types A and B) in North America. Aquatic rodents (beavers, muskrats) in North America, hares and small rodents in northern Eurasia, for *F. holarctica* (Type B). The bacterium can persist in water.

Vector: The primary vectors are ticks and biting flies (deer flies, tabanids). In central Europe: *Dermacentor reticulatus* and *Ixodes ricinus* are important vectors. In eastern USA, *D. variabilis* is the most important vector. In western USA, biting flies are the predominant vectors in arid regions. In Russia, transmission is both by ticks (Ixodes) and mosquitoes.

Transmission: By arthropod bite handling or processing of infected animal carcasses or tissues, by ingestion of contaminated water, soil or food, or by inhalation of contaminated dust or aerosols.

Cycle: Generally enzootic cycles of *F. tularensis* are unnoticed, humans are accidental hosts.

Incubation period: 1–14 days; most commonly 3–5 days.

Clinical findings: Tularemia has six characteristic clinical syndromes, depending on the site of infection: ulceroglandular (commonest), glandular, oropharyngeal, pneumonic, oculoglandular, and typhoidal. Clinical signs include sudden onset of high fever, chills, generalized aches, and chronic ulcer at the bite site (ulceroglandular). From the primary site, lymphatic spread to regional lymphnodes. Further hematogeneous dissemination to other organs. CFR for Type A (ulcero) glandular disease is < 2% if treated promptly (5 to 30% if not treated). In the acute septic form (typhoidal) of the disease, lymphadenopathy and ulcer are absent, and the CFR is high (30–60%). Oculoglandular disease is rare. Ingestion of infected material may result in oropharyngeal or GI

tularemia. In the oropharyngeal form signs are: throat pain, large tonsils, pseudomembrane, and enlarged cervical lymph nodes. Symptoms in GI tularemia range from mild persistent diarrhea to extensive intestinal ulcers and death. Pneumonic tularemia occurs after inhalation of bacteria, or secondary from other entry sites and may progress to severe pneumonia, respiratory failure, and death.

Diagnostic tests: Culture (cysteine-enriched media) or PCR on specimens of affected tissues. Blood cultures are often negative. Testing should be done in a BSL-3 facility. Serology on acute and convalescent sera.

Therapy: Streptomycin is recommended, with gentamicin as an alternative. Tetracyclines may be used for less severe cases.

Prevention: Wear impermeable gloves when handling or skinning rodents or lagomorphs; cook wild game well; avoid drinking water from untreated sources; wear long-sleeved clothes and use repellent to protect against arthropod bites.

Epidemiology: *F. tularensis tularensis* Type A is found in North America and the distribution is associated with wild rabbits, ticks, and tabanid flies. Type B is found throughout the northern hemisphere, mainly in Eurasia and is associated with multiple rodent species, hares, ticks, blood-feeding mosquitoes, and tabanid flies. There is also an association with water bodies (streams) and flooding. In the USA, around 200 human tularemia cases are reported each year, mostly in rural areas during summer months. In Europe, most cases are reported from Sweden, Finland, and Russia, and is recently emerging in Spain. Rural populations are most at risk (e.g. farmers, hunters). Human outbreaks often coincide with wild animal outbreaks.

Map sources: The Tularemia map was modified from P. Keim et al. (2007) with a US map inset with data from CDC, available at: www.cdc.gov/tularemia/.

Key references

Dennis DT, et al. (2001) Tularemia as a biological weapon: medical and public health management. *JAMA* **285**(21): 2763–2773.

Ellis J, et al. (2002) Tularemia. *Clin Microb Rev* **15**(4):631–646.

Keim P, et al. (2007) Molecular epidemiology, evolution, and ecology of Francisella. *Ann NY Acad Sci* **1105**:30–66.

Vogler AJ, et al. (2009) Phylogeography of Francisella tularensis: global expansion of a highly fit clone. *J Bacteriol* **191**(8):2474–2484.

Atlas of Human Infectious Diseases, First Edition. Heiman F.L. Wertheim, Peter Horby and John P. Woodall.
© 2012 Blackwell Publishing Ltd. Published 2012 by Blackwell Publishing Ltd.

Typhoid Fever

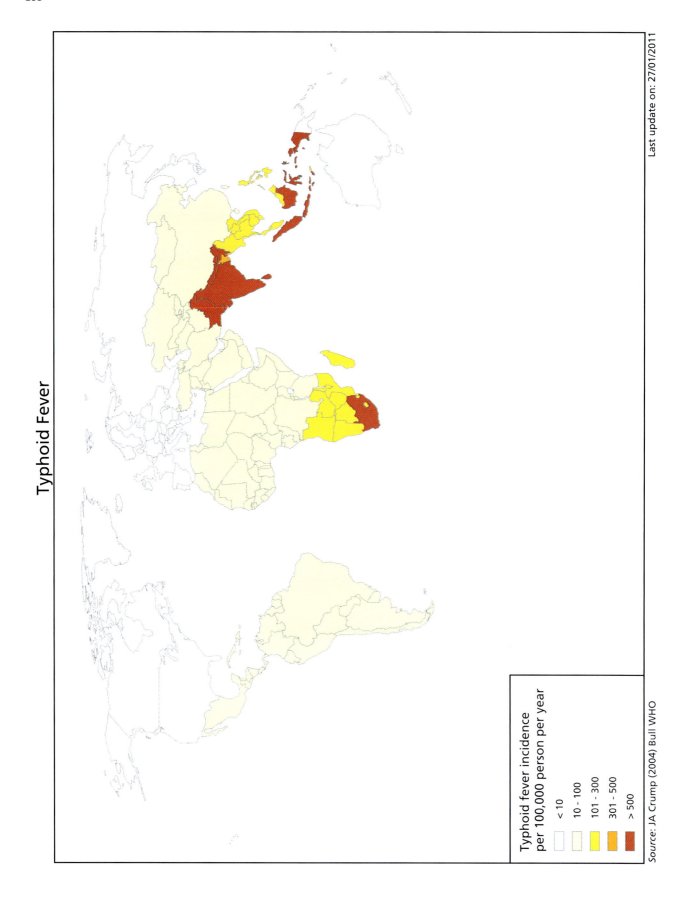

Typhoid fever incidence
per 100,000 person per year

    < 10

    10 - 100

    101 - 300

    301 - 500

    > 500

Source: JA Crump (2004) Bull WHO

Last update on: 27/01/2011

Disease: Typhoid Fever

Classification: ICD-9 002.0; ICD-10 A01

Syndromes and synonyms: Enteric fever, typhus abdominalis.

Agent: *Salmonella enterica enterica* serovar Typhi (*S.* Typhi), a Gram-negative bacillus. *S.* Typhi belongs to Salmonella serogroup D and possesses somatic antigen O9, a single flagellar antigen Hd, and virulence antigen Vi. *S.* Paratyphi A can cause similar disease.

Reservoir: Mainly humans; rarely domestic animals. Humans can be short-term carriers after an infection (10%) or become chronic carriers in the biliary tract (1–5%), shedding viable bacteria in the stool. Chronic carriers are mainly adults with pre-existing biliary tract pathology. Urinary carriage may occur in areas where *Schistosoma haematobium* is endemic.

Vector: Flies can contaminate foods.

Transmission: Via fecal contaminated water, drinks or food from infected individuals or carriers; transmission may also occur in men who have sex with men.

Cycle: Infected individuals shed bacteria into environment, contaminating water and food products that are subsequently ingested by other humans.

Incubation period: 7–14 days, may be up to 2 months.

Clinical findings: Common presenting symptoms are: influenza-like symptoms (fever, dry cough, chills, myalgia), headache, malaise, anorexia, nausea, abdominal discomfort with abdominal tenderness, coated tongue, and hepatosplenomegaly. Adults may have constipation, while young children and HIV patients more often have diarrhea. In 5–30% a rash is present on the abdomen and chest. Children <5 years regularly have unspecific symptoms and remain undiagnosed. Complications occur in 10–15%, including GI bleeding (most common), intestinal perforation, and typhoid encephalopathy. CFR is approximately 2% (range: 0–18%).

Diagnostic tests: Bone marrow culture is the gold standard; blood culture; stool culture; serology; Widal test performance is poor and should not be used.

Therapy: Fluorquinolones are recommended in the absence of resistance. Resistance to ampicillin, chloramphenicol, and cotrimoxazole is widespread and resistance to older generation quinolones and third-generation cephalosporins is rising. Both gatifloxacin and azithromycin can be recommended for the treatment of uncomplicated cases in areas with MDR or nalidixic acid resistance. Third-generation cephalosporins is used for severe cases. Surgery for abdominal complications (e.g. perforation). Dexamethason is recommended for severe cases.

Prevention: Vaccination of risk groups; eradicating carriage; hygiene; sanitation; access to clean water; pasteurization of dairy products; quality control and hygiene procedures for the food industry; exclude typhoid carriers from food handling.

Epidemiology: In 2000 it was estimated there were approximately 21,650,000 new *S.* Typhi cases and 216,500 deaths, with large regional variability. These estimates are based on limited data from mainly countries with a high incidence of disease. Typhoid fever incidence is highest among infants and children living in South Central and Southeast Asia and South Africa. Two seasonality patterns are observed: (1) higher incidence in warmer dry months leading to higher bacterial loads in the water, and (2) higher incidence in the rainy season, due to spillover from sewage to drinking water. Declines are seen in regions were living conditions have improved, mainly due to access to clean water and sanitation (see Water and Sanitation map).

Map sources: The Typhoid Fever map is modified from JA Crump (2004).

Key references
Crump JA (2004) The global burden of typhoid fever. *Bull World Health Org* **82**:346–353.

Crump JA (2010) Global trends in typhoid and paratyphoid fever. *Clin Infect Dis* **50**:241–246.

Ochiai RL (2008) A study of typhoid fever in five Asian countries: disease burden and implications for controls. *Bull World Health Org* **86**:260–268.

Parry CM, et al. (2002) Typhoid fever. *N Engl J Med* **347**(22): 1770–1782.

Atlas of Human Infectious Diseases, First Edition. Heiman F.L. Wertheim, Peter Horby and John P. Woodall.
© 2012 Blackwell Publishing Ltd. Published 2012 by Blackwell Publishing Ltd.

Fungal Infections

Blastomycosis

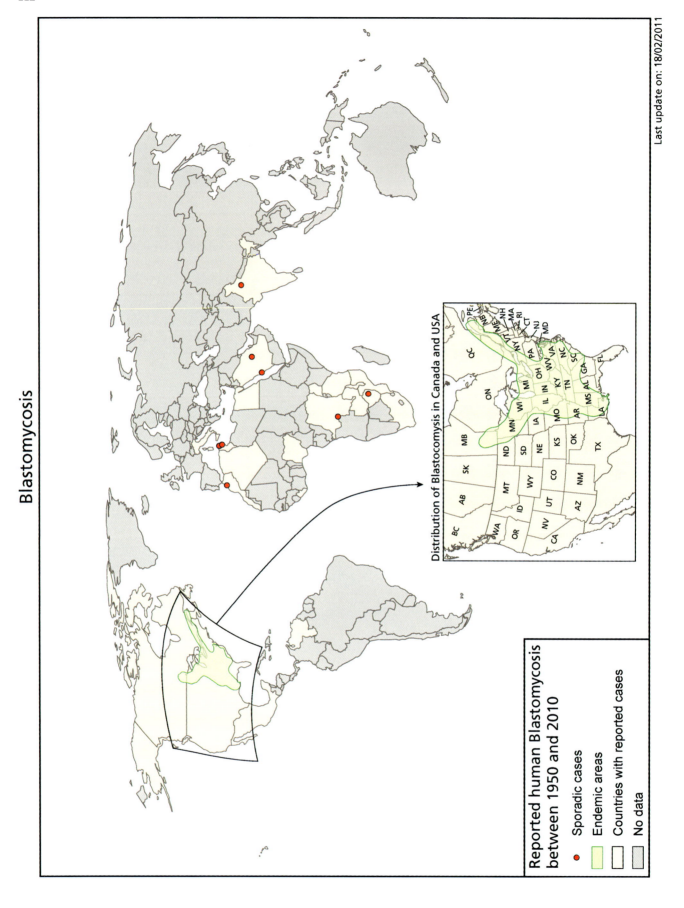

Distribution of Blastocomysis in Canada and USA

Reported human Blastomycosis
between 1950 and 2010

- Sporadic cases
- Endemic areas
- Countries with reported cases
- No data

Last update on: 18/02/2011

Disease: **Blastomycosis**

Classification: ICD-9 116.0; ICD-10 B40

Synonyms: North American blastomycosis, Gilchrist disease

Agent: *Blastomyces dermatitidis* (teleomorph *Ajellomyces dermatitidis*), a dimorphic fungus: grows as a pathogenic yeast at body temperature and as a mold in the environment.

Reservoir: Not completely understood: moist environments close to waterways, in forest or under flooring, also sandy and acidic soil and rotten vegetation. Bird excreta have also been implicated as a potential reservoir. Dogs are more commonly infected than humans but do not transmit disease.

Transmission: Inhalation of spores from disturbed soil. There is no person-to-person transmission.

Cycle: Environment (soil) to human. Fungal spores are inhaled and convert to the pathogenic yeast form in the lung from where they can disseminate to other organs.

Incubation period: Weeks to months; median 45 days.

Clinical findings: A granulomatous fungal infection of the lung, skin, bone or genitourinary tract. Pulmonary infection may be acute or chronic. Acute: fever, cough and pulmonary infiltrate, resolving in 1–3 weeks. Chronic infection is more common and characterized by erythematous papules on the face and extremities, low-grade fever, and weight loss; pulmonary infection may cavitate. Occasionally bone, prostate, epididymis and central nervous system may be affected. Untreated disseminated or chronic pulmonary disease is generally fatal. The main differential diagnosis is tuberculosis.

Diagnostic tests: Microscopy of sputum smear or material from lesions can show characteristic budding forms of the fungus; culture; serology is not routinely used.

Therapy: Amphotericin B is recommended for severe cases. Itraconazole for milder cases.

Prevention: None.

Epidemiology: Blastomycosis is a sporadic disease with a worldwide distribution, though most cases are reported from North America. It is endemic in the Mississippi and Ohio river basins and around the Great Lakes. In endemic areas blastomycosis is frequent in dogs but rare in cats and other animals. The annual incidence of blastomycosis in northern Wisconsin is estimated to be 40–100 per 100,000 in humans and 1,400 per 100,000 in dogs. In the USA outbreaks are usually seen in the spring and fall, indicating infection 1–3 months earlier. Cases are commoner in males and the disease is rare in children. Blastomycosis occurs close to rivers and lakes with changing water levels. Activities involving shores or waterways, like fishing and canoeing, are identified as risk factors for infection.

Map sources: The Blastomycosis map was made by geocoding human blastomycosis cases in the medical literature. The distribution of Blastomycosis in Canada and USA was obtained from KD Reed et al. (2008).

Key references

Pfaller MA, et al. (2010) Epidemiology of invasive mycoses in North America. *Crit Rev Microb* **36**(1):1–53.

Reed KD, et al. (2008) Ecologic niche modeling of *Blastomyces dermatitidis* in Wisconsin. *PLoS ONE* **3**(4):e2034.

Saccente M (2010) Clinical and laboratory update on blastomycosis. *Clin Microb Rev* **23**(2):367–381.

Watts B, et al. (2007) Clinical problem-solving: building a diagnosis from the ground up; a 49-year-old man came to the clinic with a 1-week history of suprapubic pain and fever. *N Engl J Med* **356**:1456–1462.

Atlas of Human Infectious Diseases, First Edition. Heiman F.L. Wertheim, Peter Horby and John P. Woodall.
© 2012 Blackwell Publishing Ltd. Published 2012 by Blackwell Publishing Ltd.

Coccidioidomycosis

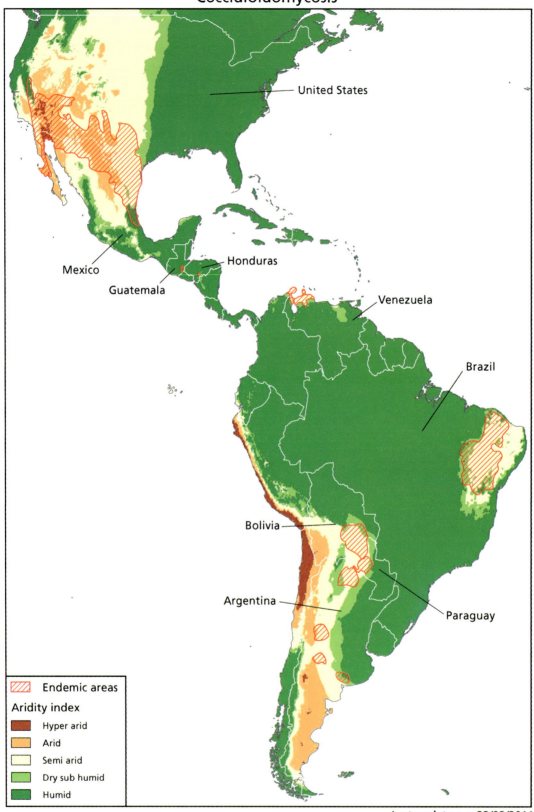

United States

Mexico

Honduras

Guatemala

Venezuela

Brazil

Bolivia

Argentina

Paraguay

Endemic areas

Aridity index

Hyper arid

Arid

Semi arid

Dry sub humid

Humid

Last update on: 23/02/2011

Disease: Coccidioidomycosis

Classification: ICD-9 114; ICD-10 B38

Synonyms: Valley fever, San Joaquin fever, Desert fever, Desert rheumatism, California disease.

Agent: *Coccidioides immitis* (Californian) and *C. posadasii* (non-Californian), dimorphic, soil-borne, ascomycete fungi unique to the western hemisphere.

Reservoir: Dry, sandy alkaline soil in the semi-arid zones of the USA–Mexico border and parts of Central and South America. In North America, the fungus is mainly found in the Lower Sonoran Life Zone with low rainfall and high temperatures *C. immitis* is present in California, and probably northern Mexico and Arizona, and *C. posadasii* is present in the remaining areas.

Transmission: Inhalation of arthroconidia (reproductive spores) from the environment or dusty fomites. Sometimes through direct inoculation or transplantation. Person-to-person transmission is extremely rare.

Cycle: The fungal agent reproduces asexually; the mold forms arthroconidia that are aerosolized and can germinate into new mycelia under appropriate conditions. Arthroconidia are infectious when inhaled by an animal or human (accidental hosts). In the lung the arthroconidia convert to spherules in which endospores can develop untill the spherule ruptures and the endospores are released, forming new spherules.

Incubation period: Primary infection: 1–4 weeks; chronic/disseminated form of disease may be months to years.

Clinical findings: About 60% of exposures result in asymptomatic infection. Symptoms range from benign pulmonary infection (fever, chills, cough, chest pain, dyspnea), night sweats, anorexia and weight loss to progressive pulmonary or extrapulmonary disease involving skin, bones and/or joints, the central nervous system, and other organ systems. Most patients with primary disease recover spontaneously and have life-long immunity to re-infection. Chronic and disseminated disease is estimated to occur in up to 5% of cases. Meningeal infection occurs in less than 1% of extrapulmonary cases and requires life-long treatment.

Diagnostic tests: Microscopy of respiratory secretions, pleural fluid, tissue or exudate in which detection of spherules containing endospores is diagnostic (double-walled structures, size 20–100 µm) fungal culture of sputum, blood, pus, and urine; coccidioidal serologic tests; cocciodin or spherulin skin test (not available in USA). Serology on CSF to diagnose meningitis.

Therapy: Amphotericin B desoxycholate and/or azole antifungals; surgery to remove foci.

Prevention: It is an occupational risk for those working in the environment in endemic regions (e.g. farmers, soldiers). Dust control where feasible (e.g. paving roads). Arthroconidia are resistant to extreme environmental conditions and can survive for many years in dust. Screening of organ donors for coccidioidomycosis in endemic areas. As the fungus is easily aerosolized it is a laboratory hazard.

Epidemiology: Infections are most frequent in a period of drought and winds (dust storms) after heavy rains that advance mold growth, usually late summer or early fall. It is estimated that more than 150,000 primary infections occur annually in the USA. Incidence in California and Arizona appears to have increased since 1991 and again since 2001, probably driven by immigration of non-immunes and wheather conditions that favor dissemination of the fungus. Prevalence of infection in northern Mexico is reported to be 10–40%. Male gender, African-American and Filipino race/ethnicity, immunosuppression, diabetes, older age and pregnancy are risk factors for chronic and disseminated disease. Infections outside the western hemisphere are extremely rare and primarily imported.

Map sources: The Coccidioidomycosis map is modified from RF Hector *et al.* (2005) and combined with aridity index data from FAO, at: www.fao.org/geonetwork/srv/en/.

Key references

Ampel NM (2010) New perspectives on coccidioidomycosis. *Proc Am Thorac Soc* **7**(3):181–185.

Center for Food Security and Public Health (2010) Coccidioidomycosis. *Factsheet*. At www.cfsph.iastate.edu.

Hector RF, et al. (2005) Coccidioidomycosis – a fungal disease of the Americas. *PLoS Med* **2**(1):e2.

Atlas of Human Infectious Diseases, First Edition. Heiman F.L. Wertheim, Peter Horby and John P. Woodall.
© 2012 Blackwell Publishing Ltd. Published 2012 by Blackwell Publishing Ltd.

Histoplasmosis

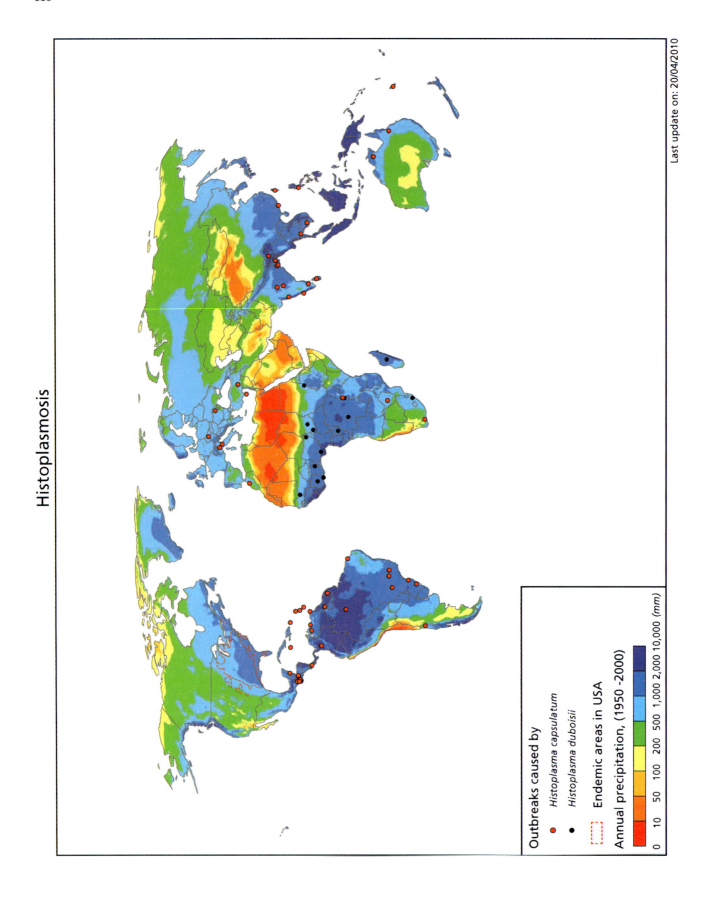

Last update on: 20/04/2010

Outbreaks caused by

○   *Histoplasma capsulatum*

●   *Histoplasma duboisii*

⌶   Endemic areas in USA

Annual precipitation, (1950 -2000)

| 0 | 10 | 50 | 100 | 200 | 500 | 1,000 | 2,000 | 10,000 | *(mm)* |

Disease: Histoplasmosis

Classification: ICD-9 115; ICD-10 B39.0-B39.4, B39.9

Synonyms: Cave disease, Ohio valley disease, reticuloendotheliosis, African histoplasmosis.

Agent: The dimorphic fungi: *Histoplasma capsulatum* (worldwide) and *H. capsulatum* var. *duboisii* (Africa). The fungi grow as a mycelium in the soil at ambient temperatures and convert to the yeast form in the lung at body temperature.

Reservoir: Soil with high nitrogen content, particularly areas with a lot of bird or bat guano, like barns and caves. Blackbird roosts can also be heavily contaminated. Unlike bats, birds are not infected by *H. capsulatum* and do not excrete the fungus in their droppings. Bird droppings are considered a nutrient source for fungal growth in the already contaminated soil.

Transmission: Through inhalation of aerosolized microconidia from disturbed soil or guano. Also by inoculation and organ transplantation.

Cycle: The fungus grows as a mycelium in the environment and in human or animal tissue it converts into a budding yeast.

Incubation period: 3 to 17 days; average 10 days.

Clinical findings: Histoplasmosis may be divided into the following four types: (1) pulmonary histoplasmosis, (2) disseminated histoplasmosis, (3) cutaneous histoplasmosis, and (4) African histoplasmosis. Most infections are asymptomatic or mild and resolve without treatment. The acute phase begins with fever, malaise, chest pains and a dry cough. Chest X-ray findings are normal in 40–70% of cases. Severe infections result in mediastinitis, hepatosplenomegaly, lymphadenopathy and adrenal enlargement. Osteomyelitis is rare. Disseminated disease occurs in patients with altered cellular immunity such as individuals with AIDS and those receiving immunosuppressive medications. It presents with systemic complaints and multiple organ involvement: lung, spleen, bone marrow, adrenals, CNS and GI tract being the most affected. Disseminated histoplasmosis is fatal unless treated. Past infection results in partial protection. Reactivation is uncommon but may occur.

Diagnostic tests: Serology is mainly used (immunodiffusion and CF tests). Detection of antigen in blood, CSF, urine or bronchoalveolar lavage fluid by radioimmunoassay. Microscopy on Giemsa stained bone-marrow or blood smear. Histoplasma skin tests indicate whether a person has been exposed. PCR-based tests are available. Fungal culture is generally slow.

Therapy: For mild cases, an oral triazole; for severe cases, amphotericin B followed by an oral triazole for at least a year.

Prevention: Avoid accumulations of bird or bat droppings such as are found in caves. The USA government provides a document, 'Histoplasmosis: Protecting Workers at Risk', with information on work practices and personal protective equipment.

Epidemiology: *H. capsulatum* grows in soil and material contaminated with bird or guano. The fungus has been found in poultry house litter, caves, areas harboring bats and in bird roosts. *Histoplasma capsulatum* is found throughout the world excluding areas of very low and very high rainfall. It is endemic in certain areas of the United States, particularly in states bordering the Ohio river valley and the lower Mississippi river, where 90% of the population have positive histoplasmin skin tests, indicating a large amount of asymptomatic infection. *H. capsulatum* var. *duboisii* is common in caves in southern and East Africa. Infection can occur outside the cave entrance without entering. Infants, young children, and older persons, in particular those with chronic lung disease, are at increased risk for severe disease. Disseminated disease is more frequently seen in people with cancer, AIDS or other forms of immunosuppression.

Map sources: The Histoplasmosis map was made by geocoding reported human Histoplasmosis cases in the medical literature up to 2010, and showing annual precipitation obtained from WorldClim – Global Climate Data, available at: www.worldclim.org.

Key references

Ashbee HR, et al. (2008) Histoplasmosis in Europe. *Med Mycol* **46**(1):57–65.

Lenhart SW, et al. (2004) Histoplasmosis: Protecting Workers at Risk. DHHS (NIOSH) Publication No. 2005–109.

Gugnani HC, et al. (1997). African histoplasmosis: a review. *Rev Iberoam Micol* **14**(4):155–159.

Knox KS, et al. (2010) Histoplasmosis. *Proc Am Thorac Soc* **7**(3):169–172.

Atlas of Human Infectious Diseases, First Edition. Heiman F.L. Wertheim, Peter Horby and John P. Woodall.
© 2012 Blackwell Publishing Ltd. Published 2012 by Blackwell Publishing Ltd.

Mycetoma

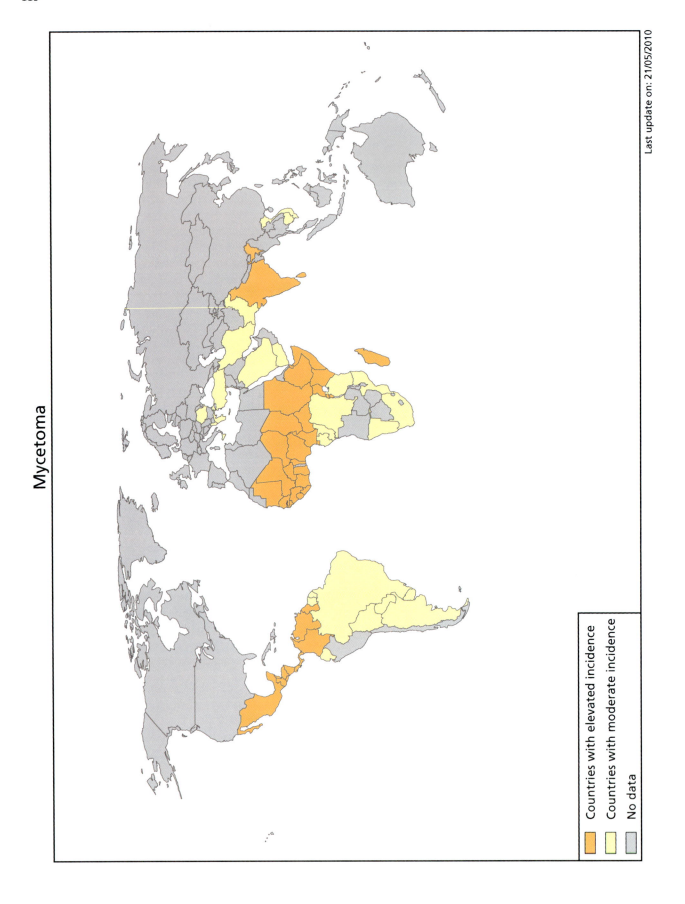

Countries with elevated incidence

Countries with moderate incidence

No data

Last update on: 21/05/2010

Disease: **Mycetoma**

Classification: ICD-9 039; ICD-10 B47

Synonyms: Maduromycosis, Madura foot

Agent: There are two different groups of etiologic agents: fungi and bacteria. Fungal mycetoma is called eumycetoma, and at least 34 fungal species have been implicated. The fungi *Madurella mycetomatis* and *Pseudallescheria boydii* are the most common fungal causative agents of eumycetoma. Bacterial mycetoma is called actinomycetoma and at least 14 actinomycetes have been implicated, of which the bacterial species of *Nocardia*, *Streptomyces* and *Actinomadura* are the most common causative agents of actinomycetoma.

Reservoir: Soil, decaying vegetation.

Transmission: Through contamination of penetrating wounds (e.g. by thorns, splinters). There is no person-to-person transmission.

Cycle: Environment with occasional spillover to humans.

Incubation period: Months to years.

Clinical findings: A chronic inflammatory process of soft tissue, with generally painless swelling and suppuration, developing sinus tracts from which pus-containing granules drains. Lesions on foot or leg below the knee, sometimes hand, shoulder, back or elsewhere. The periosteum and bones may be attacked.

Diagnostic tests: Pus contains visible granules, histopathology of biopsy, culture (slow).

Therapy: For bacteria, clindamycin, trimethoprim-sulfamethoxazole, long-acting sulfonamides; for fungi, itraconazole, ketaconazole, or voriconazole. Resection of small lesions; advanced lesions may require amputation of the hand or leg.

Prevention: Use closed footwear; thoroughly clean penetrating wounds in endemic areas.

Epidemiology: Common in tropical and subtropical areas world wide among people who go barefoot, endemic between 30°N and 15°S of the equator. Mycetoma is endemic in areas with a short rainy season of relatively low rainfall and a temperature range of 30–37 °C, followed by a long dry season with low relative humidity temperatures ranging from a night-time low of as little as 15 °C to a daytime maximum of up to 60 °C. This extreme alteration in weather conditions might be necessary to the survival of the causative organism in its natural niche in soil or plant material. Cases have been exported from the endemic region to many non-endemic countries. World wide, about 60% of cases are caused by actinomycetes; the rest are caused by fungi. In Africa, eumycetomas are more frequently observed than actinomycetomas; in India, actinomycetes are found in more than half of the cases reported. In South America, 90% of the cases are caused by actinomycetes. Infection is most often seen in herdsmen, farmers, and other field laborers. Males are 4–5 times more often affected than females, even in areas where both sexes spend a lot of time in the fields. Mycetoma is seen in all age groups, but usually in adults 20–40 years old. The disease progresses faster in HIV-positive and other immunocompromised patients.

Map sources: The Mycetoma map is modified from the thesis of W. van de Sande (2007), with permission.

Key references

Lopez Martinez LJ, et al. (1992) Epidemiology of mycetoma in Mexico: study of 2105 cases. *Gac Med Mex* **128**:477–481.

Van de Sande W (2007) *Genetic variability, antigenicity, and antifungal susceptibility of* Madurella mycetomatis. Thesis, Erasmus University, Rotterdam.

Welsh O, et al. (2007) Mycetoma. *Clin Dermatol* **25**(2):195–202.

Paracoccidioidomycosis

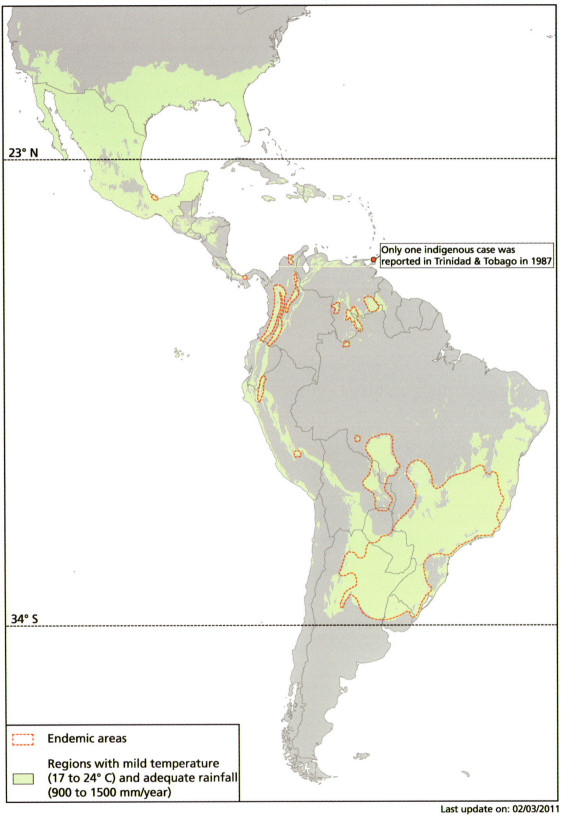

23° N

Only one indigenous case was
reported in Trinidad & Tobago in 1987

34° S

Endemic areas

Regions with mild temperature
(17 to 24° C) and adequate rainfall
(900 to 1500 mm/year)

Last update on: 02/03/2011

Disease: Paracoccidioidomycosis

Classification: ICD-9 116.1; ICD-10 B41

Synonyms: South American blastomycosis, Brazilian blastomycosis, Lutz–Splendore–Almeida disease.

Agent: *Paracoccidioides brasiliensis*, a dimorphic fungus. At room temperature, *P. brasiliensis* is a mold and at body temperature (37 °C) a yeast.

Reservoir: The natural reservoir is unclear. The fungus can be isolated from nine-banded armadillos (*Dasypus novemcinctus*). The disease has also been reported in dogs and other animals. Culturing the fungus from soil is difficult and regularly negative. As armadillos have close contact with soil, it is expected that soil is a reservoir. By using nine-banded armadillos as sentinel animals, it has been shown that the habitat of *P. brasiliensis* is likely humid vegetation close to water sources.

Transmission: Not completely understood. Possibly in the soil the fungus produces infective propagula that can become airborne, inhaled, and lead to respiratory infection. Infections may also occur through traumatic lesions, but this has not been demonstrated.

Cycle: Unknown.

Incubation period: Months to years.

Clinical findings: Paracoccidioidomycosis is a chronic progressive systemic mycosis. There are two disease forms: (1) an acute/subacute form in children that mainly involves the reticulo-endothelial system, and (2) a chronic or adult form with a long latent period, that mainly affects men and generally is a pulmonary infection. The disease can disseminate to mucous membranes, skin, and lymph nodes. Relapses occur in immune-compromised patients and in those with disseminated disease. CFR can be up to 10%, highest in children with underlying conditions, and lowest in adults.

Diagnostic tests: Demonstration of multiple-budding cells in body fluid aspirates or tissue biopsy specimens by microscopy. Isolation of the fungus. Serology and histopathology.

Therapy: Mild disease: oral itraconazole or trimethoprim-sulfamethoxazole. For severe cases: iv amphotericin B or trimethoprim-sulfamethoxazole. Treatment is long and is monitored by clinical and radiological signs.

Prevention: Avoid contact with armadillos or their habitat.

Epidemiology: Most South and several Central American countries between 23°N and 34°S have paracoccidioidomycosis endemic regions, particularly Brazil, Colombia, Venezuela, and Argentina. The prevalence of paracoccidioidomycosis in endemic areas can be up to 75% in adults, with active disease developing in approximately 2% of infected individuals. The endemic areas are generally forest areas with many water streams, mild temperatures, a short winter, and a summer with moderate rain. The disease mainly affects active rural workers (coffee, cotton, and tobacco farmers), probably due to environmental exposure. This explains why the disease is more common in men aged 30 to 60 years. Postpubertal women are partially protected by estrogen that prevents the fungus from transitioning to the yeast form. Contact with nine-banded armadillos has also been shown to be a risk factor for paracoccidioidomycosis.

Map sources: The Paracoccidioidomycosis map was made by mapping endemic regions stated in the medical literature. We used climate data from www.worldclim.org to show regions suitable for paracoccidioidomycosis: mild temperature (17 to 24 °C) and rainfall between 900 and 1,500 mm/year. The 23°N and 34°S lines indicate the geographic limits of the disease.

Key references

Bagagli E, et al. (2006) Phylogenetic and evolutionary aspects of *Paracoccidioides brasiliensis* reveal a long coexistence with animal hosts that explain several biological features of the pathogen. *Infect Genet Evol* **6**(5):344–351.

Blotta MHSL, et al. (1999) Endemic regions of paracoccidioidomycosis in Brazil: A clinical and epidemiologic study of 584 cases in the southeast region. *Am J Trop Med Hyg* **61**(3):390–394.

Nucci M, et al. (2009) Paracoccidioidomycosis. *Curr Fung Infect Rep* **3**(1):15–20.

Restrepo A, et al. (2001) The habitat of *Paracoccidioides brasiliensis*: how far from solving the riddle? *Med Mycol* **39**:233–241.

Travassos LR, et al. (2008) Treatment options for paracoccidioidomycosis and new strategies investigated. *Expert Rev Anti Infect Ther* **6**(2):251–262.

Atlas of Human Infectious Diseases, First Edition. Heiman F.L. Wertheim, Peter Horby and John P. Woodall.
© 2012 Blackwell Publishing Ltd. Published 2012 by Blackwell Publishing Ltd.

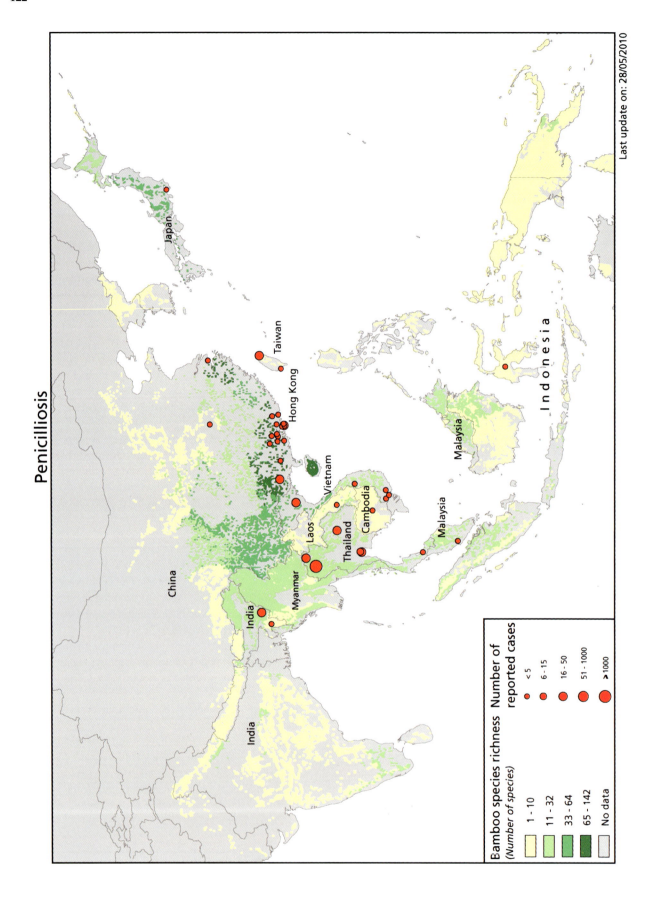

Penicilliosis

Last update on: 28/05/2010

Bamboo species richness
(Number of species)

1 - 10
11 - 32
33 - 64
65 - 142
No data

Number of
reported cases

< 5
6 - 15
16 - 50
51 - 1000
> 1000

China

India

Japan

Taiwan

Hong Kong

Vietnam

Laos

Myanmar

Thailand

Cambodia

Malaysia

Malaysia

Indonesia

India

Disease: Penicilliosis

Classification: ICD-9 117.3; ICD-10 B48.4

Synonyms: None.

Agent: *Penicillium marneffei*, a dimorphic fungus. It is the only *Penicillium* species that is dimorphic: at body temperature or 37 °C it is a yeast form and at cooler temperature it grows as a mold.

Reservoir: Unclear. Bamboo rats (*Rhizomys sinensis, R. pruinosus, R. sumatrensis,* and *Cannomys badius*) are natural hosts and the fungus is detected in the soil of their burrows. *P. marneffei* can survive in sterile soil for several weeks and only a few days in non-sterile soil. *P. marneffei* has not been recovered from environments not associated with bamboo rats. Bamboo rats (except *C. badius*) eat principally bamboo.

Transmission: Unclear, but likely through inhalation of *P. marneffei* conidia from the environment; cutaneous inoculation may also occur. There is no human-to-human transmission.

Cycle: Unknown. It has been proposed that bamboo rats may amplify infectious dispersal stages for human infections.

Incubation period: Few weeks to months.

Clinical findings: Clinical presentation depends on level of immune suppression. *P. marneffei* is most often an opportunistic infection in HIV patients with low CD4 counts (<100 cells/μL). Most present with fever and typical skin lesions. Other findings are anemia, generalized lymphadenopathy, weight loss, and hepatosplenomegaly. Respiratory signs can also be observed. Skin lesions are often papules with central necrosis on the face and neck, but other body sites can also have lesions. Other opportunistic infections also need to be excluded in these patients.

Diagnostic tests: Microscopy of infected tissue in which typical intracellular yeast cells are found; culture of blood, bone marrow, skin lesion, or lymph node.

Therapy: Amphotericin B iv or itraconazole. Long-term azole maintenance treatment is required in HIV patients to prevent relapses.

Prevention: Secondary prophylaxis with itraconazole. HIV patients with low CD4 counts should avoid endemic areas.

Epidemiology: Together with tuberculosis and cryptococcosis, penicilliosis is a common opportunistic infection in HIV patients in Southeast Asia. Though we could not find a report from Myanmar, it is expected to be present there. In northern Thailand it causes 15% of the HIV-related diseases. Before the HIV epidemic it was a rare disease in immunocompromised patients residing in endemic areas in Asia. Cases of penicilliosis have been described world wide, mainly in HIV patients with a travel history to endemic regions. A single case has been described from Ghana where there was no clear travel history to Southeast Asia. The association between bamboo rats and human infection is unclear. There is an association between infection risk and doing agricultural work, suggesting that soil exposure is a risk factor. The disease has a seasonal pattern with more cases during the rainy season.

Map sources: The Penicilliosis map was made by geocoding reported human cases in the medical literature up to 2010. Bamboo richness data is obtained from N. Bystriakova et al. (2010), with permission. Bamboo richness serves as a proxy for the distribution of the bamboo rat for which we could not find data.

Key references

Bystriakova N, et al. (2003) Distribution and conservation status of forest bamboo biodiversity in the Asia-Pacific Region. *Biodiv Conserv* **12**:1833–1841.

Cao C, et al. (2011) Common reservoirs for *Penicillium marneffei* infection in humans and rodents, China. *Emerg Infect Dis* **17**(2):209–214.

Pryce-Miller E, et al. (2008) Environmental detection of *Penicillium marneffei* and growth in soil microcosms in competition with *Talaromyces stipitatus*. *Fungal Ecol* **1**:49–56.

Ustianowski AP, et al. (2008) *Penicillium marneffei* infection in HIV. *Curr Opin Infect Dis* **21**(1):31–36.

Vanittanakom N, et al. (2006) *Penicillium marneffei* infection and recent advances in the epidemiology and molecular biology aspects. *Clin Microbiol Rev* **19**(1):95–110.

Atlas of Human Infectious Diseases, First Edition. Heiman F.L. Wertheim, Peter Horby and John P. Woodall.
© 2012 Blackwell Publishing Ltd. Published 2012 by Blackwell Publishing Ltd.

Parasitic Infections

Amebiasis, *Entamoeba histolytica*

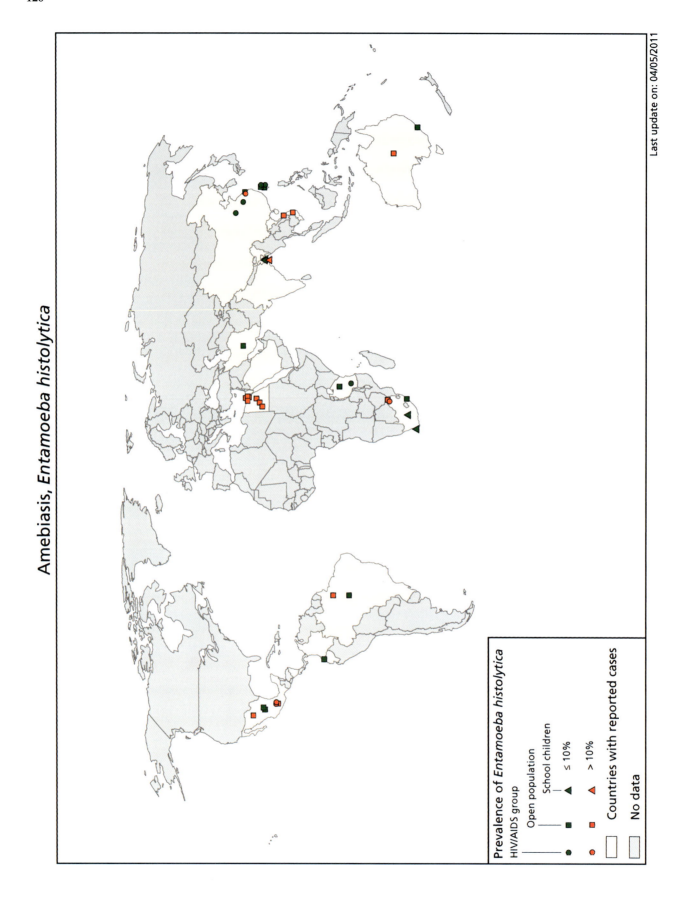

Prevalence of *Entamoeba histolytica*

HIV/AIDS group

Open population

School children

▲ ≤ 10%

▲ > 10%

■ ■

● ●

Countries with reported cases

No data

Last update on: 04/05/2011

Disease: Amebiasis, *Entamoeba histolytica*

Classification: ICD-9 006; ICD-10 A06

Synonyms: Amebiasis, amebic dysentery, amebic liver abscess, ameboma, amoebiasis.

Agent: A protozoan parasite, *Entamoeba histolytica*, that exists in two forms: non-motile cyst and motile trophozoite. *E. histolytica* needs to be distinguished from the non-pathogenic *E. dispar*. *E. moshkovskii* is a common cause of non-invasive diarrhea.

Reservoir: Humans; the parasite has also been detected in non-human primates (cynomolgus monkeys, macaques). *E. moshkovskii* can be found in varying wet environments: clean river sediments, sewage, and brackish coastal pools.

Transmission: Fecal–oral route, mainly exposure to food or water contaminated with infectious cysts. Direct human-to-human transmission occurs via oral and anal sexual activities.

Cycle: Ingested *E. histolytica* non-motile cysts will excyst in the gastrointestinal tract and develop to motile trophozoites that can penetrate the gut mucosa. In the colon, the trophozoites encyst and the cysts are excreted with the feces.

Incubation period: Days to months.

Clinical findings: 90% of the cases will be self-limited and asymptomatic; 10% develop invasive intestinal disease (colitis), and <1% extra-intestinal disease (liver abscess). Amebic colitis presents with abdominal cramps, weight loss, and watery or sometimes bloody diarrhea; most patients are afebrile. Amebic colitis rarely progresses to necrotizing colitis, ameboma, and toxic megacolon. Amebic colitis affects children and adults equally, but mainly males. Amebic liver-abscess mainly occurs in men aged 18 to 50 years, for unknown reasons. *E. moshkovskii* can cause non-invasive diarrhea.

Diagnostic tests: Microscopy of stool specimens cannot distinguish between *E. histolytica*, *E. moshkovskii*, and *E. dispar*; PCR is able to distinguish between these species; stool antigen tests can identify *E. histolytica*.

Therapy: Invasive disease: tinidazole or metronidazole. For severe amebic colitis antibiotics are added to prevent and treat bacterial peritonitis. Surgery for intra-abdominal complications (e.g. bleeding, perforation). Aspiration for liver abscesses. Intraluminal parasites and asymptomatic infection are treated with paromomycin.

Prevention: Sanitation and access to clean water. Personal hygiene during food preparation and sexual activities. Screening and treatment of close contacts.

Epidemiology: *E. histolytica* is distributed world wide, especially in countries with poor sanitation and little access to clean water (see Water and Sanitation maps). It is estimated that *E. histolytica* is responsible for 40,000 to 100,000 deaths per year. Most prevalence studies in the past did not distinguish between *E. histolytica* and the non-pathogenic *E. dispar*, and therefore little is known of the current disease prevalence of the pathogenic *E. histolytica*. *E. histolytica* infection is endemic in Mexico, India, South Africa, some Central and South American countries, and Asian Pacific countries. Community-based studies in urban slums in Bangladesh showed that: 9% of preschool children suffer from amebic diarrhea each year, with 2% requiring a hospital visit. In developed countries, amebiasis is seen in travelers and immigrants from developing countries, and cases may also be found in closed psychiatric institutions. MSM are also a risk group, since they are more exposed.

Map sources: The Amebiasis map was made with data from C. Ximenez et al. (2009) and shows data from prevalence surveys of various populations. There is a lack of data on the amebiasis disease burden since the discovery of *E. dispar*. Global burden data is urgently needed.

Key references
Ali IKM, et al. (2003) *Entamoeba moshkovskii* infections in children in Bangladesh. *Emerg Infect Dis* **9**(5):580–584.

Haque R, et al. (2003) Amebiasis. *N Engl J Med* **348**:1565–1573.

Haque R, et al. (2009) Association of common enteric protozoan parasites with severe diarrhea in Bangladesh. *Clin Infect Dis* **48**:1191–1197.

Stanley Jr, SL (2003) Amoebiasis. *Lancet* **361**:1025–1034.

Ximenez C, et al. (2009) Reassessment of the epidemiology of amebiasis: state of the art. *Infect Genet Evol* **9**:1023–1032.

Atlas of Human Infectious Diseases, First Edition. Heiman F.L. Wertheim, Peter Horby and John P. Woodall.
© 2012 Blackwell Publishing Ltd. Published 2012 by Blackwell Publishing Ltd.

Anisakidosis

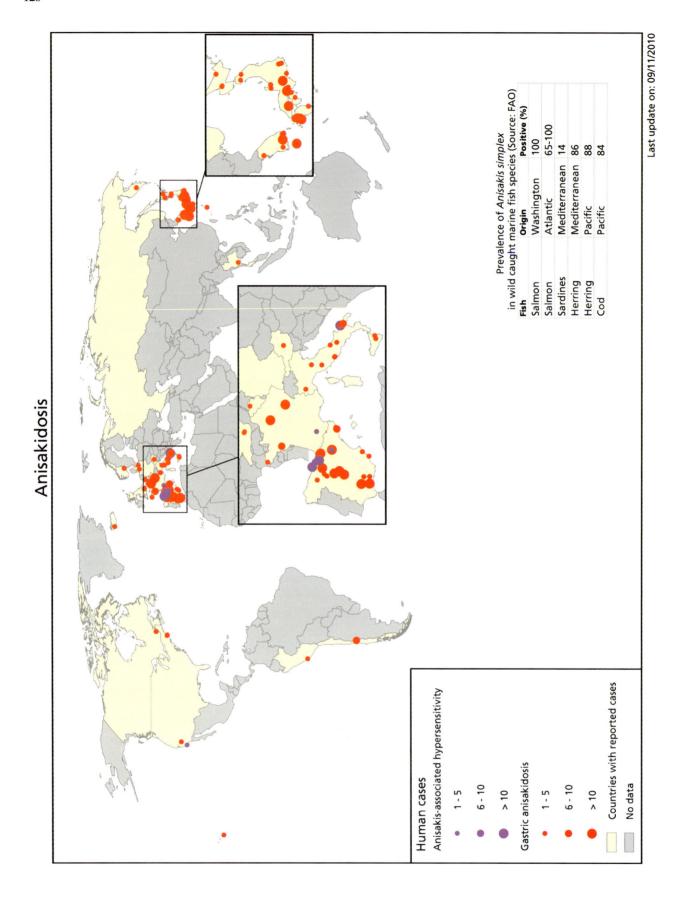

Human cases

Anisakis-associated hypersensitivity

•	1 - 5
●	6 - 10
●	> 10

Gastric anisakidosis

•	1 - 5
●	6 - 10
●	> 10

	Countries with reported cases
	No data

Prevalence of *Anisakis simplex*
in wild caught marine fish species (Source: FAO)

Fish	Origin	Positive (%)
Salmon	Washington	100
Salmon	Atlantic	65-100
Sardines	Mediterranean	14
Herring	Mediterranean	86
Herring	Pacific	88
Cod	Pacific	84

Last update on: 09/11/2010

Disease: Anisakidosis

Classification: ICD-9 127.1; ICD-10 B81.0

Synonyms: Anisakiasis, pseudaterranovosis, Cod worm disease, Herring worm disease, Whaleworm disease, and Sealworm disease.

Agent: The nematodes: *Anisakis simplex*, *A. physeteris*, *Pseudoterranova decipiens*, and *Contracaecum* spp. *A. simplex* and *P. decipiens* are the most important species for human disease. Anisakis larvae are whitish, tightly coiled, 1.5–2 cm in length, and difficult to see in fish flesh. Pseudoterranova larvae are 2–3 cm in length and red to brown in color.

Reservoir: Marine mammals (definitive host), marine invertebrates (intermediate host), and fish (intermediate host). Fish are frequently infected: tuna, cod, mackerel, herring, red snapper, pike, sardines, salmon. *A. simplex* and *A. physeteris* are parasites of whales, seals, walruses, sea lions, and related mammals. *P. decipiens* is found in Pinnipeds (seals, sea lions, walruses). *Contracaecum* spp. are parasites of sea eels and whiting, and have been associated with human anisakiasis.

Transmission: Ingestion of raw or undercooked fish. There is no person-to-person transmission.

Cycle: Ova are excreted with the feces of infected animals, and develop into larvae which are ingested by squid and other invertebrates – these in turn are ingested by fish which may be eaten raw by humans. Humans are accidental hosts.

Incubation period: Few hours for gastric anisakiasis, several weeks for intestinal anisakiasis. Immediate for anisakis-associated hypersensitivity after eating (either raw or cooked) food containing the allergen.

Clinical findings: Gastric anisakidosis: findings depend on where in the gastrointestinal tract the ingested larvae embed. Gastric anisakidosis is the predominant form with acute severe gastric pain, nausea, and vomiting and sometimes hematemesis. Intestinal anisakiasis can cause abdominal pain, obstruction, peritonitis, ulceration, and bleeding. Anisakis-associated hypersensitivity is increasingly being reported and varies from acute urticaria to anaphylaxis. Pharyngeal anisakiasis is rare with pharyngeal irritation as the main symptom.

Diagnostic tests: Endoscopic identification of larvae. Eggs and larvae are not found in the feces. Specific antibody tests are available for anisakis-associated hypersensitivity.

Therapy: Endoscopic removal of larvae; albendazole; surgery for complications. Allergic patients: symptomatic treatment.

Prevention: Avoid consumption of inadequately cooked marine fish. Clean the fish early after they are caught as larvae migrate from viscera into fish flesh after death. Freezing at $-20\,°C$ for at least 7 days kills larvae. Larvae can survive 50 days in vinegar. For allergic patients: avoid food that may contain allergen.

Epidemiology: Anisakidosis occurs world wide, mainly in coastal regions, and in cultures where consumption of raw fish occurs. Risky fish dishes are sushi, sashimi, Filipino bagoong, salted or smoked herring, gravlax, Hawaiian lomi-lomi and palu, South American ceviche, and Spanish pickled anchovies. Anisakidosis is increasingly common in western European countries and the USA due to the increasing popularity of eating raw fish (usually Sashimi). In the USA most cases are related to Pacific salmon consumption and in Europe to herring consumption. It is unclear why anisakidosis is common in Japan, but rarely reported in Taiwan or coastal China where similar fish products are eaten. Overall there is underdiagnosis of the disease due to the physicians' inexperience of the disease. Pseudoterranovosis (codworm) is relatively more common in North America than in Europe or Japan. Most allergic cases are reported from Mediterranean Europe. In Spain it is mainly related to the consumption of cooked hake and anchovies.

Map sources: The Anisakidosis map was made by geocoding reported cases in the medical literature up to 2009.

Key references

Audicana MT, et al. (2008) *Anisakis simplex*: from obscure infectious worm to inducer of immune hypersensitivity. *Clin Microbiol Rev* **21**(2):360–379.

Huss HH, et al. (2003) *Assesment and Management of Seafood Safety and Quality*. FAO Fisheries Technical Paper 444.

Sakanari JA, et al. (1989) Anisakiasis. *Clin Microbiol Rev* **2**(3):278–284.

Atlas of Human Infectious Diseases, First Edition. Heiman F.L. Wertheim, Peter Horby and John P. Woodall.
© 2012 Blackwell Publishing Ltd. Published 2012 by Blackwell Publishing Ltd.

Babesiosis

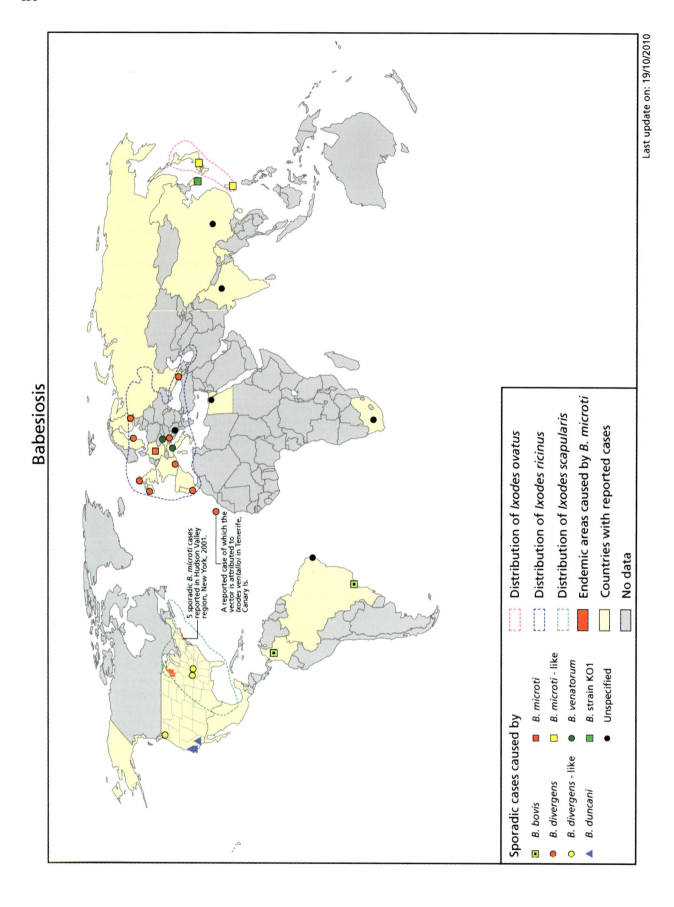

5 sporadic *B. microti* cases reported in Hudson Valley region, New York, 2001.

A reported case of which the vector is attributed to *Ixodes ventalloi* in Tenerife, Canary Is.

Sporadic cases caused by

■	*B. bovis*	●	*B. microti*
■	*B. divergens*	■	*B. microti - like*
○	*B. divergens - like*	●	*B. venatorum*
○	*B. duncani*	■	*B. strain KO1*
◄		●	Unspecified

Distribution of *Ixodes ovatus*

Distribution of *Ixodes ricinus*

Distribution of *Ixodes scapularis*

Endemic areas caused by *B. microti*

Countries with reported cases

No data

Last update on: 19/10/2010

Disease: **Babesiosis**

Classification: ICD-9 088.8; ICD-10 B60.0

Synonyms: Nantucket fever, Piroplasmosis.

Agent: Intraerythrocytic, protozoan parasites, *Babesia* spp.: *B. microti* in North America, *B. duncani* on the west coast of the USA and *B. divergens*-like in four states; *B. divergens* in Cape Verde, western Europe, and Finland; *B. venatorum* in Switzerland, Italy, and Austria; *B. microti*-like in Taiwan and Japan; *Babesia* strain KO1 in South Korea. Species are uncertain in China, Egypt, India, and South Africa.

Reservoir: Rodents, voles (*B. microti*), cattle (*B. divergens*), lagomorphs (*B.divergens*-like), possibly horses (*B. duncani*, formerly type WA1), or sheep (*Babesia* type KO1).

Vector: Minute hard ticks: *Ixodes ricinus* in Eurasia, possibly *Hemaphysalis longicornis* in Korea, *I. ovatus* in Japan. *I. scapularis* (formerly *I. dammini*) in eastern North America, possibly *I. dentatus* in the central USA, *I. pacificus* in California and Washington state, USA.

Transmission: By tick bite; rarely by blood transfusion and transplacental/perinatal. Ticks must feed for more than 24 hours for transmission to occur.

Cycle: Ticks introduce *Babesia* spp. sporozoites from the ticks' salivary glands into small mammals/humans during feeding. The sporozoites infect erythrocytes in which they asexually reproduce by budding and develop through various stages into gametocytes. Ticks can take up circulating gametocytes during feeding on an infected animal. The gametocytes fertilize in the tick gut and develop into sporozoites in their salivary glands.

Incubation period: 1–9 weeks; relapses up to more than a year.

Clinical findings: Often asymptomatic in healthy individuals. Symptomatic cases: fever, chills, myalgia, fatigue, and jaundice, hemolytic anemia; severe cases: retinal infarctions, ecchymoses and petechiae, acute respiratory failure, congestive heart failure, DIC, liver and renal failure, and splenic rupture, with a mortality rate of 5–9%, higher in immunocompromised patients. The differential diagnosis is chloroquine-resistant malaria, Lyme disease, or human granulocytic anaplasmosis.

Diagnostic tests: Microscopy on Giemsa-stained thick or thin film blood smear; PCR; isolation in hamsters (2–4 weeks for result); serology (IFA) on paired acute and convalescent sera.

Therapy: Combination of atovaquone and azithromycin for mild-to-moderate illness, clindamycin and quinine for severe disease. Exchange transfusion for life-threatening infection, dialysis in case of renal failure. Chloroquine is ineffective.

Prevention: Control deer population; avoid areas with ticks; tick bite precautions: cover skin, repellent on skin and clothing (permethrin, DEET), check daily for attached ticks and remove.

Epidemiology: Immunocompromised, asplenic, and elderly people are at higher risk of symptomatic disease. The number of cases diagnosed in the USA has increased markedly since 1975 due to an increase in the white-tailed deer population, hosts of the adult vector ticks. Nearly all patients with *Babesia divergens* infection in Europe had been splenectomized and exposed to cattle. The *B. divergens*-like parasite in the USA has a reservoir in cottontail rabbits, and is not infectious for cattle; it has been found in only 3 patients. All 3 patients with *B. venatorum* (EU1) infection had also been splenectomized. Cape Verdean, Egyptian, and Asian cases lie outside the range of *Ixodes ricinus*; *B. duncani* and *B. divergens*-like cases in west coast states of USA lie outside the range of *I. scapularis*. Possible vectors for these cases are *I. dentatus* in the central USA, and *I. pacificus* on the west coast. Infection is seasonal (summer), coinciding with abundance of nymphal ticks in warmer months.

Map sources: The Babesiosis map was made by geocoding reported cases in the medical literature up to 2010. The tick distributions are obtained from G.V. Kolonin (2009).

Key references

Kolonin GV (2009) *Fauna of Ixodid Ticks of the World*; available at www.kolonin.org.

Saito-Ito A, et al. (2000) Transfusion-acquired, autochthonous human babesiosis in Japan: isolation of Babesia microti-like parasites with hu-RBC-SCID mice. *J Clin Microbiol* **38**:4511–4516.

Vannier E, et al. (2008) Human babesiosis. *Infect Dis Clin N Am* **22**:469–488.

Vannier E, et al. (2009) Update on babesiosis. *Interdisc Persp Infect Dis* 984568.

Atlas of Human Infectious Diseases, First Edition. Heiman F.L. Wertheim, Peter Horby and John P. Woodall.
© 2012 Blackwell Publishing Ltd. Published 2012 by Blackwell Publishing Ltd.

Capillariasis, Intestinal

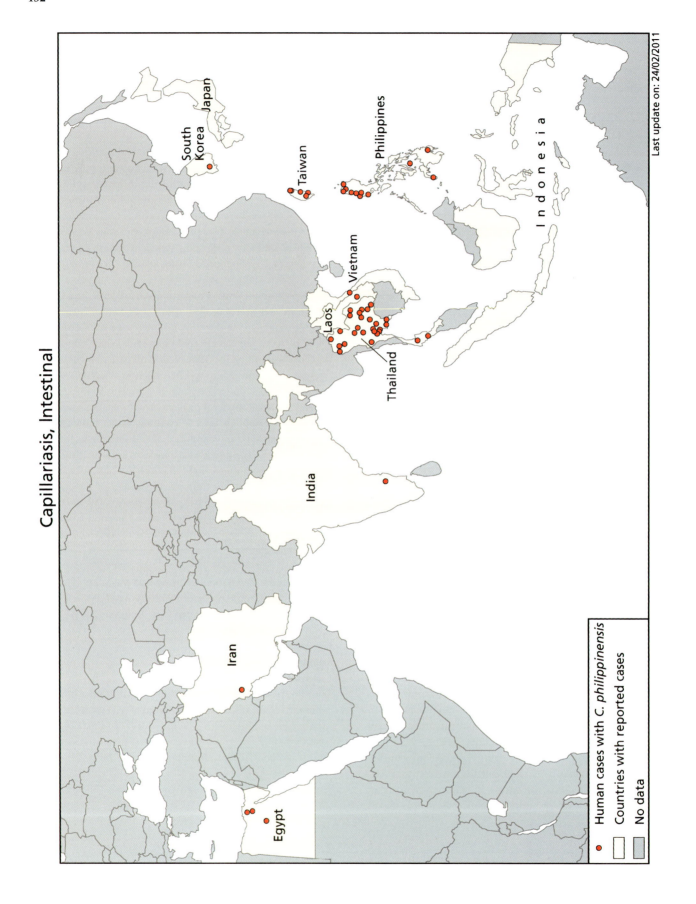

South Korea

Japan

Taiwan

Philippines

Indonesia

Vietnam

Laos

Thailand

India

Iran

Egypt

Last update on: 24/02/2011

- Human cases with *C. philippinensis*
- Countries with reported cases
- No data

Disease: Capillariasis, Intestinal

Classification: ICD-9 127.5; ICD-10 B81.1.

Syndromes and synonyms: Intestinal capillariasis, Pudoc mystery disease, wasting disease.

Agent: The agent of intestinal capillariasis is *Capillaria philippinensis* (or *Paracapillaria philippinensis*), a small nematode roundworm (males 2.3 to 3.2 mm; females 2.5 to 4.3 mm). Two other *Capillaria* species that can cause rare human infections: hepatic (*C. hepatica* or *Calodium hepaticum*) and pulmonary capillariasis (*C. aerophila*). The map only shows intestinal capillariasis.

Reservoir: For *C. philippinensis*: fish-eating birds. Freshwater fish are intermediate hosts.

Transmission: Consumption of raw or undercooked uneviscerated fish that have ingested infected feces of humans or waterfowl. There is no person-to-person transmission.

Cycle: For *C. philippinensis*: eggs are passed in the stools of humans and fish-eating birds; after ingestion by freshwater fish, larvae hatch, penetrate the intestinal wall and migrate to the tissues. Ingestion of raw or undercooked fish results in infection of the human and bird host. The adults of *C. philippinensis* reside in the mucosa of the human small intestine, where the females lay eggs. Released larvae can cause autoinfection, which may progress to hyperinfection.

Incubation period: At least 2 weeks.

Clinical findings: Intestinal capillariasis starts with mild abdominal pain, borborygmus, and diarrhea, that develops to profuse watery diarrhea. If untreated: chronic diarrhea, vomiting, malabsorption, leading to weight loss, muscle wasting, cachexia, and eventually death. Hepatic capillariasis (*C. hepatica*) is a (sub)acute hepatitis with eosinophilia, that may disseminate to other organs and can be fatal. Pulmonary capillariasis (*C. aerophila*) may present with fever, cough, asthma, and pneumonia and may also be fatal.

Diagnostic tests: Microscopy for eggs, larvae and/or adult worms in the stool, or in intestinal biopsies for *C. philippinensis* (eggs resemble those of *Trichuris trichiura*).

Therapy: Albendazole or mebendazole.

Prevention: For *C. philippinensis*: sanitation and avoid consumption of raw or improperly cooked fish.

Epidemiology: Intestinal capillariasis is generally found in countries where raw freshwater fish is eaten. The parasite was first reported in 1963 in the northern Philippines. *C. philippinensis* is endemic in the Philippines, Laos, and Thailand. Rare cases have been reported from other Asian countries and the Middle East. A single case has been reported in Spain imported from Colombia, but there are no other reports of cases in the Americas. Rare cases of human infection with *C. hepatica* and *C. aerophila* have been reported world wide. Infected fish may be exported from endemic areas to non-endemic countries.

Map sources: The Capillariasis map was made by geocoding reported human cases infected with *Capillaria philippinensis* up to 2010. There is no detailed information on where the human cases occurred in Indonesia.

Key references

Cross J (1992) Intestinal capillariasis. *Clin Microb Rev* **5** (2):120–129.

Belizario VJ Jr, et al. (2010) Intestinal capillariasis, western Mindanao, the Philippines. *Emerg Infect Dis* **16**(4):736.

Dronda F, et al. (1993) Human intestinal capillariasis in an area of nonendemicity: case report and review. *Clin Infect Dis* **17**(5):909–912.

Saichua P, et al. (2008) Human intestinal capillariasis in Thailand. *World J Gastroent* **14**(4):506–510.

Atlas of Human Infectious Diseases, First Edition. Heiman F.L. Wertheim, Peter Horby and John P. Woodall.
© 2012 Blackwell Publishing Ltd. Published 2012 by Blackwell Publishing Ltd.

Clonorchiasis

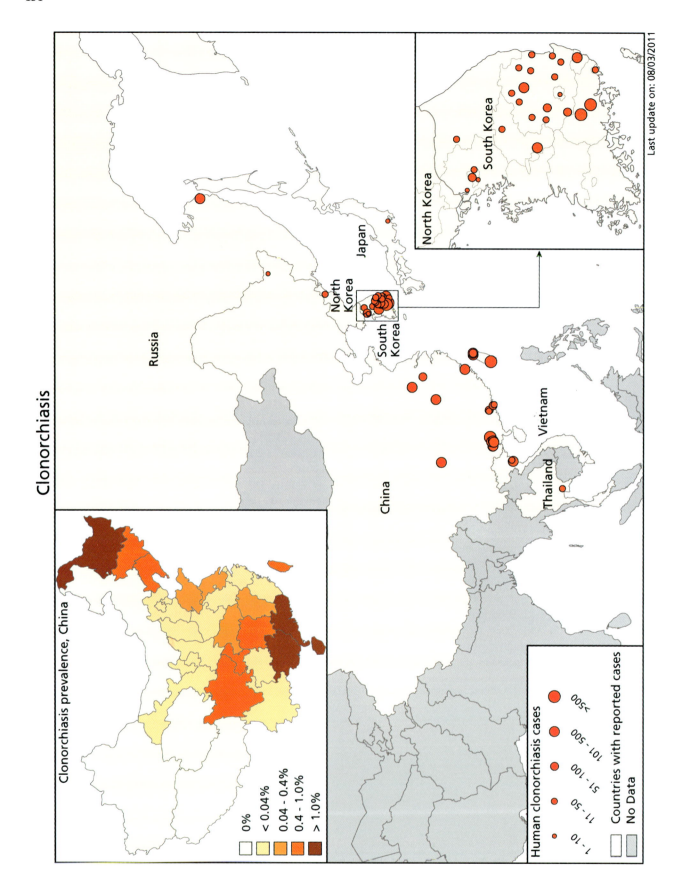

Clonorchiasis prevalence, China

- 0%
- < 0.04%
- 0.04 - 0.4%
- 0.4 - 1.0%
- > 1.0%

Human clonorchiasis cases

- 1 - 10
- 11 - 50
- 51 - 100
- 101 - 500
- >500

Countries with reported cases

No Data

Last update on: 08/03/2011

Disease: **Clonorchiasis**

Classification: ICD-9 121.1; ICD-10 B66.1

Syndromes and synonyms: Chinese liver fluke, Oriental liver fluke.

Agent: *Clonorchis sinensis*, a trematode (fluke) 10–25 mm long and 3–5 mm wide.

Reservoir: Piscivorous (fish-eating) mammals, including: humans, dogs, cats, pigs, rats, and several species of wild animals. Humans can remain infected for several decades.

Vector: Freshwater operculate snails (mainly *Parafossarulus* sp. and *Bithynia* sp.).

Transmission: Consumption of raw or undercooked infected freshwater fish, mainly Cyprinidae (carp and minnows) or shrimp.

Communicability: None.

Cycle: Fish-eating mammals (including humans) shed *C. sinensis* eggs into the environment that are ingested by snails, where they develop into cercariae. The motile cercariae are released into water and infect freshwater fish and encyst in meat and skin as metacercariae. When ingested by mammals, the metacercariae migrate into the bile ducts where they develop into adult flukes that produce and excrete eggs into feces. The cycle takes approximately 3 months.

Incubation period: Depends on infecting dose. Larvae reach adult fluke stage in less than one month.

Clinical findings: Loss of appetite, epigastric discomfort, rarely jaundice due to bile duct obstruction, cirrhosis, liver enlargement, ascites and edema. After years of chronic infection there is a risk of cholangiocarcinoma.

Diagnostic tests: Visualizing characteristic eggs in feces or duodenal fluid by microscopy.

Therapy: Praziquantel; surgery in case of biliary obstruction.

Prevention: Proper cooking, or freezing of fish at −20 °C for 7 days destroys the parasite. Abandon use of human feces to fertilize fish ponds.

Epidemiology: Clonorchiasis is the most common liver fluke in humans. Estimates show that approximately 35 million people are infected world wide, of which 15 million are in China. In endemic areas, the highest prevalence is in adults over 30 years of age. The intensity of human infection depends on the eating habits of the population. In Asia, eating raw fish is common together with alcohol consumption and, therefore, men are more often infected than women. The incidence is low in children. In China the prevalence in some regions is increasing, probably due to increased consumption of raw freshwater fish. The geographical extent of the disease is determined by snail distribution, the eating habits of the local population, and contamination of freshwater with egg-containing feces. In southern China the disease is maintained by the practice of using human feces in carp raising ponds to promote plankton growth, on which the fish feed. In non-endemic areas it appears in Asian immigrants, and in people who consume raw, dried, smoked or pickled fish imported from endemic areas.

Map sources: The Clonorchiasis map was made by geocoding human cases reported in the medical literature up to 2010.

Key references

Lun ZR, et al. (2005) Clonorchiasis: a key foodborne zoonosis in China. *Lancet Infect Dis* **5**(1):31–41.

Marcos LA, et al. (2008) Update on hepatobiliary flukes: fascioliasis, opisthorchiasis and clonorchiasis. *Current Opinion Infect Dis* **21**(5):523–530.

Rim HJ (2005) Clonorchiasis, an update. *J Helminth* **79**:269–281.

Atlas of Human Infectious Diseases, First Edition. Heiman F.L. Wertheim, Peter Horby and John P. Woodall.
© 2012 Blackwell Publishing Ltd. Published 2012 by Blackwell Publishing Ltd.

Cysticercosis

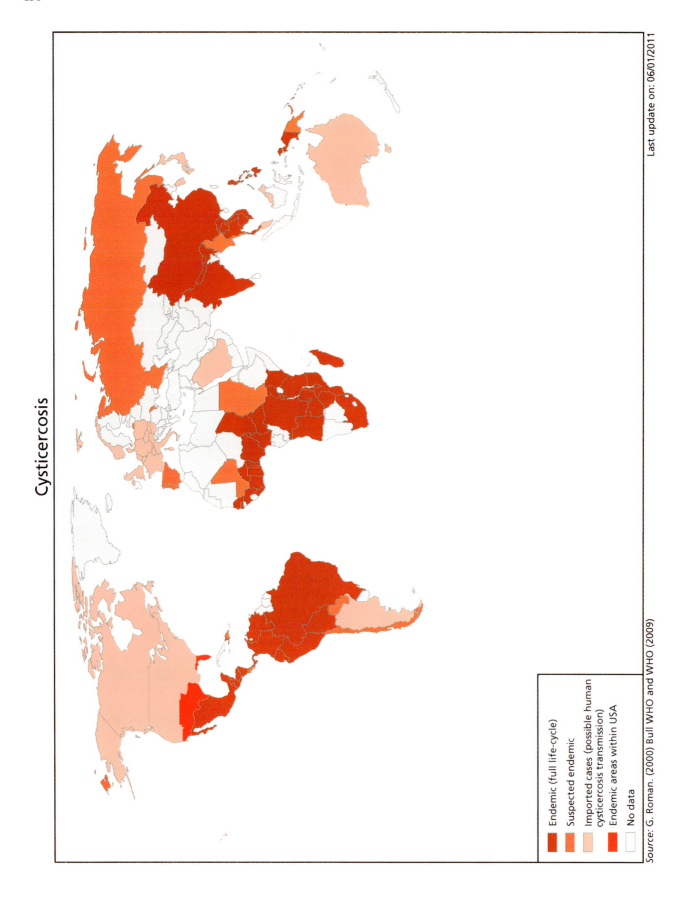

Endemic (full life-cycle)

Suspected endemic

Imported cases (possible human
cysticercosis transmission)

Endemic areas within USA

No data

Source: G. Roman. (2000) Bull WHO and WHO (2009)

Last update on: 06/01/2011

Disease: **Cysticercosis**

Classification: ICD-9 123.1; ICD-10 B 69.0

Syndromes and synonyms: *Taenia solium* infection, neurocysticercosis, cerebral cysticercosis, taeniosis, taeniasis.

Agent: Larval stage of the pork tapeworm *T. solium*. Adult *T. solium* can be 2–5 meters in length and lives in the small intestine of human host.

Reservoir: Humans are the definitive host; pigs are an intermediate host.

Transmission: Cysticercosis develops after ingesting *T. solium* eggs; Taeniasis (tapeworm carriage) occurs after ingestion of raw or undercooked pork meat with cysticerci; human to human transmission is by the feco–oral route.

Cycle: Pigs or humans ingest eggs from contaminated environment. Adult tapeworms will only develop in humans after eating raw or undercooked pork containing cysticerci. It takes 2 months for larvae to become an adult worm and produce eggs (up to 300,000 eggs per day). In pigs, eggs invade the general circulation via the intestinal wall and migrate to skeletal and heart muscles where they form cysticerci.

Incubation period: It takes 2 months (range: 5–12 weeks) to mature to an adult worm in the intestine. The incubation period of neurocysticercosis (time from infection to first symptom) is extremely variable from months to several years.

Clinical findings: Taeniosis is *T. solium* infection of the small intestine and varies from asymptomatic (the most frequent) to weight loss, anorexia and abdominal pain. Cysticercosis is a tissue infection with *T. solium* larvae with findings depending on where cysticerci develop (subcutaneous, eye, heart, CNS). Its localization in the CNS, causing neurocysticercosis, is the most severe form of the disease: seizures, headache, focal neurologic signs, epilepsy, and hydrocephalus may develop. The CFR is low.

Diagnostic tests: Taeniosis: detection of eggs in stool by microscopy; *T. solium* eggs can not be distinguished from *T. saginata* eggs; serology; Neurocysticercosis: histology; CT or MRI scan brain; serology is not sensitive or specific for neurocysticercosis.

Therapy: Taeniosis: praziquantel. Neurocysticercosis: Treatment must be individualized case by case but could include cestocidal drugs (albendazole or praziquantel), symptomatic measures (antiepileptic drugs, oedema reducing drugs, ventriculoperitoneal shunt) and removal by neurosurgery (limited indications).

Prevention: Sanitation (particularly use of latrine and maintaining pigs enclosed); hygiene; meat inspection; thorough cooking of pig meat before consumption; treatment of tapeworm carriers. A vaccine has been developed for cattle.

Epidemiology: Cysticerosis has a worldwide distribution, mainly where pigs are consumed and sanitation is substandard (see *Streptococcus suis* map for pig density and Sanitation map). In endemic countries it is an important cause of epilepsy, causing a high disease burden in mainly poor families. In several countries neurocysticercosis is the cause of 10–50% of seizures. Neurocysticercosis is common in Latin America and non-Muslim African and Asian countries where pig is eaten and traditional pig rearing is practiced. Regions with the habit of eating raw or undercooked pig meat are at increased risk. In Europe, cysticercosis has largely disappeared due to strong health system and good sanitation. In several developed nations, like the USA and Spain, there is an increase in certain regions where lots of migrants live who have come from high endemic countries. Tapeworm carriers can cause small outbreaks, as was observed in a Jewish community in New York that employed cooks from Latin America.

Map sources: The Cysticercosis map is modified from G. Roman et al. (2000) and WHO (2009) at: http://gamapserver.who.int/mapLibrary/Files/Maps/Global_cysticercosis_2009.png.

Key references

Carpio A (2002) Neurocysticercosis: an update. *Lancet Infect Dis* **2**:751–762.

Carpio A, et al. (2008) Effects of albendazole treatment on neurocysticercosis: a randomised controlled trial. *J Neurol Neurosurg Psychiat* **79**(9):1050–1055.

Dixon HB, et al. (1961) Cysticercosis: an analysis and follow-up of 450 cases. *Spec Rep Ser Med Res Coun* **299**:1–58.

Engels D, et al. (2003) The control of human (neuro)cysticercosis: which way forward? *Acta Trop* **87**:177–182.

Roman G, et al. (2000) A proposal to declare neurocysticercosis an international reportable disease. *Bull World Health Organ* **78**(3):399–406.

Atlas of Human Infectious Diseases, First Edition. Heiman F.L. Wertheim, Peter Horby and John P. Woodall.
© 2012 Blackwell Publishing Ltd. Published 2012 by Blackwell Publishing Ltd.

Diphyllobothriasis

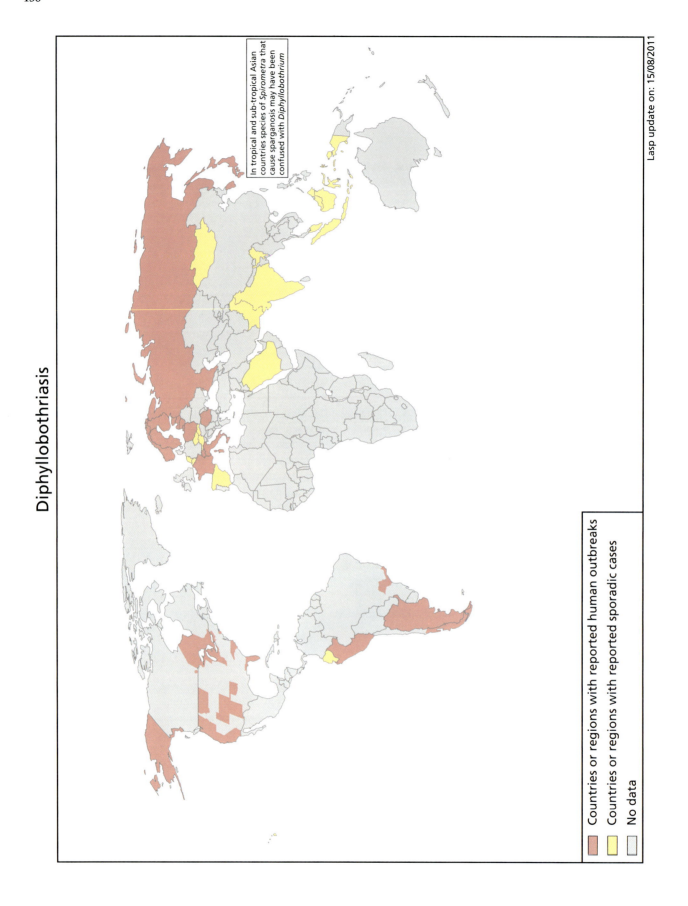

In tropical and sub-tropical Asian countries species of *Spirometra* that cause sparganosis may have been confused with *Diphyllobothrium*

Lasp update on: 15/08/2011

Countries or regions with reported human outbreaks

Countries or regions with reported sporadic cases

No data

Disease: **Diphyllobothriasis**

Classification: ICD-9 123.4; ICD-10 B70.0

Syndromes and synonyms: Diphyllobothriosis, Dibothriocephaliasis, broad or fish tapeworm infection

Agent: The cestode *Diphyllobothrium latum* (fish or broad tapeworm), the largest human tapeworm (up to 25 meters long). In Japan and eastern Russia *D. nihonkaiense* is common. At least 13 other *Diphyllobothrium* species have been reported to infect humans, but less frequently.

Reservoir: In addition to humans, dogs and fish-eating terrestrial and marine mammals can also serve as definitive hosts for *D. latum*.

Transmission: Consumption of raw or undercooked freshwater fish containing infectious larvae. There is no direct person-to-person transmission.

Cycle: Eggs are passed in feces into freshwater bodies, mature in about 2 to 3 weeks, depending on water temperature, and hatch ciliated larvae (coracidia). Coracidia develop into procercoid larvae after ingestion by freshwater crustaceans (copepods). The copepods are eaten by a second intermediate host, typically small fish. The larvae migrate into the musculature where they develop into the human infectious plerocercoid larvae. Larger predator fish (e.g. pike, burbot, perch) ingest the smaller infected fish upon which the plerocercoid larvae migrate to the flesh of these larger fish that serve as third intermediate hosts harboring larvae. Humans and larger mammals acquire the disease by eating these larger fish raw or undercooked. The larvae mature into adult tapeworms that attach to the small intestinal wall by scolex and develop egg-filled proglottids that detach. Up to 1 million eggs per day per worm are passed in the feces, 2–6 weeks after infection.

Prepatent period: 2–6 weeks.

Clinical findings: Most infections are asymptomatic or mild. Symptoms are: abdominal discomfort, diarrhea, vomiting and weight loss, rarely anemia. Massive infections may result in intestinal obstruction. Migration of proglottids can cause cholecystitis or cholangitis. Proglottids can be seen in the stool.

Diagnostic tests: Microscopic identification of eggs in the stool, visualization of proglottids passed in the stool.

Therapy: Praziquantel and niclosamide are the drugs of choice. In untreated cases the worms can live up to 25 years and produce eggs.

Prevention: Avoid ingesting raw freshwater fish. Adequate cooking, freezing at −20 °C for at least 7 days, or irradiation of fish or meat will kill encysted larvae. Sanitation.

Epidemiology: Human infection is associated with cold waters in the northern hemisphere. A 2005 estimate stated that 20 million people were infected world wide. It is common in communities, as in Japan, that have a habit of eating raw or undercooked fish. Risky fish dishes are sushi, sashimi, South American ceviche, fish carpaccio, salmon tartare, and salted or marinated fillets in Scandinavia or Baltic region. Historically, Finland and Alaska had a high disease prevalence, but this has decreased due to preventive measures. Women seem more at risk, probably due to being involved in meal preparation. The disease incidence is increasing in some countries such as Russia, South Korea, Japan, and Brazil. Cases are also reported from regions where diphyllobothriasis was expected to have been eliminated, such as Alpine lakes in Switzerland, northern Italy, and eastern France. It is not clear whether the cases reported in Hawaii and Brazil are autochthonous or from imported fish. *D. nihonkaiense*, present in Japan and far eastern Russia, has been reported from a patient who ate raw Pacific sockeye salmon (*Oncorhynchus nerka*) from British Columbia, Canada. *D. pacificum* (formerly *D. arctocephalinum*) is increasingly reported as a human parasite along the coast of South America. Infected fish can be transported to any part of the world for consumption.

Map sources: The Diphyllobothriasis map was made by visualizing regions or countries were cases have been reported in the medical literature up to 2010.

Key references

Rausch RL, et al. (2010) Identity of *Diphyllobothrium* spp. (Cestoda: Diphyllobothriidae) from sea lions and people along the Pacific Coast of South America. *J Parasit* **96**(2):359–365.

Scholz T, et al. (2009) Update on the human broad tapeworm (genus *Diphyllobothrium*), including clinical relevance. *Clin Microbiol Rev* **22**(1):146–160.

Atlas of Human Infectious Diseases, First Edition. Heiman F.L. Wertheim, Peter Horby and John P. Woodall.
© 2012 Blackwell Publishing Ltd. Published 2012 by Blackwell Publishing Ltd.

Dracunculiasis

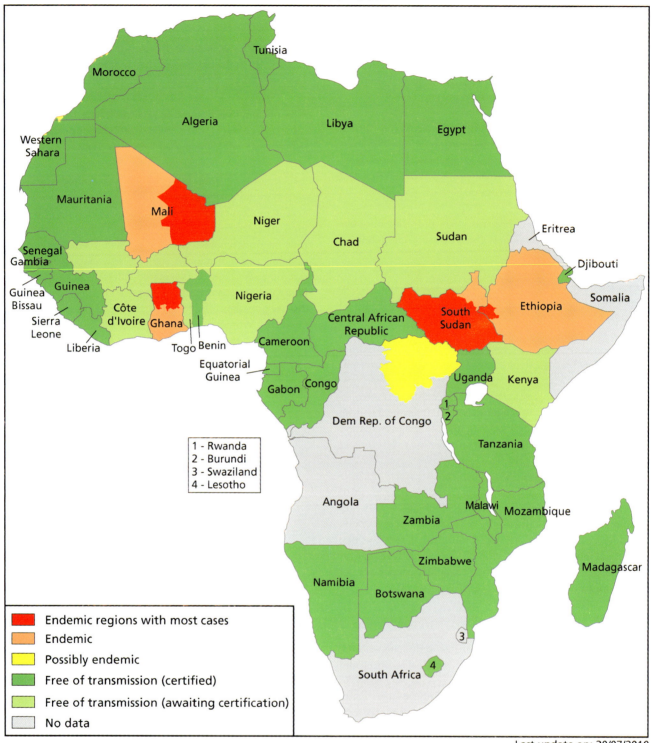

1 - Rwanda
2 - Burundi
3 - Swaziland
4 - Lesotho

Legend:
- Endemic regions with most cases
- Endemic
- Possibly endemic
- Free of transmission (certified)
- Free of transmission (awaiting certification)
- No data

Last update on: 20/07/2010

Disease: Dracunculiasis

Classification: ICD-9 125.7; ICD-10 B72

Syndromes and synonyms: Guinea worm disease, Medina worm disease, Pharaoh worm disease, serpent worm disease, dracontiasis.

Agent: *Dracunculus medinensis*, a nematode roundworm. The longest adult female recorded is 80 cm, and adult male 40 cm.

Reservoir: Humans.

Vector: *Cyclops* spp., microscopic copepods (crustaceans) commonly known as water fleas.

Transmission: By ingestion of infected copepods, usually with drinking water.

Cycle: Human–copepod–human. Adult female worm expels larvae through a hole in the skin of the leg or foot of an infected person into stagnant water where they are ingested by the vectors. The larvae become infectious in 2 weeks and when the vectors are ingested and digested, the larvae are freed and migrate into the subcutaneous tissue of the abdomen and thorax. There they mature into adults. Larvae are shed for 2–3 weeks, are viable in water for up to 5 days, and develop in the copepod for 2 weeks.

Incubation period: About 12 months (10 to 18 months).

Clinical findings: Blister, usually on the leg or foot, which burns or itches, fever, nausea, vomiting, diarrhea, dyspnea, dizziness and generalized urticaria. Multiple and repeat infections occur, there is no protective immunity. Painful and infected ulcers can incapacitate patients for months. Secondary bacterial infection can lead to abscesses, synovitis, ankylosis and limb contractures, septic arthritis, and life-threatening sepsis.

Diagnostic tests: Visual inspection for adult worm protruding from the skin lesion; microscopic identification of larvae released when lesion is immersed in water.

Therapy: Adult worm can be extracted by carefully and slowly winding the worm around a stick over a period of days. Metronidazole or thiabendazole can facilitate the extraction process, but should be used with caution.

Prevention: Use of safe water by filtering or boiling or disinfection with temephos (insecticide). Avoid wading in contaminated water, especially people with an apparent worm. There is no vaccine, but tetanus toxoid may be given to prevent tetanus. The Global Guinea Worm Eradication Programme is led by the Carter Center, CDC, WHO, UN Children's Fund and the individual efforts of endemic nations.

Epidemiology: Historically, dracunculiasis was endemic in 20 countries in Sub-Saharan Africa and Asia, with an incidence of 3.5 million cases per year (1986). An international control effort reduced that to just over 1,785 cases detected in five African countries by 2010: Mali, Ghana, South Sudan, Chad, and Ethiopia. Nearly 95% of the cases are reported from South Sudan. Additionally, Niger reported 3 imported cases from Mali. Chad did not report cases for more than 10 years when an outbreak occurred with 10 cases in 2010. In Mali and Southern Sudan, violence has interfered with the eradication campaign, but Ghana and Ethiopia are close to eradication. Ghana diagnosed their last indigenous case in May 2010. Dracunculiasis mainly affects poor communities without a safe portable water supply and is mainly limited to remote nomadic communities. There is a marked increase in infection in the dry season when stagnant pools are the only source of water. Most cases are young (working) adults who may be exposed to contaminated water sources more frequently. There is no particular age or sex predilection. Countries free of transmission neighboring endemic countries should remain alert for imported cases and take adequate preventive measures.

Map sources: The Dracunculiasis map was made with data obtained from WHO (http://apps.who.int/dracunculiasis/dradata/) and the CDC's Guinea Worm Wrap Up Nr. 202 (2011).

Key references

Centers for Disease Control and Prevention (2010) Progress toward global eradication of dracunculiasis, January 2009–June 2010. *Morb Mortal Wkly Rep* **59**(38):1239–1242.

Centers for Disease Control and Prevention (2011) Guinea Worm Wrap Up nr 202. *Memorandum*.

Glenshaw MT, et al. (2009) Guinea worm disease outcomes in Ghana: determinants of broken worms. *Am J Trop Med Hyg* **81**(2):305–312.

Iriemenam NC, et al. (2008) Dracunculiasis – the saddle is virtually ended. *Parasitol Res* **102**(3):343–347.

Lodge M (2010) And then there were four: more countries beat guinea worm disease. *Brit Med J* **340**:c496.

Atlas of Human Infectious Diseases, First Edition. Heiman F.L. Wertheim, Peter Horby and John P. Woodall.
© 2012 Blackwell Publishing Ltd. Published 2012 by Blackwell Publishing Ltd.

142

Echinococcosis, *Echinococcus multilocularis*

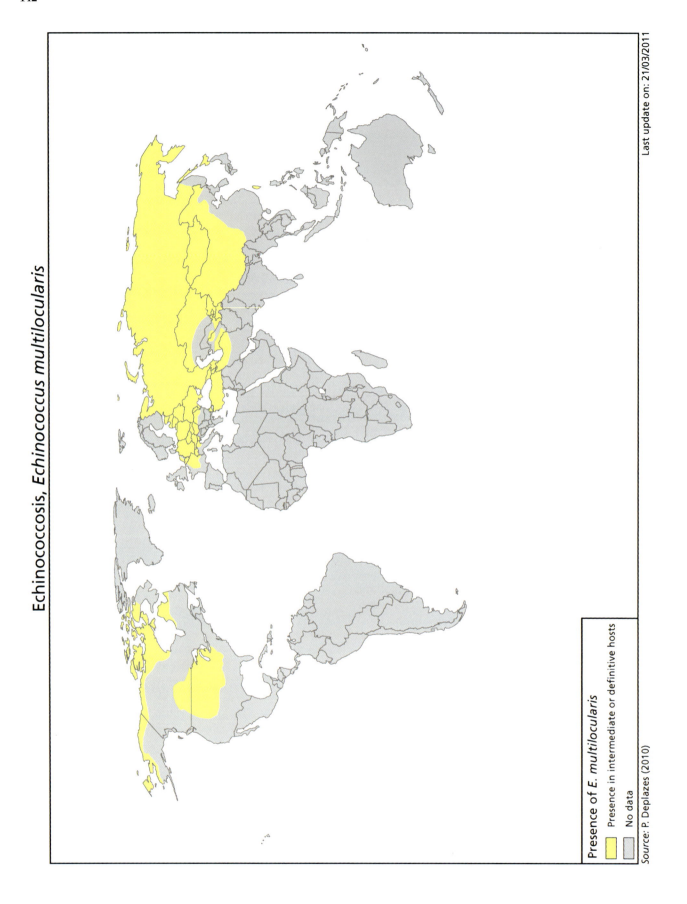

Presence of *E. multilocularis*

■ Presence in intermediate or definitive hosts

■ No data

Source: P. Deplazes (2010)

Last update on: 21/03/2011

Disease: Echinococcosis, *Echinococcus multilocularis*

Classification: ICD-9 122.7; ICD-10 B67.5–B67.7

Syndromes and synonyms: Alveolar or multilocular echinococcosis.

Agent: *Echinococcus multilocularis*, a small (3–6 mm long) cyclophyllid cestode (tapeworm).

Reservoir: Foxes (including urban foxes) are the definitive hosts, wild rodents (mainly Arvicolidae), voles and lemmings are intermediate hosts. Foxes have extended their distribution into urban areas, partly due to a decrease in rabies deaths in foxes since rabies vaccination.

Transmission: Ingestion of tapeworm eggs from feces of foxes, dogs, and cats or contaminated fomites. There is no person-to-person transmission.

Cycle: Fox–rodent–fox (sylvatic cycle). Foxes are the definitive hosts of the adult worm. Eggs are excreted with the feces and ingested by humans or the intermediate rodent host, where they hatch. The larvae penetrate the intestinal wall and via the blood they reach the liver, lungs, brain, and heart. There they form metacestodes in which protoscolices develop. When the rodent is eaten by the definitive host, these attach to the small intestine and grow into adult worms. Occasionally wild carnivores (e.g. coyotes or wolves) can be definitive hosts. In some rural areas there is a synanthropic cycle in which dogs or cats are definitive hosts, acquiring the parasite from wild rodents.

Incubation period: 5–15 years in humans (5–7 weeks in dogs).

Clinical findings: Headache, nausea, vomiting, abdominal pain, and hepatomegaly. In the later stage of the disease, the metacestode may grow into neighboring organs (e.g. through the diaphragm into the lungs), and metastases can form anywhere. The differential diagnosis is hepatic cirrhosis or carcinoma. The disease can be fatal.

Diagnostic tests: Histopathology; imaging tests; serodiagnosis with purified *E. multilocularis* antigen; PCR.

Therapy: Mebendazole or albendazole; radical surgical excision.

Prevention: Avoid exposure to feces of reservoir species wash hands, fruit and vegetables, periodically treat high-risk dogs, eliminate ownerless dogs. Praziquantel-containing baits have reduced infection in urban foxes and water voles in Switzerland and Germany. Eggs are highly sensitive to elevated temperatures and desiccation, but survive for months at freezing temperatures and are not affected by common disinfectants or ethanol.

Epidemiology: Echinococcosis is restricted to the northern hemisphere, and is most commonly found in adults. The distribution of infected foxes is highly uneven; sandy soils, dry habitats and large forests are unfavorable for the parasite. In Europe, foxes have adapted well to urban life and urban fox densities now can exceed rural fox densities. However, there is no clear correlation between fox densities and cases of human alveolar echinococcosis. In some areas there is a shift from a sylvatic to a synantropic cycle, including domestic dogs, as was seen in China and Alaska. Such a shift leads to a higher risk of infection in humans. The prevalence in dogs and cats is still very low in Europe, even in areas highly endemic for infection in foxes.

Map sources: The Echinococcosis (*E. multilocularis*) map was modified from a map provided by Peter Deplazes, University of Zurich, Switzerland. The map shows areas where there is convincing parasite detection in intermediate or definitive hosts, including humans.

Key references

Deplazes P, et al. (2004) Wilderness in the city: the urbanization of *Echinococcus multilocularis*. *Trends Parasit* **20**(2):77–84.

Hegglin D, et al. (2003) Anthelmintic baiting of foxes against urban contamination with *Echinococcus multilocularis*. *Emerg Infect Dis* **9**(10):1266–1272.

Romig T, et al. (2006) The present situation of echinococcosis in Europe. *Parasit Int* **55**:S187–S191.

Tackmann T, et al. (1998) Spatial distribution patterns of *Echinococcus multilocularis* (Leuckart 1863) (Cestoda: Cyclophyllidea: Taeniidae) among red foxes in an endemic focus in Brandenburg, Germany. *Epidemiol Infect* **120**:101–109.

Veit P, et al. (1995) Influence of environmental factors on the infectivity of *Echinococcus multilocularis* eggs. *Parasitology* **110**:79–86.

Atlas of Human Infectious Diseases, First Edition. Heiman F.L. Wertheim, Peter Horby and John P. Woodall.
© 2012 Blackwell Publishing Ltd. Published 2012 by Blackwell Publishing Ltd.

Eosinophilic Meningitis, Angiostrongylus cantonensis

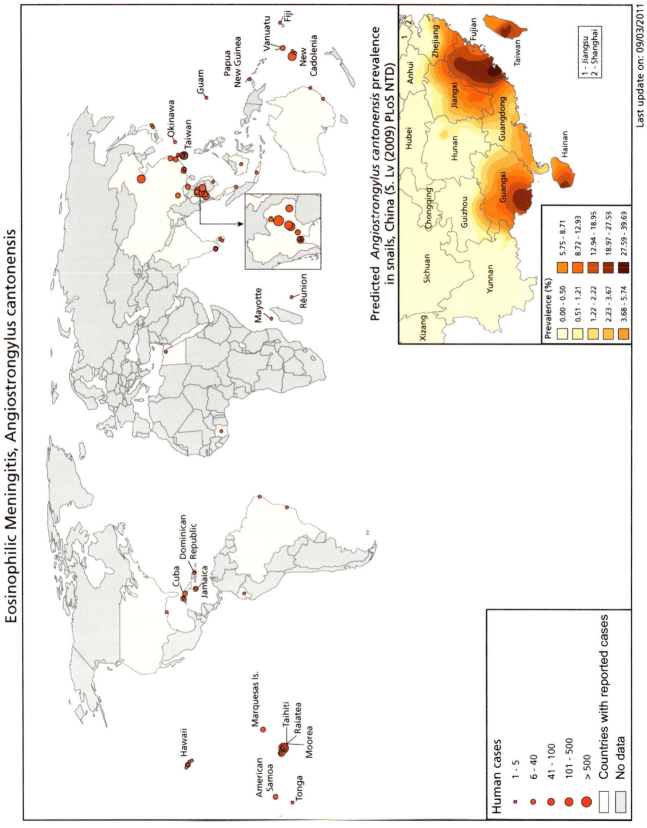

Predicted *Angiostrongylus cantonensis* prevalence in snails, China (S. Lv (2009) PLoS NTD)

Last update on: 09/03/2011

Disease: Eosinophilic Meningitis, *Angiostrongylus cantonensis*

Classification: ICD-9 128.8; ICD-10 B83.2

Syndromes and synonyms: Eosinophilic meningoencephalitis, angiostrongyliasis

Agent: *Angiostrongylus cantonensis*, a nematode lungworm of rats. Adult worms are 17 to 25 mm long. *Angiostrongylus costaricensis* is the causal agent of abdominal, or intestinal, angiostrongyliasis and is not shown on the map. Other pathogens, like *Gnathostoma spinigerum*, are able to cause eosinophilic meningitis, but are not shown on the map.

Reservoir: Rats (*Rattus*, particularly *R. norvegicus* and *Bandicotta* spp.). Infected dogs, wild mammals, and marsupials have been found, but do not contribute to the spread of the disease.

Vector: Snails, slugs, and land planarians. The giant African snail, *Achatina fulica*, is the major source of infection world wide; but has been replaced by the imported South American golden apple snail, *Pomacea canaliculata*, in Taiwan and mainland China.

Transmission: Consumption of raw or undercooked vector molluscs, infested vegetables or vegetable juice, or other fresh water related food.

Cycle: Rat–mollusc–rat; humans are incidental dead-end hosts. Larvae are excreted with rat feces, ingested by vector molluscs, in which they develop into the infecting third stage larvae in about 12 days. When ingested by a rat, the larvae enter the brain, mature into adults, and migrate through the bloodstream to the lungs. There, female worms lay eggs (about 15,000 per day) that hatch into larvae, which in 6–8 weeks migrate through the bronchial system up the trachea to the pharynx, are swallowed and excreted. When ingested by a human, the third stage larvae also migrate to the CNS, but the worm does not mature.

Incubation period: 1 day to several months, depending on parasite load; usually 1–3 weeks.

Clinical findings: Cough, rhinorrhea, sore throat, malaise, and fever can develop when the worms move through the lungs. In about 5 to 14 days the larvae reach the central nervous system, leading to subacute meningitis. Eosinophilic meningitis is defined as meningitis with $> = 10$ eosinophils/µL in CSF or at least 10% eosinophils in the total CSF leukocyte count. Some cases have low-grade fever and temporary facial paralysis. Signs of raised intracranial pressure, like diplopia. Worms occasionally enter the eye. The course of the illness ranges from a few days to several months. Death is rare.

Diagnostic tests: Mainly a clinical diagnosis: subacute eosinophilic meningitis in an endemic area. Most common test is serology, but there are often false-positives due to cross-reactivity with other parasites. Worms are rarely seen in CSF by microscopy. MRI or CT scan of the brain is not diagnostic.

Therapy: Mebendazole or albendazole with adjunctive corticosteroids. Lumbar puncture relieves the headache. Ocular infection requires surgery.

Prevention: Avoid eating raw slugs, snails, other molluscs, freshwater prawns, land crabs, and uncooked vegetables grown in ponds (e.g. watercress) from endemic areas. Washing of vegetables does not guarantee absence from larval contamination. Boil snails and crustaceans for 5 minutes or freeze at $-15\,°C$ for 24 hours.

Epidemiology: An estimated 650 million people are at risk in 10 provinces of China. The distribution is closely correlated with the habit of consuming raw terrestrial molluscs, reptiles, or amphibians. The majority of cases are in adults, except in Taiwan where most cases are in children. *Pomacea canaliculata*, a snail native to South America, was imported into Taiwan in 1981 as a food source and then into mainland China. It has replaced *A. fulica* as the main intermediate host of *A. cantonensis* and has become the main source of human infection in Taiwan and mainland China. Depending on the region, up to 70% of *P. canaliculata* can be infected.

Eating raw frogs also lead to human infections in China, and the USA. Consumption of lizards caused several cases in Thailand, Sri Lanka, and India. Cases have been seen in at least five countries in Europe and New Zealand in travelers returning from endemic regions. Malnutrition and debilitating diseases can exacerbate the infection.

Map sources: The Eosinophilic meningoencephalitis map was made by geocoding reported cases in the medical literature. The inset map with *A. cantonensis* prevalence in snails is obtained from S. Lv et al. (2009).

Key references

Wang Q-P, et al. (2008) Human angiostrongyliasis. *Lancet Infect Dis* **8**(10):621–630.

Lv S, et al. (2009) Invasive snails and an emerging infectious disease. *PLoS Negl Trop Dis* **3**(2):e368.

Ramirez-Avila L, et al. (2009) Eosinophilic meningitis due to Angiostrongylus and Gnathostoma species. *Clin Infect Dis* **48**(3):322–327.

Atlas of Human Infectious Diseases, First Edition. Heiman F.L. Wertheim, Peter Horby and John P. Woodall.
© 2012 Blackwell Publishing Ltd. Published 2012 by Blackwell Publishing Ltd.

Fascioliasis

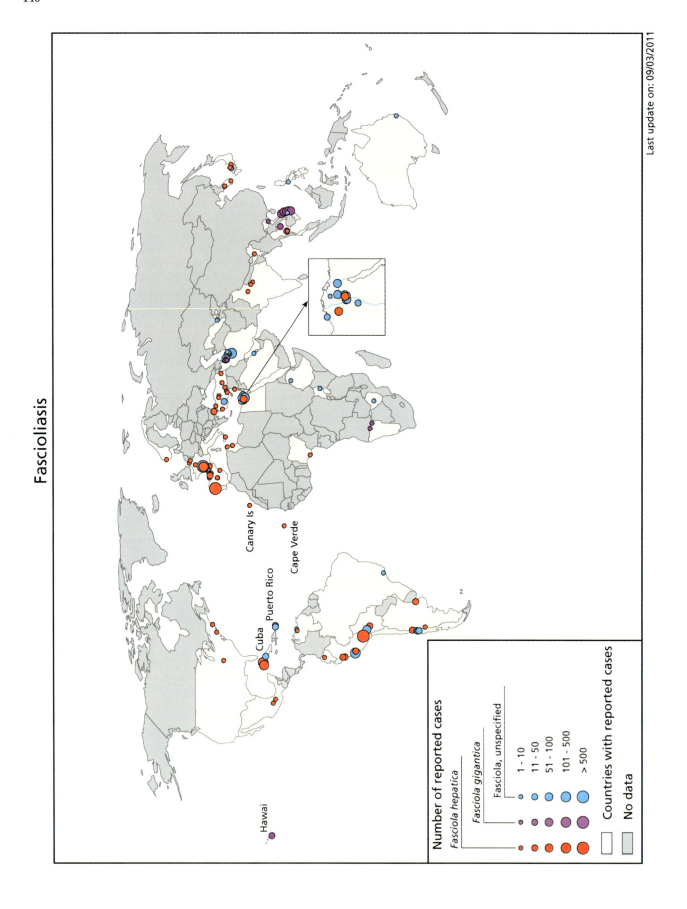

Canary Is

Cape Verde

Cuba

Puerto Rico

Hawai

Number of reported cases

Fasciola hepatica

Fasciola gigantica

Fasciola, unspecified

1 - 10
11 - 50
51 - 100
101 - 500
> 500

Countries with reported cases

No data

Last update on: 09/03/2011

Disease: **Fascioliasis**

Classification: ICD-9 121.3; ICD-10 B66.3

Syndromes and synonyms: Sheep liver fluke disease, pharyngeal fascioliasis.

Agent: Large trematode liver flukes living in blile ducts: *Fasciola hepatica* and *Fasciola gigantica*. *F. hepatica* is 20 to 30 mm long and *F. gigantica* can be up to 75 mm long.

Reservoir: Sheep, cattle, water buffalo, and other large herbivores. Occasionally humans.

Vector: Freshwater (pond) snails (Lymnaeidae).

Transmission: Accidental ingestion of metacercariae via contaminated water, watercress, or other contaminated plants (lettuce, alfalfa juice, etc.). Rarely via consumption of raw sheep or goat liver (pharyngeal fascioliasis). There is no person-to-person transmission.

Cycle: Eggs hatch in water and release miracidia larvae that penetrate the snail, where they develop to cercariae that encyst on aquatic plants (e.g. watercress) and become desiccation-resistant metacercariae. After the plants are eaten by herbivores (e.g. sheep, cattle), or water containing metacercariae is drunk, the larvae pass through the intestinal wall into the peritoneal cavity, enter the liver, and lay eggs in the bile duct, which are then excreted in the feces. The whole cycle takes 3 to 4 months.

Incubation period: 3 to 4 months, but is highly variable.

Clinical findings: Acute: hepatomegaly, prolonged fever, anorexia, weight loss, nausea, vomiting, cough, diarrhea, urticaria, lymphadenopathies, and arthralgias. Significant clinical improvement 3–5 days after specific treatment is diagnostic. Chronic (which may be asymptomatic and last for more than 10 years): biliary obstruction with upper abdominal pain, cholecystitis, cholangitis, and extrahepatic cholestasis. Liver fibrosis may be a complication of the infection.

Diagnostic tests: Microscopy for eggs on stool samples by the Kato–Katz or rapid sedimentation techniques (RSTs) are diagnostic for the chronic infection. Serological tests (Fas2-ELISA) is recommended for acute infection. The intradermal test is rapid and sensitive, but as it is not sufficiently specific it is no longer used. Radiology, such as computed tomography, can demonstrate liver lesions (only in acute infection) similar to metatastic lesions. For chronic infections, a cholangiogram can detect bile duct pathology caused by the adult parasites.

Therapy: Above 95% cure rate with a single dose triclabendazole. Albendazole or praziquantel are not effective.

Prevention: Sanitation to avoid contamination of vector snail habitat with human or animal feces. Improve water drainage, use molluscicides and avoid eating uncooked aquatic plants in endemic areas and drinking untreated water.

Epidemiology: It is estimated that 17 million people are infected world wide and 91 million are at risk of infection. *F. hepatica* is endemic on all continents but is of particular public health importance in the Andean countries (especially Peru and Bolivia), Ecuador, Chile, Argentina, Brazil, Venezuela, Cuba, Mexico, the Islamic Republic of Iran, Egypt, Philippines, and western Europe (e.g. France, Portugal, and Spain). Infections with *F. gigantica* are restricted to Africa and Asia. Both species of fluke overlap in many areas of Africa and Asia, whereas *F. hepatica* is the major concern in the Americas, Europe, and Oceania. The rural areas of the Andean region of Peru and Bolivia have prevalence rates of up to 68%. Women are affected more than men, with higher prevalence rates, more severe infections, and more reported liver or biliary complications; children are affected more than adults. The main source of infection is the consumption of raw vegetables contaminated with metacercariae, such as watercress, salads, and contaminated water from irrigation channels. Pharyngeal fascioliasis may occur after ingestion of raw goat or sheep liver – a dish in some Middle Eastern countries.

Map sources: The Fascioliasis map was made by geocoding reported human cases in the medical literature up to 2009. *F. gigantica* could be more widespread than shown, because it could be the species reported as unspecified *Fasciola*. We were only able to find a few reports of human cases with *F. gigantica* in Africa, but it is probably underreported.

Key references

Keiser J, et al. (2009) Food-borne trematodiasis. *Clin Microbiol Rev* **22**(3):466–483.

Marcos LA, et al. (2008) Update on hepatobiliary flukes: fascioliasis, opisthorchiasis and clonorchiasis. *Curr Opin Infect Dis* **21**(5):523–530.

Atlas of Human Infectious Diseases, First Edition. Heiman F.L. Wertheim, Peter Horby and John P. Woodall.
© 2012 Blackwell Publishing Ltd. Published 2012 by Blackwell Publishing Ltd.

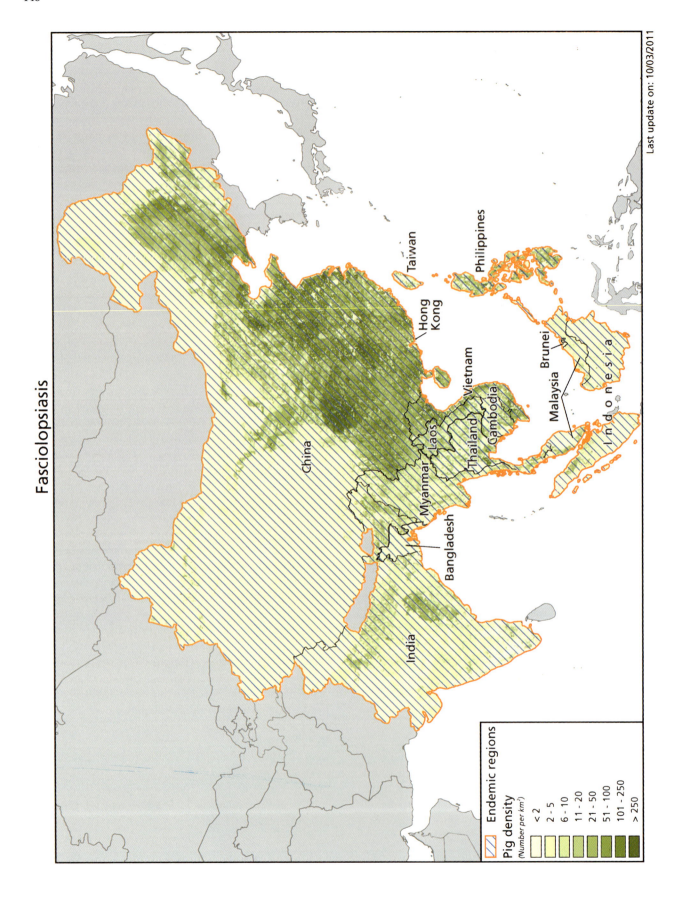

Fasciolopsiasis

Last update on: 10/03/2011

Endemic regions

Pig density
(Number per km²)

<2
2 - 5
6 - 10
11 - 20
21 - 50
51 - 100
101 - 250
> 250

China

India

Bangladesh

Myanmar

Laos

Thailand

Cambodia

Vietnam

Hong Kong

Taiwan

Philippines

Malaysia

Brunei

Indonesia

Disease: Fasciolopsiasis

Classification: ICD-9 121.4; ICD-10 B66.5

Syndromes and synonyms: Giant intestinal fluke infection.

Agent: *Fasciolopis buski*, a large trematode worm that can be up to 75 mm long.

Reservoir: Pigs and humans are definitive hosts; less often dogs.

Transmission: Eating contaminated water plants. There is no person-to-person transmission.

Cycle: Eggs develop in water in 3–7 weeks, hatch producing miracidia which enter the intermediate snail hosts, in which they develop into cercariae. The cercariae encyst on water plants and develop to metacercariae. When ingested, the metacercariae excyst in the duodenum, where the flukes attach to the mucosa of the small intestine, mature, and start egg production in 2 to 3 months.

Incubation period: Varies from 1 to 3 months.

Clinical findings: Usually asymptomatic or mild. Diarrhea alternating with constipation, vomiting and anorexia, edema of the face, abdominal wall and legs, ascites. Heavy worm loads may cause bowel obstruction. Eosinophilia, vitamin B12 deficiency, and secondary anemia may occur.

Diagnostic tests: Detection of eggs in feces (eggs resemble those of *Fasciola hepatica*). Adult flukes may be seen in the stools or vomit.

Therapy: Praziquantel or niclosamide.

Prevention: Sanitation. Avoid eating uncooked water plants in endemic areas. Do not fertilize water plants for consumption with human or pig feces. Abandon practice of feeding water plants to pigs. Health education. The eggs can resist low temperatures and can be maintained at 4 °C for 3 to 4 months; they are killed at 50 °C in 4 hours. Water can be chemically treated to kill the flukes.

Epidemiology: Especially prevalent in pig-rearing regions of Southeast Asia, where it is estimated that 10 million people are infected. The disease is most common in lowlands where the snail host is present and it is common practice to fertilize water plants with pig or human feces. Disease spread is facilitated by heavy rainfall and extensive flooding, leading to fecal contamination of the water. Highest incidence and intensity of infection is found in 10 to 14 year old children (no sex difference), probably because they pick and consume water plants when they play. In foci of parasite transmission, the prevalence of infection in children ranges from 57% in mainland China to 25% in Taiwan, and from 50% in Bangladesh and 60% in India to 10% in Thailand. Water morning glory (*Ipomoea aquatica*), water caltrop (*Trapa bicornis*), lotus (*Nymphaea lotus*), water cress (*Neptunia oleracea*), and water hyacinth (*Eichhornia speciosa*) are most responsible for human infection, but cysts also float on the surface and may be drunk.

Map sources: The Fasciolopsiasis map is made by showing the countries that have reported human fasciolopsiasis cases, as reported in the medical literature up to 2010. We also show pig density data as the disease is endemic in pig-rearing regions in Asia. The pig density data is obtained from FAO available at: www.fao.org/ag/againfo/resources/en/glw/home.html.

Key references

Graczyk TK, et al. (2001) Fasciolopsiasis: is it a controllable food-borne disease? *Parasitol Res* **87**(1):80–83.

Keiser J, et al. (2009) Food-borne trematodiases. *Clin Microbiol Rev* **22**(3):466–483.

Sripa B, et al. (2010) Food-borne trematodiases in Southeast Asia epidemiology, pathology, clinical manifestation and control. *Adv Parasitol* **72**:305–350.

Yoshihara S, et al. (1999) Helminths and helminthiosis of pigs in the Mekong Delta Vietnam with special reference to ascariosis and *Fasciolopsis buski* infection. *Jap Agric Res Qtly* **33**(3):193–199.

Atlas of Human Infectious Diseases, First Edition. Heiman F.L. Wertheim, Peter Horby and John P. Woodall.
© 2012 Blackwell Publishing Ltd. Published 2012 by Blackwell Publishing Ltd.

Filariasis

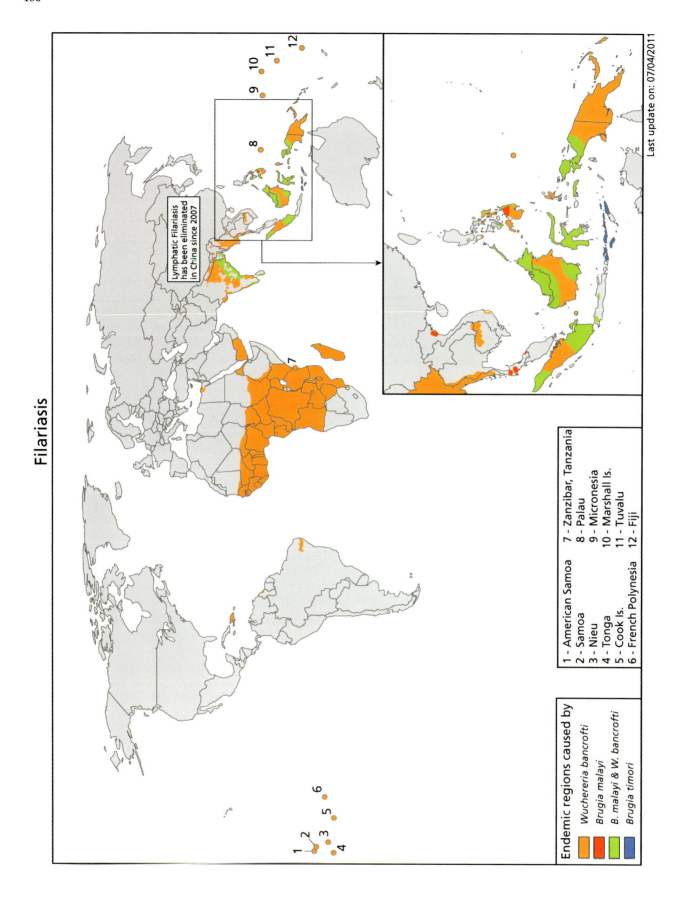

Lymphatic Filariasis has been eliminated in China since 2007

Endemic regions caused by

▮	*Wuchereria bancrofti*
▮	*Brugia malayi*
▮	*B. malayi & W. bancrofti*
▮	*Brugia timori*

1 - American Samoa
2 - Samoa
3 - Nieu
4 - Tonga
5 - Cook Is.
6 - French Polynesia
7 - Zanzibar, Tanzania
8 - Palau
9 - Micronesia
10 - Marshall Is.
11 - Tuvalu
12 - Fiji

Last update on: 07/04/2011

Disease: Filariasis

Classification: ICD-9 125.0, 125.1, 125.6; ICD-10 B74.0, B74.1, B74.2

Syndromes and synonyms: Bancroftian filariasis, Brugian filariasis, lymphatic filariasis, Malayan filariasis, Timorean filariasis.

Agent: *Wuchereria bancrofti, Brugia malayi,* and *B. timori,* threadlike nematode worms 80 to 100 mm long (*W. bancrofti*), or 43 to 55 mm long (*B. malayi*).

Reservoir: Mainly humans. In Southeast Asia, monkeys, wild carnivores, dogs, and cats may also be infected with *B. malayi. W. bancrofti* has no known reservoir host.

Vector: For *W. bancrofti: Culex quinquefasciatus, Anopheles* spp., and *Aedes* spp. in the Pacific Islands; for *B. malayi: Mansonia, Anopheles,* and *Aedes;* for *B. timori, An. barbirostris. Anopheles* spp. transmit parasites less efficiently than *Culex* spp., and *Culex* spp. are more abundant in urban settings.

Transmission: A large number of infective mosquito bites are necessary to establish infection.

Cycle: Microfilariae in human blood are ingested by a vector mosquito, and develop in 2 weeks into larvae that enter the mouth-parts. Larvae are deposited onto the skin and invade through the wound made at the next mosquito feed. In humans, they travel via the lymphatics, when adults they form 'nests' and produce microfilariae, which migrate to the blood and display periodicity coinciding with the peak vector biting times.

Incubation period: 3–6 months for *B. malayi* worms to mature and produce microfilariae that appear in the blood; 6–12 months for *W. bancrofti* and *B. timori.*

Clinical findings: Infection is often asymptomatic but as the adult worms live for 5–10 years, some will develop painful swelling (sometimes enormous) of legs or arms, and, in cases of Bancroftian filariasis, the breasts or scrotum (hydrocele). Up to 40% have renal involvement. Acute cases may have high fever, recurrent lymphadenitis, and retrograde lymphangitis.

Diagnostic tests: Microscopy to detect microfilariae in finger-prick blood smears; immunochromatic test cards; ultrasound to locate 'nests.'

Therapy: For interrupting transmission: mass treatment with a single dose of albendazole or ivermectin combined with diethyl-carbamazine citrate (DEC) once a year for at least 5 years; or the regular intake of DEC-fortified salt for at least one year; individual treatment: DEC can worsen onchocercal eye disease and cause serious adverse reactions in patients with loiasis. Pathogenicity of filarial nematodes is largely due to the immune response to their endosymbiotic *Wolbachia* bacteria, therefore doxycycline may be used. The treatment for hydrocele is surgery.

Prevention: In 2000, WHO started the Global Programme to Eliminate Lymphatic Filariasis that aims to interrupt transmission and reduce morbidity. Endemic areas are mapped with subsequent mass treatment for the population at-risk (see Therapy) for 5 years. Care needs to be taken in loiasis endemic areas to prevent adverse events (see Loiasis map); vector control (e.g. bed nets, repellent).

Epidemiology: WHO (2010) estimates that there are over 120 million infections world wide, with 40 million patients incapacitated or disfigured by the disease, principally in India and Sub-Saharan Africa. 90% of the infections are due to *W. bancrofti.* Chronic manifestations mainly occur in the elderly. About 27 million have hydrocele (men) and 16 million have lymphedema or elephantiasis of the leg (mostly women). Asia and South America have lower Bancroftian filariasis prevalences (below 8%) than Sub-Saharan Africa (up to 37%) and Pacific Island (up to 48%) regions. Within areas of low prevalence, pockets of high prevalence may exist (e.g. Reciffe, Brazil). In the Americas there is only active transmission in four countries and mainly affects the poor and slum inhabitants. China has been declared non-endemic for lymphatic filariasis since 2007 and Korea in 2008, achieved by extensive control efforts. The vectors are still present and therefore there remains a risk of re-emergence.

Map sources: The Lymphatic filariasis map was made with information obtained from WHO, CIESIN, and medical literature. Useful distribution data are available at: www.filariasis.org.

Key references

Addiss DG (2010) Global elimination of lymphatic filariasis. *PloS Negl Trop Dis* **4**(6):e471.

Taylor MJ, et al. (2010) Lymphatic filariasis and onchocerciasis. *Lancet* **376**(9747):1175–1185.

World Health Organization (2010) *Lymphatic Filariasis. Progress Report 2000–2009 and Strategic Plan 2010–2020.*

Atlas of Human Infectious Diseases, First Edition. Heiman F.L. Wertheim, Peter Horby and John P. Woodall.
© 2012 Blackwell Publishing Ltd. Published 2012 by Blackwell Publishing Ltd.

Hookworm

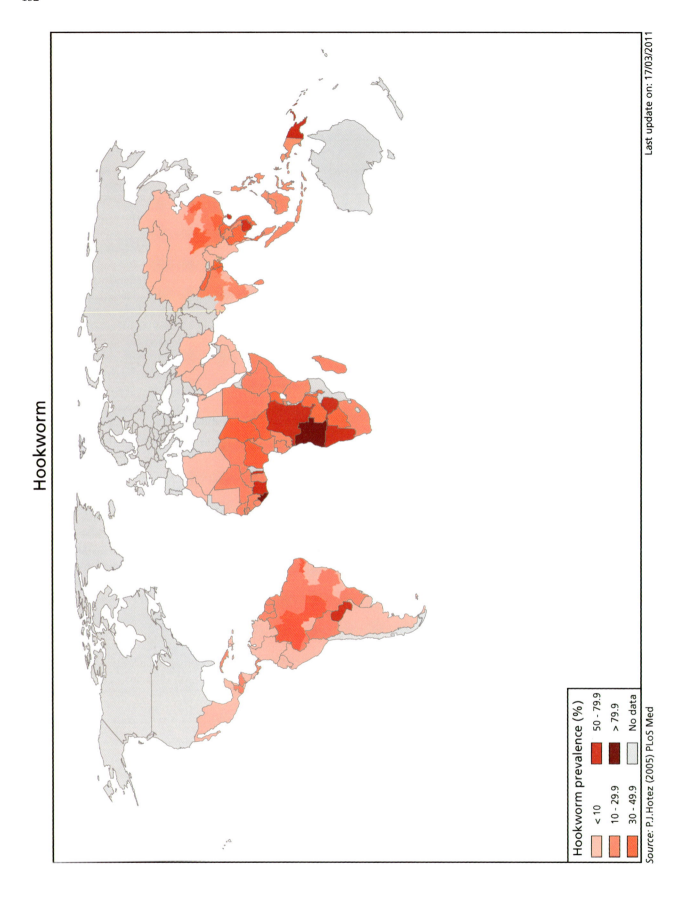

Hookworm prevalence (%)

	<10		50 - 79.9
	10 - 29.9		> 79.9
	30 - 49.9		No data

Source: P.J.Hotez (2005) PLoS Med

Last update on: 17/03/2011

Disease: Hookworm

Classification: ICD-9 126; ICD-10 B76

Syndromes and synonyms: Ancylostomiasis, Necatoriasis, Uncinariasis, ground itch.

Agent: The blood-feeding nematodes *Ancylostoma duodenale* and *Necator americanus*, also known as soil-transmitted helminths (STHs). *A. ceylanicum* has a limited distribution. The adult nematodes are up to 10 mm long.

Reservoir: Humans.

Transmission: Infective larvae in soil invade the skin; *A. duodenale* larvae can also infect via oral ingestion.

Cycle: Hookworm eggs hatch in the soil and develop to infective larvae (L3) that can penetrate the skin. After entering the host, the larvae migrate to the lungs, move up the trachea and swallowed. In the gastrointestinal tract the larvae mature to adult worms (both sexes). After mating, the female hookworms produce up to 30,000 eggs per day that are shedded with the stools into the environment.

Incubation period: Varies from weeks to several months, depending on infection intensity.

Clinical findings: Hookworm morbidity is higher in patients infected with large numbers of adult parasites. Attachment of the hookworm to the intestinal mucosa results in loss of blood, eventually resulting in anemia and malnutrition in chronic cases. Chronic hookworm infection can impair cognitive and growth development in children.

Diagnostic tests: Microscopy (Kato-Katz method). Quantitative fecal egg counts are a marker for worm burden: 2,000 to 4,000 eggs per gram of feces is considered to be moderate infection, and ≥4,000 eggs is heavy infection.

Therapy: Deworming with mebendazole or albendazole; repeat treatment in case eggs are still detected in feces. Iron supplementation to correct anemia.

Prevention: The impact of sanitation, footwear, and health education is minimal. To reduce the disease burden of STHs, mass treatment campaigns with benzimidazoles and praziquantel are undertaken, and sanitation and access to clean water improved. As most STHs occur in children, control efforts are targeted at schools. Infective larvae can survive in soil for several months.

Epidemiology: The global number of hookworm disease cases is estimated to be 740 million individuals, with the highest prevalence in Sub-Saharan Africa and eastern Asia. The majority (85%) of the hookworm infections are caused by *Necator americanus*, which is the predominant hookworm of Latin America, the Caribbean, Sub-Saharan Africa, and Southeast Asia. There is strong association between hookworm prevalence and poverty (see Human Development map). The remaining 15% infections by *Ancylostoma duodenale* are in focal pockets in India, especially around Uttar Pradesh and West Bengal, and in China north of the Yangtze river. Mixed infections may also occur. Hookworm disease prevalence rises with age and plateaus in adults. Disease is more prevalent where individuals walk barefoot in regions lacking sanitation (see Sanitation map). Hookworm larvae prefer sandy soil in mild humid climates, resulting that individuals living in coastal areas have the highest infection intensity.

Map sources: The Hookworm map is modified from P.J. Hotez et al. (2005). For more detailed information on the distribution of STHs, see www.thiswormyworld.org.

Key references

Hotez PJ, et al. (2005) Hookworm: 'the great infection of mankind.' *PLoS Med* **2**(3):e67.

Hotez PJ, et al. (2004) Current concepts: Hookworm infection. *N Engl J Med* **351**:799–807.

De Silva NR, et al. (2003) Soil-transmitted helminth infections: updating the global picture. *Trends Parasitol* **19**:547–551.

Leishmaniasis, Cutaneous and Mucosal, New World

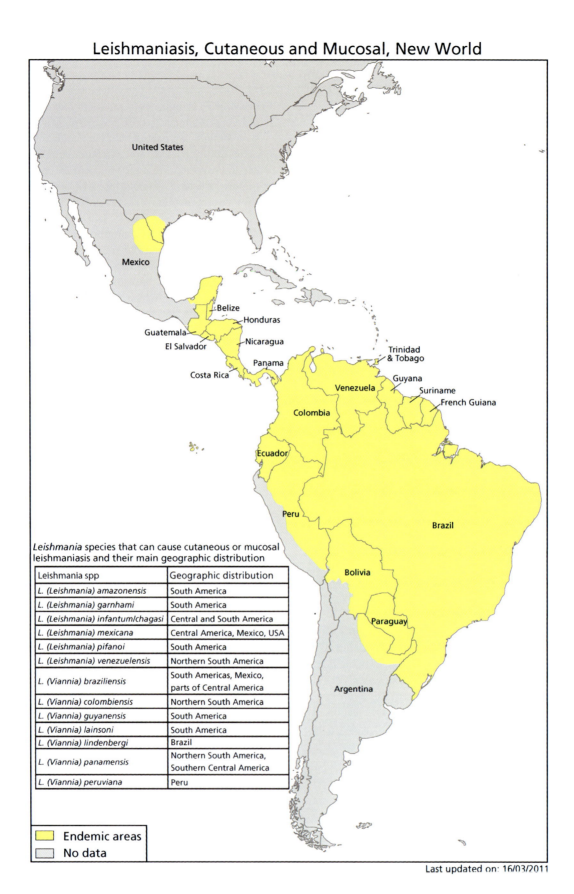

Leishmania species that can cause cutaneous or mucosal leishmaniasis and their main geographic distribution

Leishmania spp	Geographic distribution
L. (Leishmania) amazonensis	South America
L. (Leishmania) garnhami	South America
L. (Leishmania) infantum/chagasi	Central and South America
L. (Leishmania) mexicana	Central America, Mexico, USA
L. (Leishmania) pifanoi	South America
L. (Leishmania) venezuelensis	Northern South America
L. (Viannia) braziliensis	South Americas, Mexico, parts of Central America
L. (Viannia) colombiensis	Northern South America
L. (Viannia) guyanensis	South America
L. (Viannia) lainsoni	South America
L. (Viannia) lindenbergi	Brazil
L. (Viannia) panamensis	Northern South America, Southern Central America
L. (Viannia) peruviana	Peru

Endemic areas
No data

Last updated on: 16/03/2011

Disease: Leishmaniasis, Cutaneous and Mucosal, New World

Classification: ICD-9 085; ICD-10 B55

Syndromes and synonyms: Cutaneous and mucosal leishmaniasis (CL): Espundia, Uta, Chiclero ulcer, forest yaws.

Agent: *Leishmania* species, protozoa, members of the Trypanosomatidae family, order Kinetoplastida. Based on development characteristics in the sandfly, *Leishmania* species are classified into the subgenera *Viannia* and *Leishmania*, within which there are various species complexes. *Leishmania* species causing (muco)cutaneous disease in the Americas are: *L. (Viannia) braziliensis* (espundia), *L. (Viannia) colombiensis*, *L. (Leishmania) mexicana* (chiclero ulcer), *L. (Leishmania) pifanoi*, *L. (Viannia) liansoni*, *L. (Leishmania) garnhami*, *L. (Leishmania) amazonensis*, *L. (Viannia) panamensis*, *L. (Viannia) guyanensis* (forest yaws), and *L. (Viannia) peruviana* (Uta). *L. infantum/chagasi* can cause both visceral and cutaneous leishmaniasis. *L. chagasi* is considered to be the same species as *L. infantum*, and will be referred to as *L. infantum/chagasi*.

Reservoir: Mainly rodents and other sylvatic mammals. Canines are a reservoir for *L. infantum/chagasi* and possible reservoir for *L. (Viannia)* spp.

Vector: Female phlebotomine sandflies (*Lutzomyia* spp.).

Transmission: By bite of an infected phlebotomine sandfly.

Cycle: During bloodmeal, the sandfly ingests infected blood with amastigotes. The amastigotes develop to motile promastigotes that multiply in the sandfly gut, and finally motile promastigotes travel to the mouth parts and are injected into another host during feeding. In the host cell the promastigotes develop into amastigotes.

Incubation period: Varies from one week to several months.

Clinical findings: Painless cutaneous lesions appear at the site of sandfly bite and typically these develop into ulcers with a raised border. Occasionally nodular and rarely verrucous lesions. Multiple lesions and regional lymphadenopathy may be present. Lesions may resolve spontaneously or remain for several months to years. Rarely dissemination to mucosa occurs of the upper respiratory tract with local tissue destruction leading to disfigurement (most often by *L. braziliensis*, known as espundia), with risk of severe and sometimes fatal secondary infections.

Diagnostic tests: Demonstration of intracellular amastigotes in Giemsa stained slit skin smear or biopsy specimen by microscopy; PCR tests have been developed for the different *Leishmania* species; culture of promastigotes with special media is laborious and requires experience. The Montenegro skin test is simple, sensitive and specific, but does not aid in differentiating between past and present infections.

Therapy: Systemic treatment to prevent dissemination with pentavalent antimonials. Depending on the infecting *Leishmania* species, alternative systemic treatment can be administered with: amphotericin B, pentamidine, or miltefosine. Topical treatment options are: paramomycin, ketoconazole, and thermotherapy.

Prevention: Personal protection from sandfly bites (e.g. protective clothing, insecticide-treated bednets, residual insecticiding of breeding places).

Epidemiology: The highest global burden of CL is in the Old World. In the Americas, Bolivia, Brazil, and Peru have the highest burden of CL. In the New World, CL mainly occurs in forested areas, whereas in the Old World it is associated with semi-arid and desert regions. Transmission can also occur in deforested areas. Disease mainly occurs in those living or working in the forests of endemic areas. Outbreaks can occur during military training in the jungle or infrastructural projetcs in endemic areas. Also, travelers acquire the disease during visits to rural or jungle regions. Disease prevalence increases with age and then plateaus, likely due to acquired immunity. Clusters of leishmaniasis are seen in households, which is probably related to the short flight range of sandflies.

Map sources: This map was made by reconciling maps from WHO: (www.who.int/leishmaniasis/leishmaniasis_maps/en/index. html) and R. Reithinger et al. (2007).

Key references

Campbell-Lendrum D, et al. (2001) Domestic and peridomestic transmission of American cutaneous leishmaniasis. *Mem Inst Oswaldo Cruz* **96**(2):159–162.

Reithinger R, et al. (2007) Cutaneous leishmaniasis. *Lancet Infect Dis* **7**(9):581–596.

World Health Organization (2010) *Control of the Leishmaniases.* WHO Expert Technical Report Series, Nr 949.

Atlas of Human Infectious Diseases, First Edition. Heiman F.L. Wertheim, Peter Horby and John P. Woodall.
© 2012 Blackwell Publishing Ltd. Published 2012 by Blackwell Publishing Ltd.

Leishmaniasis, Cutaneous and Mucosal, Old World

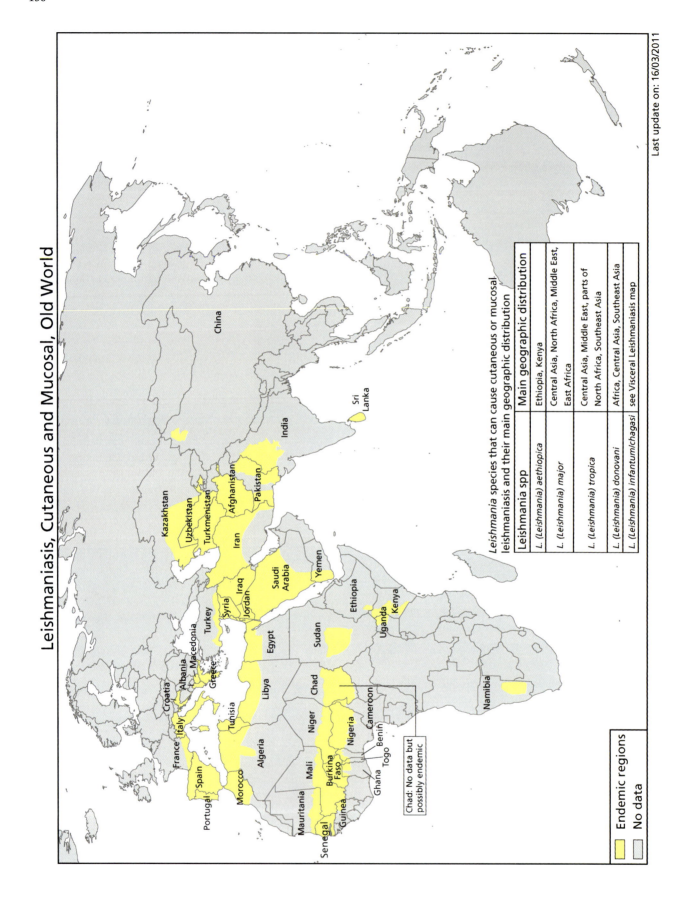

Last update on: 16/03/2011

Leishmania species that can cause cutaneous or mucosal leishmaniasis and their main geographic distribution

Leishmania spp	Main geographic distribution
L. (Leishmania) aethiopica	Ethiopia, Kenya
L. (Leishmania) major	Central Asia, North Africa, Middle East, East Africa
L. (Leishmania) tropica	Central Asia, Middle East, parts of North Africa, Southeast Asia
L. (Leishmania) donovani	Africa, Central Asia, Southeast Asia
L. (Leishmania) infantum/chagasi	see Visceral Leishmaniasis map

Chad: No data but possibly endemic

Endemic regions
No data

Disease: Leishmaniasis, Cutaneous and Mucosal, Old World

Classification: ICD-9 085; ICD-10 B55

Syndromes and synonyms: Cutaneous and mucosal leishmaniasis (CL): Aleppo evil, Baghdad boil, Delhi boil, Oriental sore, Delhi boil, and others.

Agent: *Leishmania* species, protozoa, members of the Trypanosomatidae family, order Kinetoplastida. *Leishmania* species that cause CL in the old world are: *Leishmania major, L. tropica*, and *L. aethiopica. L. killicki* is synonymous to *L. tropica. L. infantum/chagasi* and *L. donovani* can cause both visceral and cutaneous leishmaniasis. *L. chagasi* is considered the same species as *L. infantum*, and are referred to as *L. infantum/chagasi.*

Reservoir: Wild rodents (gerbils) that live in burrows together with sandfly vector. Hyraxes for *L. aethiopica.*

Vector: Female phlebotomine sandflies (*Phlebotomus papatasi, P. sergenti, P.chadaudi, P. longipes, P. pedifer*)

Transmission: By bite of an infected phlebotomine sandfly.

Cycle: During bloodmeal, the sandfly ingests infected blood with amastigotes. The amastigotes develop to motile promastigotes that multiply in the sandfly gut, and finally motile promastigotes travel to the mouth parts and are injected into another host during feeding. In the host cell the promastigotes develop into amastigotes.

Incubation period: Varies from a week to several months.

Clinical findings: Mainly presents as a dry skin lesion that is covered with a crust and is smaller than the classic wet leishmania skin lesions in the New World. Lesions may persist for months or years. Diffuse cutaneous leishmaniasis may be seen with *L. aethiopica*; leishmaniasis recidivans may be seen with *L. tropica*. Mucosal leishmaniasis is rare in the Old World, and more common in the Americas.

Diagnostic tests: Demonstration of intracellular amastigotes in Giemsa stained slit skin smear or biopsy specimen by microscopy; PCR tests have been developed for the different *Leishmania* species; culture of promastigotes with special media is laborious and requires experience. The Montenegro skin test is simple, sensitive and specific, but does not aid in differentiating between past and present infections.

Therapy: Intravenous, intramuscular, and intralesional application of pentavalent antimonials; also miltefosine is being tested for its efficacy. Topical treatment options are: paramomycin, ketoconazole, and thermotherapy.

Prevention: Personal protection from sandfly bites (e.g. protective clothing, insecticide-treated bednets, residual insecticide of breeding places). There is no vaccine for human use.

Epidemiology: World wide there are approximately 1.5 million new cases of CL per year, with most cases reported from Afghanistan, Algeria, Pakistan, Saudi Arabia, and Syria in the Old World. The highest burden of CL in the Old Word is in rural semi-arid and desert regions, but transmission is being increasingly seen in peri-urban and urban environments. Disease prevalence increases with age and then plateaus, likely due to acquired immunity. Clusters of leishmaniasis are seen in households, which is likely related to the short flight range of sandflies.

Map Sources: The Cutaneous and Mucosal Leishmaniasis, Old World, map was made by reconciling maps from WHO (www.who.int/leishmaniasis/leishmaniasis_maps/en/index.html), EU (http://bioval.jrc.ec.europa.eu/products/glc2000/products.php), and R. Reithinger et al. (2007). The map was updated with medical literature and expert opinion.

Key references

Ready PD (2010) Leishmaniasis emergence in Europe. *Euro Surveill* **15**(10):19505.

Lukes J. (2007) Evolutionary and geographical history of the Leishmania donovani complex. *PNAS* **104**(22):9375–9380.

World Health Organization (2010) *Control of the Leishmaniases.* WHO Expert Technical Report Series, Nr 949.

Pratlong F, et al. (2009) Geographical distribution and epidemiological features of Old World cutaneous leishmaniasis. *Trop Med Int Health* **14**(9):1071–1085.

Reithinger R (2007) Cutaneous leishmaniasis. *Lancet Infect Dis* **7**(9):581–596.

Atlas of Human Infectious Diseases, First Edition. Heiman F.L. Wertheim, Peter Horby and John P. Woodall.
© 2012 Blackwell Publishing Ltd. Published 2012 by Blackwell Publishing Ltd.

Leishmaniasis, Visceral

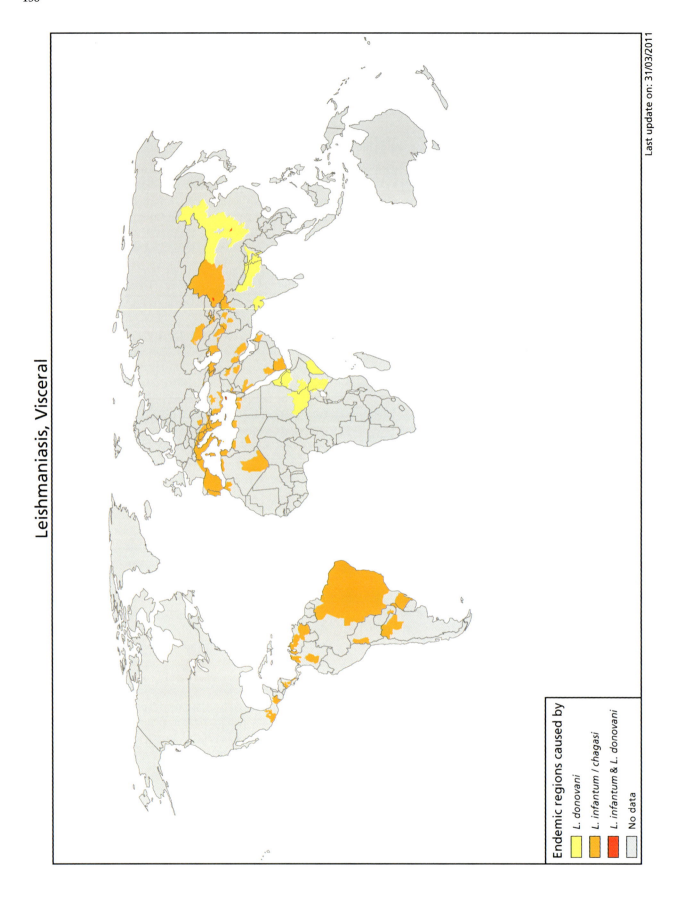

Endemic regions caused by

L. donovani

L. infantum / chagasi

L. infantum & L. donovani

No data

Last update on: 31/03/2011

Disease: **Leishmaniasis, Visceral**

Classification: ICD-9 085.0; IDC-10 B55.0

Syndromes and synonyms: Kala-azar (Hindi for black sickness), black disease, dum-dum fever.

Agent: Parasite, kinetoplastida. *Leishmania donovani* and its subspecies *donovani* and *infantum*. *L. chagasi* is considered to be the same species as *L. infantum*, and are referred to as *L. infantum/chagasi*. Occasionally, other *Leishmania* spp. can cause visceral disease, usually in immunocompromised individuals.

Reservoir: Humans (mainly *L. donovani*), wild Canidae (foxes, raccoon dogs, jackals, wolves), domestic dogs (mainly *L. infantum/chagasi*), and rodents.

Vector: Phlebotomine sandfly: *Lutzomyia* spp. (New World) and *Phlebotomus* spp. (Old World).

Transmission: Bite of infective female sandfly. Rare reports exist of non-vector transmission, including transmission by blood transfusion, sharing of syringes, venereal contact, and possibly transplacentally; potential transmission via organ transplantation.

Cycle: During blood meal, the sandfly ingests infected blood with amastigotes. The amastigotes develop to motile promastigotes that multiply in the sandfly gut, and finally motile promastigotes travel to the mouth parts and are injected into another host during feeding. In the host cell the promastigotes develop into amastigotes.

Incubation period: Usually 2–6 months (range: 10 days to years).

Clinical findings: Infection may be asymptomatic or progressive and fatal, if untreated. Onset is often insidious. Common symptoms include fever, malaise, weight loss, and sweats. Cough may be prominent. Symptoms can come and go. Splenomegaly, hepatomegaly, and lymphadenopathy are common findings. HIV-infected individuals are at increased risk for symptomatic infection. Bacterial co-infections, including tuberculosis, may occur. Anemia, leucopenia, and thrombocytopenia are common laboratory findings.

Diagnostic tests: Identification of intracellular amastigotes in stained smears from blood, bone marrow, spleen, liver, lymph nodes. PCR is sensitive and specific. Serologic tests can be useful, though they may be negative in HIV-infected patients with leishmaniasis. Rapid diagnostic tests (rK39) are available.

Therapy: Pentavalent antimonials; pentamidine; amphotericin. Other drugs and regimens are being tested (including paramomycin, miltefosine).

Prevention: Vector control; personal protection from sandfly bites (e.g. protective clothing, insecticide-treated bednets, residual insecticiding of breeding places); use of deltamethrin-impregnated dog collars and dog vaccination; there is no vaccine for human use.

Epidemiology: VL is found in 62 countries where an estimated 500,000 cases occur annually and 120 million persons are at risk. Approximately 90% of VL cases occur in rural and suburban areas of five countries: Bangladesh, India, Nepal, Sudan, and Brazil. During epidemics, >5% of a population may develop symptomatic infection. Persons who are under age of 5 years, malnourished and immunocompromised (including HIV-infected individuals) are more likely to develop symptomatic, often severe, infection. There are indications that VL is spreading to historically non-endemic areas, like northern parts of Europe and Western Upper Nile Sudan. Clearly the distribution of VL is dynamic and adapts to changes in demographics, human behavior, environment (deforestation, urbanization), and host factors (HIV). VL is reported in Chad, DRC, and Zambia, but the infectious agent is unknown. *L. donovanis* has been found in Sri Lanka, but only as a cause of cutaneous leishmaniasis.

Map sources: The Leishmaniasis (visceral) map was made with multiple sources from the medical literature and WHO.

Key references

Alvar J, et al. (2006) Leishmaniasis and poverty. *Trends Parasit* **22**(12):552–557.

Gramiccia M, et al. (2007) The leishmaniases in Southern Europe. In: *Emerging Pests and Vector-Borne Diseases: Ecology and Control of Vector-Borne Diseases*, Vol. **1**, pp. 75–95 (eds Takken W and Knols BGJ). Wageningen Academic Publishers.

Guerin P, et al. (2002) Visceral leishmaniasis: current status of control, diagnosis, and treatment, and a proposed research and development agenda. *Lancet Infect Dis* **2**:494–501.

Herwaldt BL (1999) Leishmaniasis. *Lancet* **354**:1191–1199.

Ready PD (2010) Leishmaniasis emergence in Europe. *Euro Surveill* **15**(10):19505.

World Health Organization (2010) *Control of the Leishmaniases*. WHO Expert Technical Report Series, Nr 949.

Atlas of Human Infectious Diseases, First Edition. Heiman F.L. Wertheim, Peter Horby and John P. Woodall.
© 2012 Blackwell Publishing Ltd. Published 2012 by Blackwell Publishing Ltd.

Loiasis

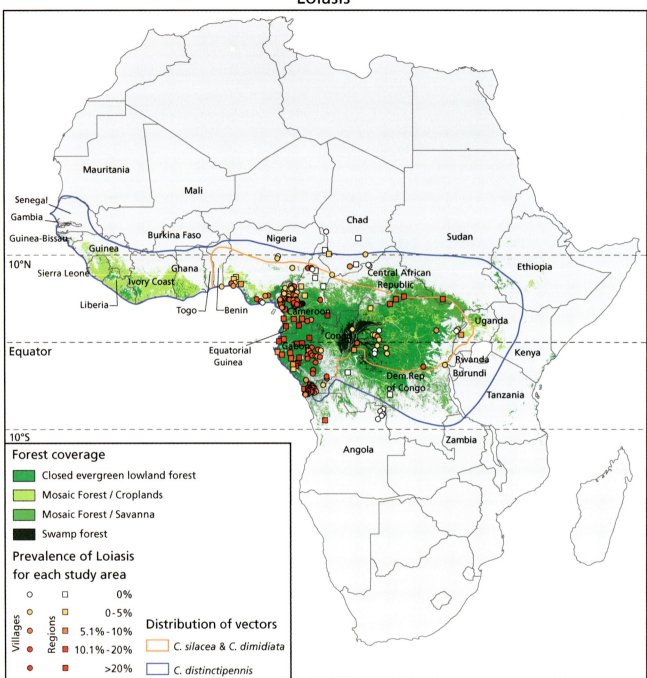

Forest coverage

- Closed evergreen lowland forest
- Mosaic Forest / Croplands
- Mosaic Forest / Savanna
- Swamp forest

Prevalence of Loiasis for each study area

Villages	Regions	
○	□	0%
○	□	0 - 5%
○	□	5.1% - 10%
●	■	10.1% - 20%
●	■	>20%

Distribution of vectors

- C. silacea & C. dimidiata
- C. distinctipennis

Last update on: 15/02/2011

Disease: **Loiasis**

Classification: ICD-125.2; ICD-10 B74.3

Syndromes and synonyms: Loa loa filariasis, loiasis, African eyeworm, Calabar swelling

Agent: Filarial nematode (roundworm), *Loa loa*. Adult worms are nematodes that live freely in subcutaneous tissue. Adult females are 40–70 mm long and males are 30–34 mm long.

Reservoir: Humans. Loa loa also infects some monkeys but the human and simian cycles seem to be independent.

Vector: Tabanid adult female flies, mainly *Chrysops silacea*, *C. dimidiata*, and *C. distinctipennis*. These day-biting and blood-sucking flies breed in forested and damp environments (e.g. swamps or rotten vegetation). Other favorable environments are cocoa plantations. *Chrysops* are attracted by movement, dark objects, and smoke. The vector does not enter structures like homes or barns. Up to 18% of the vector population can be infected with *L. loa* in endemic areas.

Transmission: Infective larvae migrate out of the mouth part of the fly during bite onto the skin and subsequently enter the wound. The tabanid bite is painful with blood loss.

Cycle: Human-deer fly-human. After infective larvae enter the wound they migrate and develop into adult worms in subcutaneous tissue. Adult worms produce microfilariae, that circulate in the peripheral blood in daytime and can be taken up by the next fly during feeding. In the fly they develop into larvae in 10–12 days and enter the proboscis, and the cycle repeats. An infected human can remain infectious to the vector for up to 15 years. Transmission is facilitated by the fact that microfilaremia and the vector-biting activity occur in daytime.

Incubation period: 4 months to several years.

Clinical findings: Loiasis is not as severe as other filarial diseases. Typical finding is transient subcutaneous swellings (Calabar swellings) which are angiedemas. These swellings are itchy and mainly occur on the limbs, especially forearms and when close to joints may restrict movement. Less frequently: giant urticaria, arthritis, and fever. The adult worm sometimes migrates across the subconjunctiva of the eye. Encephalopathic reactions may occur during mass ivermectin treatment campaigns to control onchocerciasis. These SAEs mainly occur in those with heavy infection (>30,000 microfilariae per ml blood).

Diagnostic tests: Microscopy of stained thick blood smears taken around noon; membrane filtration; PCR. Eosinophilia and high IgE levels are indicators of active infection.

Therapy: Surgical extraction of adult worms from the eye. Diethylcarbamazine (DEC) is filaricidal but can cause SAEs in patients with heavy infection. SAEs can be reduced by co-administering antihistamines or steroids. Alternative: albendazole with a lower risk of SAEs in case of heavy infection.

Prevention: Protection from vector bites by wearing permethrin-treated light-colored clothes and fly repellent on exposed skin. DEC can be used as prophylaxis, but should not be used routinely.

Epidemiology: Loiasis occurs in areas where the *Chrysops* vectors breed in the tropical rainforest of Central Africa, where it is estimated that 12–13 million humans are infected. The prevalence of microfilaremia increases with age, and is more common in men as they are more exposed. Loiasis has gained attention because of the serious adverse events that can occur during mass ivermectin treatment campaigns for onchocerciasis control. It has been proposed that areas where the Loiasis prevalence is >20%, are at increased risk for adverse events during mass ivermectin treatment.

Map sources: The Loiasis map was made with data from Boussinesq et al. (1997) and Thomson et al. (2004) and updated with medical literature. The distribution of the vectors was reproduced from WHO (1989).

Key references

Boussinesq M, et al. (1997) Prevalences of Loa loa microfilaraemia throughout the area endemic for the infection. *Ann Trop Med Parasitol* **91**(6):573–589.

Boussinesq M. (2006) Loiasis. *Ann Trop Med Paras* **100**(8): 715–731.

Padget JJ, et al. (2008) Loiasis: African eye worm. *Trans R Soc Trop Med Hyg* **102**:983–989.

World Health Organization (1989) *Geographical distribution of arthropod-borne diseases and their principal vectors*. Unpublished report.

Atlas of Human Infectious Diseases, First Edition. Heiman F.L. Wertheim, Peter Horby and John P. Woodall.
© 2012 Blackwell Publishing Ltd. Published 2012 by Blackwell Publishing Ltd.

162

Malaria, *Plasmodium falciparum*

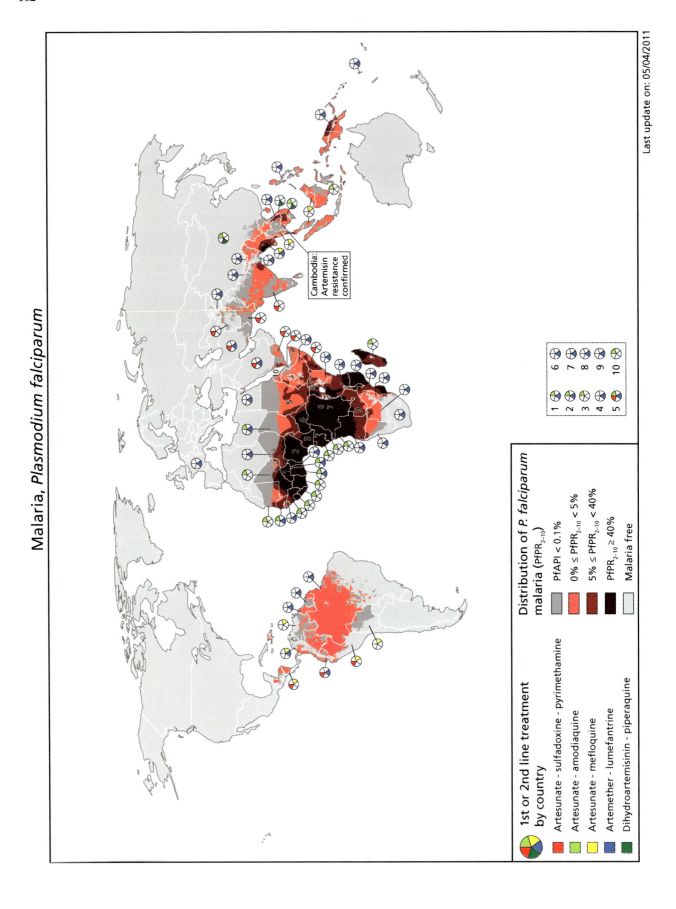

Cambodia: Artemisin resistance confirmed

1st or 2nd line treatment by country

- Artesunate - sulfadoxine - pyrimethamine
- Artesunate - amodiaquine
- Artesunate - mefloquine
- Artemether - lumefantrine
- Dihydroartemisinin - piperaquine

Distribution of *P. falciparum* malaria (PfPR$_{2-10}$)

- PfAPI < 0.1%
- 0% ≤ PfPR$_{2-10}$ < 5%
- 5% ≤ PfPR$_{2-10}$ < 40%
- PfPR$_{2-10}$ ≥ 40%
- Malaria free

Last update on: 05/04/2011

Disease: Malaria, *Plasmodium falciparum*

Classification: ICD-9 084; ICD-10 B50

Syndromes and synonyms: Falciparum malaria, malaria tropica, tropical fever, blackwater fever, paludism, marsh fever.

Agent: *Plasmodium falciparum*, an intracellular protozoan parasite in the Phylum Apicomplexa. Among the malaria parasites, *P. falciparum* causes the vast majority of mortality.

Reservoir: Humans.

Vector: Mosquito (*Anopheles* spp.), mainly bites between dusk and dawn (see Anopheles map).

Transmission: By mosquito bite (*Anopheles* spp.). Transmission has been described in needle sharing IVDUs and through blood transfusion.

Cycle: There is an asexual phase in humans and a sexual phase in the vector mosquito. The mosquito injects sporozoites that invade human liver cells where they reproduce and develop to merozoites, which, after release, infect erythrocytes. The erythrocytic stages multiply around 10-fold every 48-hours. Erythrocytes can release gametocytes which infect mosquitoes during a blood meal. In the mosquito, gametocytes develop into sporozoites.

Incubation period: 7 to 15 days, but can be longer.

Clinical findings: Uncomplicated malaria: acute febrile illness with headache, chills, sweats, nausea, and vomiting; hepatosplenomegaly. Findings of severe malaria can be: cerebral malaria (confusion, seizures, impaired consciousness to coma), hemolysis, severe anemia, hypotension, renal failure, metabolic acidosis and death. Often high parasite counts are found in patients with severe malaria (>5% infected erythrocytes).

Diagnostic tests: Light microscopy of Giemsa stained thick and thin blood smears; rapid diagnostic tests (RDTs) based on immunochromatography on blood; PCR.

Therapy: Malaria requires urgent treatment and type of treatment depends on disease severity and drug resistance in the region. Artemisinin resistance has been confirmed in the Thai–Cambodian border region. Uncomplicated *P. falciparum* malaria: artemisinin-based combination therapies (ACTs); the choice of ACTs is based on the resistance levels of the partner medicine in the combination. Artemisinin and its derivatives should not be used as monotherapy. Severe malaria: artesunate iv or im; complete treatment with an ACT or artesunate plus doxycycline or clindamycin.

Prevention: Vector control; mosquito repellent; insecticide-treated bed nets; residual spraying of insecticides; treatment of infected humans. Recently control measures are being upscaled in a malaria elimination effort. Morocco, United Arab Emirates, and Turkmenistan have been certified malaria free by WHO.

Epidemiology: The limits of *P. falciparum* malaria is determined by the presence of vector species and control measures within a certain region. *P. falciparum* malaria causes approximately 500 million cases each year and around one million deaths in Sub-Saharan Africa. In 2007 almost 60% of the 2.4 billion people at risk of malaria were living in areas with a stable risk of *P. falciparum*. High endemicity was most common and widespread in the African region. In the Americas, those at risk were all in the low endemicity class. In Asia 88% are in the low endemicity class, 11% in the intermediate class, and 1% in the high endemicity class. Recent progress is being made by the Global Malaria Action Plan to reduce malaria morbidity and mortality world wide and have a vision for malaria elimination. Ranking countries on the possibility of elimination shows that it is most feasible in the Americas and several countries in Asia and the west Pacific. It is least feasible in Africa, where much of west and central Africa need more than 90% reduction in transmission.

Map sources: The Malaria (*Plasmodium falciparum*) map is reproduced with permission from the Malaria Atlas Project, S. I. Hay et al. (2009). Data on first and second line drugs for malaria were obtained from WHO's *Global Report on Antimalarial Drug Efficacy and Drug Resistance 2000–2010* (2010).

Key references

Hay SI, et al. (2009) A world malaria map: *Plasmodium falciparum* endemicity in 2007. *PloS Med* **6**(3):e1000048.

Lancet Series (2010) Malaria elimination. *Lancet* **376** (9752):1566–1615.

World Health Organization (2010) *Guidelines for the Treatment of Malaria*, 2nd edition. Geneva.

Atlas of Human Infectious Diseases, First Edition. Heiman F.L. Wertheim, Peter Horby and John P. Woodall.
© 2012 Blackwell Publishing Ltd. Published 2012 by Blackwell Publishing Ltd.

Malaria, *Plasmodium knowlesi*

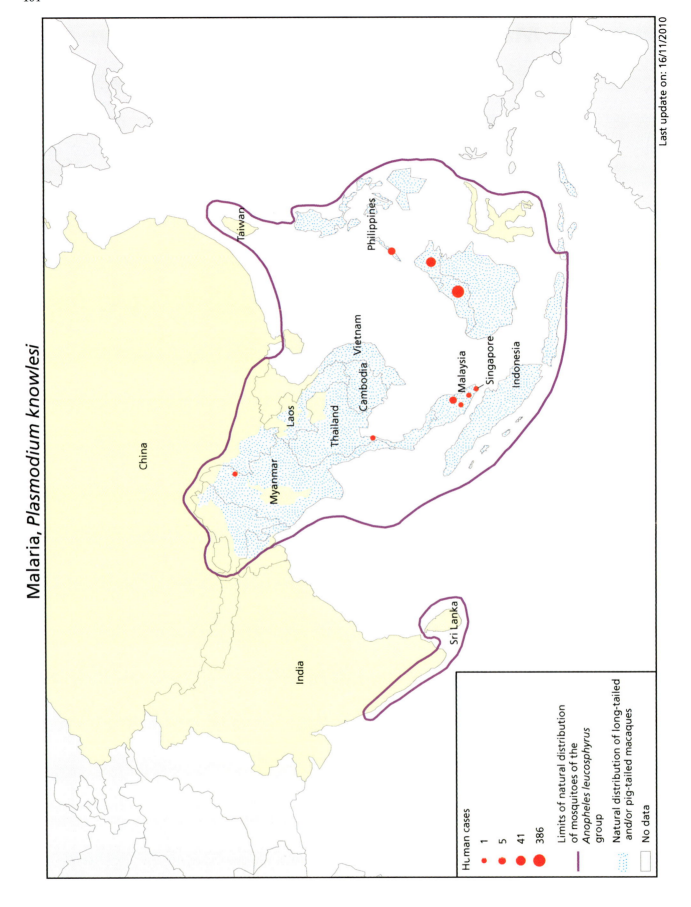

Last update on: 16/11/2010

Human cases
- 1
- 5
- 41
- 386

Limits of natural distribution of mosquitoes of the *Anopheles leucosphyrus* group

Natural distribution of long-tailed and/or pig-tailed macaques

No data

China

India

Sri Lanka

Taiwan

Myanmar

Laos

Thailand

Cambodia

Vietnam

Malaysia

Singapore

Indonesia

Philippines

Disease: Malaria, *Plasmodium knowlesi*

Classification: ICD-9 84.4; IDC-10 B53.1

Synonym: Knowlesi malaria, simian malaria

Agent: *Plasmodium knowlesi*, an intacellular protozoan parasite in the Phylum Apicomplexa. *P. knowlesi* is an Old World simian malaria parasite.

Reservoir: Long-tailed and pigtailed macaques, and banded leaf monkeys. *P. knowlesi* can also infect other primates, including New World marmosets (*Callithrix jacchus*), African olive baboons (*Papio anubis*), Old World macaques, and humans by blood passage and mosquito bites.

Vector: *P. knowlesi* transmission is restricted to the Leucosphyrus group of anophelines, consisting of 20 species.

Transmission: By mosquito bite. Experiments demonstrated human to human transmission with the mosquito as vector, but there is no direct human-to-human transmission.

Cycle: Monkey–mosquito–monkey; *P. knowlesi* has a short (24-hour) asexual lifecyle; humans are incidental hosts.

Incubation period: About 12 days.

Clinical findings: Headache, fever, chills. Abdominal pain, renal impairment, jaundice, and thrombocytopenia may occur. Coma and death are rare.

Diagnostic tests: Often misidentified as *P. malariae*, but skilled microscopists are able to make the distinction. A relatively severe illness with a microscopic diagnosis of *P. malariae* should alert clinicians to the possibility of *P. knowlesi* because *P. malariae* malaria is almost invariably mild. Species can be confirmed by PCR if needed.

Therapy: Chloroquine is effective; primaquine is likely unnecessary as a gametocidal drug since gametocytes appear to be sensitive to chloroquine.

Prevention: Early detection and containment of human-to-human *P. knowlesi* transmission in the event of a complete emergence into the human population; vector control; anti-mosquito measures.

Epidemiology: The first human *P. knowlesi* case acquired in nature was detected in 1965 in Malaysia. *P. knowlesi* malaria is widely distributed across Sarawak and Sabah in Malaysian Borneo and extends to the state of Pahang in Peninsular Malaysia. *P. knowlesi* malaria cases have also been acquired in Thailand, Myanmar, Singapore, and the Philippines. The distribution and incidence of *P. knowlesi* malaria is yet unknown. Bases on current knowledge on the vector and reservoir, human knowlesi malaria is likely not rare in areas inhabited by the natural macaque hosts and the vectors. Humans working in the vicinity of forests are considered at risk. Deforestation now also brings humans in semi-urban areas into contact with reservoir hosts. Interestingly, *P. knowlesi* has been used in the past as a pyretic agent for the treatment of patients with neurosyphilis.

Map sources: The Malaria, *Plasmodium knowlesi* map is modified from in J. Cox-Singh et al. (2008).

Key references

Cox-Singh J, et al. (2008) Knowlesi malaria: newly emergent and of public health importance? *Trends Parasitol* **24** (9):406–410.

Daneshvar C, et al. (2010) Clinical and parasitological response to oral chloroquine and primaquine in uncomplicated human Plasmodium knowlesi infections. *Malar J* **9**:238.

Atlas of Human Infectious Diseases, First Edition. Heiman F.L. Wertheim, Peter Horby and John P. Woodall.
© 2012 Blackwell Publishing Ltd. Published 2012 by Blackwell Publishing Ltd.

Malaria, *Plasmodium ovale*

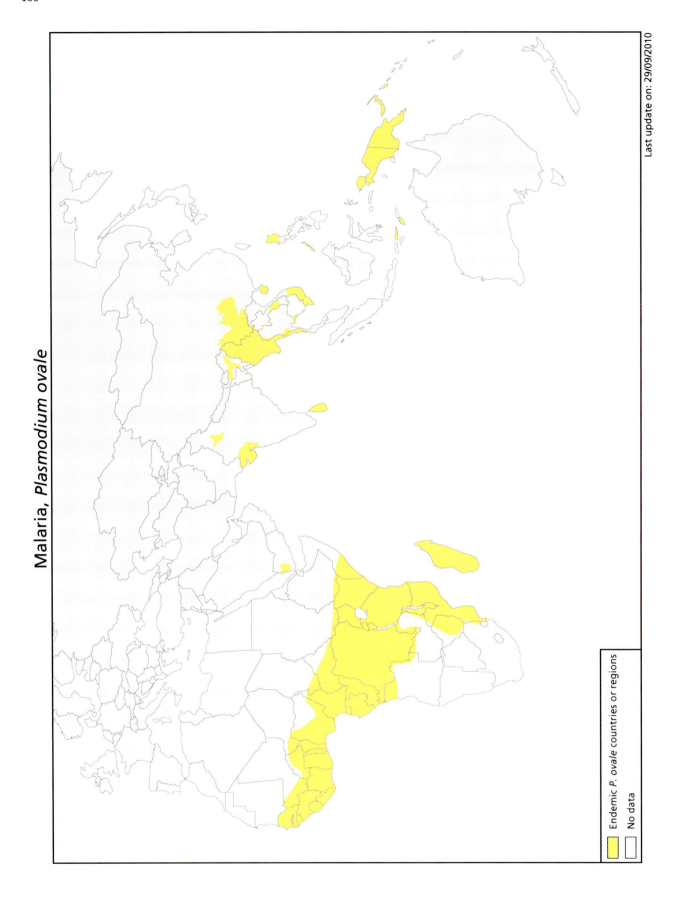

Last update on: 29/09/2010

Endemic *P. ovale* countries or regions

No data

Disease: Malaria, *Plasmodium ovale*

Classification: ICD-9 084.3; ICD-10 B53.0

Synonyms: malaria, paludism, tropical fever.

Agent: *Plasmodium ovale*, an intacellular protozoan parasite in the Phylum Apicomplexa. Phylogenetically, *P. ovale* clusters with other *Plasmodium* species affecting simian primates.

Reservoir: Humans and possibly other primates (chimpanzees). Evidence of naturally occurring *P. ovale* in chimpanzees has been reported.

Vector: Female mosquito of the genus *Anopheles* (see *Anopheles* map).

Transmission: By mosquito bite (*Anopheles* spp.).

Cycle: Infective sporozoites are inoculated by the bite of anopheles mosquitoes and through the bloodstream and lymphatics reach the liver where they differentiate into tissue schizonts that release merozoites, or to a dormant stage (hypnozoite) that can become active after months or years, causing relapse. Merozoites released from liver infect erythrocytes that develop to schizonts, rupture and release merozoites that will infect new erythrocytes (this cycle takes 48 hours). Some merozoites develop into gametocytes that are able to infect mosquitoes during a blood meal.

Incubation period: 12 to 20 days, up to to several months

Clinical findings: Acute febrile illness with chills, sweats, nausea, headache, and vomiting. Usually does not last longer than 2 weeks.

Diagnostic tests: Microscopy of Giemsa-stained blood film; differentiation from *P. vivax* can be difficult and result in misidentification; parasite load is generally low and may be undetectable by light microscopy; in regions where *P. falciparum* / *P. vivax* predominate, *P. ovale* is frequently overlooked; parasitemia is present for about 2 weeks; PCR.

Therapy: Need to treat both *P. ovale* blood and liver stage with chloroquine (blood stage) and primaquine (liver stage).

Prevention: Vector control; mosquito repellent; insecticide-treated bed nets; treatment of infected humans.

Epidemiology: *P. ovale* initally was thought to be limited to Sub-Saharan Africa, Papua New Guinea, eastern Indonesia, and the Philippines. It is actually more widely distributed, and is reported in the Middle East, the Indian Subcontinent, and various parts of Southeast Asia. *P. ovale* has not yet been reported in South America. In general, *P. ovale* is relatively uncommon, though in West Africa prevalences above 10% are observed. Also, infections are most common in children <10 years. There is likely underreporting due to underdiagnosis. Due to the short duration of parasitemia and low parasite loads, *P. ovale* is regularly 'missed' in cross-sectional surveys.

Map sources: The Malaria (*Plasmodium ovale*) map is modified from A.J. Lysenko et al. (1969) and updated with recent literature. Interestingly, no global map of the geographical distribution of *P. ovale* has been produced since that of Lysenko et al. in 1969.

Key references

Collins WE (2005) Plasmodium ovale: parasite and disease. *Clin Microbiol Rev* **18**:570–581.

Duval L, et al. (2009) Chimpanzee malaria parasites related to *Plasmodium ovale* in Africa. *PLoS ONE* **4**(5):e5520.

Lysenko AJ, et al. (1969) An analysis of the geographical distribution of *Plasmodium ovale*. *Bull World Health Org* **40**:383–394.

Mueller I, et al. (2007) *Plasmodium malariae* and *Plasmodium ovale* – the 'bashful' malaria parasites. *Trends Parasitol* **23** (6):278–283.

WHO (2010) *Guidelines for the Treatment of Malaria*, 2nd edn. Geneva.

Atlas of Human Infectious Diseases, First Edition. Heiman F.L. Wertheim, Peter Horby and John P. Woodall.
© 2012 Blackwell Publishing Ltd. Published 2012 by Blackwell Publishing Ltd.

168

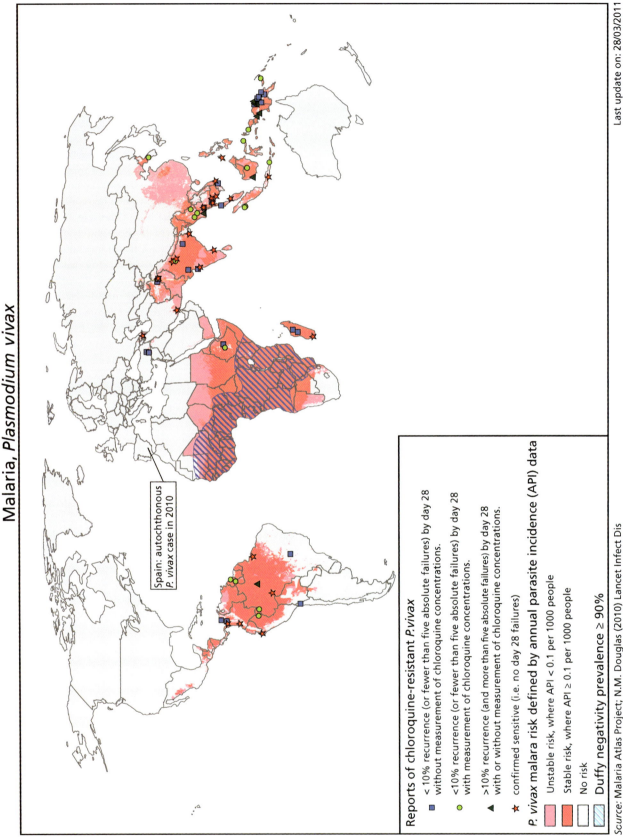

Malaria, *Plasmodium vivax*

Spain: autochthonous
P. vivax case in 2010

Reports of chloroquine-resistant *P.vivax*

- ■ < 10% recurrence (or fewer than five absolute failures) by day 28 without measurement of chloroquine concentrations.
- ○ <10% recurrence (or fewer than five absolute failures) by day 28 with measurement of chloroquine concentrations.
- ▲ >10% recurrence (and more than five absolute failures) by day 28 with or without measurement of chloroquine concentrations.
- ✶ confirmed sensitive (i.e. no day 28 failures)

P. vivax malara risk defined by annual parasite incidence (API) data

- Unstable risk, where API < 0.1 per 1000 people
- Stable risk, where API ≥ 0.1 per 1000 people
- No risk
- Duffy negativity prevalence ≥ 90%

Source: Malaria Atlas Project; N.M. Douglas (2010) Lancet Infect Dis

Last update on: 28/03/2011

Disease: Malaria, *Plasmodium vivax*

Classification: ICD-9 084.1; ICD-10 B51.0–B51.9.

Synonyms: Vivax malaria; recurring malaria; tertian malaria; paludism; marsh fever; ague.

Agent: *Plasmodium vivax*, an intacellular protozoan parasite in the Phylum Apicomplexa.

Reservoir: Humans.

Vector: Female mosquito of the genus *Anopheles*; mainly bites between dusk and dawn (see *Anopheles* map).

Transmission: By mosquito bite (*Anopheles* spp.); transmission has been described in needle sharing IVDUs and blood transfusion.

Cycle: Infective sporozoites are inoculated by bite from anopheles mosquitoes and through the bloodstream and lymphatics reach the liver where they differentiate into tissue schizonts that release merozoites, or to a dormant stage (hypnozoite) that can become active after months or years, causing relapse. Merozoites released from liver mostly infect reticulocytes that develop to schizonts, rupture and release merozoites that will infect new reticulocytes (this cycle takes 48 hours) Gametocytes are able to infect mosquitoes during a blood meal.

Incubation period: 12 days to several months

Clinical findings: Common unspecific symptoms are acute febrile illness with chills, sweats, nausea, headache, and vomiting; high fever with chills is more common in *P. vivax* than in *P. falciparum* malaria. Recent reports provide evidence that vivax malaria is not as benign as previously thought. *P. vivax* can lead to severe anemia, acute respiratory distress, liver failure, renal failure, and even cerebral malaria.

Diagnostic tests: Microscopy: in Giemsa-stained blood smears Schüfner's dots are seen; rapid diagnostic tests (RDTs); PCR.

Therapy: Need to treat both *P. vivax* blood and liver stage. Uncomplicated *P. vivax* malaria: Chloroquine combined with primaquine (liver stage). In case of resistance: ACTs combined with primaquine. For severe vivax malaria: prompt treatment and case management as *P. falciparum* malaria. Treatment needs to be modified in case of G6PD deficiency

(see Inheritable Blood Disorder map). *P. vivax* chloroquine resistance is established in Papua New Guinea and eastern Indonesia.

Prevention: Vector control; mosquito repellent; insecticide-treated bed nets; treatment of infected humans.

Epidemiology: Vivax malaria is the second most important malaria species after *P. falciparum* and accounts for 25–40% of the cases world wide with 132–391 million cases per year. Outside Africa it is the dominant species, mainly in Asia. The distribution is wider than *P. falciparum* as it is able to develop at lower temperatures and can form hypnozoites in human liver. The high prevalence of Duffy negativity in western Africa has influenced the epidemiology of *P. vivax*, as Duffy-negative people are apparently resistant to vivax malaria, although several reports suggest that Duffy-negative people can be infected with *P. vivax*. The disease burden is greatest in infants. In 2010, an autochtonous *P. vivax* case was diagnosed in north-eastern Spain. Malaria was declared eradicated from Spain in 1964. *P. vivax* may have been transmitted by the local vector *Anopheles atroparvus*, which can transmit Asiatic *P. vivax* strains.

Map sources: The Malaria (*Plasmodium vivax*) map is reproduced with permission from the Malaria Atlas Project, C.A. Guerra et al. (2010). The *P. vivax* resistance data was obtained from N.M. Douglas et al. (2010).

Key references

Douglas NM, et al. (2010) Artemisinin combination therapy for vivax malaria. *Lancet Infect Dis* **10**:405–416.

Guerra CA, et al. (2010) The international limits and population at risk of *Plasmodium vivax* transmission in 2009. *PloS Negl Trop Dis* **4**(8):e774.

Mueller I, et al. (2009) Key gaps in the knowledge of *Plasmodium vivax*, a neglected human malaria parasite. *Lancet Infect Dis* **9**:555–566.

Mercereau-Puijalon O, et al. (2010) *Plasmodium vivax* and the Duffy antigen: a paradigm revisited. *Transf Clin Biol* **17**:176–183.

Price RN, et al. (2007) Vivax malaria: neglected and not benign. *Am J Trop Med Hyg* **77** (6 Suppl):79–87.

Santa-Olalla Peralta P, et al. (2010) First autochthonous malaria case due to *Plasmodium vivax* since eradication, Spain, October 2010. *Euro Surveill* **15**(41):19684.

World Health Organization (2010) *Guidelines for the Treatment of Malaria*, 2nd edition, Geneva.

Atlas of Human Infectious Diseases, First Edition. Heiman F.L. Wertheim, Peter Horby and John P. Woodall.
© 2012 Blackwell Publishing Ltd. Published 2012 by Blackwell Publishing Ltd.

Onchocerciasis

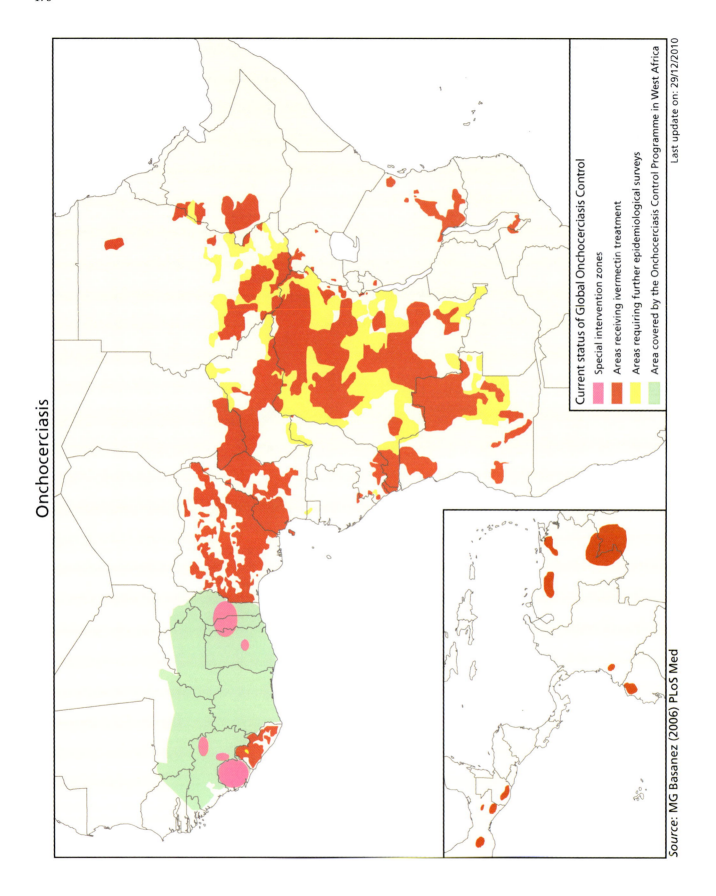

Current status of Global Onchocerciasis Control

Special intervention zones

Areas receiving ivermectin treatment

Areas requiring further epidemiological surveys

Area covered by the Onchocerciasis Control Programme in West Africa

Last update on: 29/12/2010

Source: MG Basanez (2006) PLoS Med

Disease: Onchocerciasis

Classification: ICD-9 125.3; ICD-B73

Syndromes and synonyms: River blindness, onchodermatitis.

Agent: *Onchocerca volvulus*, a filarial nematode (roundworm). Adult female worm is approximately 50 cm long.

Reservoir: Humans are the only natural host. The parasite can be experimentally transferred to chimpanzees.

Vector: Female blackflies (*Simulium*). Transmission by *S. damnosum* complex in Africa is responsible for >95% onchocerciasis cases. *S. neavei* complex in East Africa and *S. rasyani* in Yemen. In Latin America: *S. ochraceum* (Mexico and Guatemala), *S. exiguum* (Colombia and Ecuador), *S. metallicum* (northern Venezuela), and *S. guianeense* (southern Venezuela and Brazil). Blackfly larvae develop in fast-flowing rivers and the adult fly's flight range is up to 40 miles, explaining the patchy distribution of the disease. Aided by wind, blackflies can fly up to 500 km, explaining reinvasion of areas under control.

Transmission: By bite of the vector.

Cycle: Microfilariae ingested by the fly develop in about 7 days into infective L3 stages and migrate to the head and escape into the skin during feeding. In the subcutaneous tissues the L3 larvae moult into L4 stages and produce nodules within which they develop in 10 months into adult filariae and can live there for 14–15 years. The female worms can produce microfilariae for ±10 years. Microfilariae are typically found in the skin, skin lymphatics, and ocular tissues. They have a lifespan of up to 2 years. Humans remain infectious for about 10 years, the time the female worm remains fertile, but reinfection occurs in endemic areas.

Incubation period: It takes about 10 months for L3 to develop into adults. After 12–18 months microfilariae are found in the skin.

Clinical findings: Fibrous subcutaneous nodules in the head and shoulders (Americas), pelvic girdle and legs (Africa), a pruritic rash, disfiguring skin lesions (chronic papular and lichenified onchodermatitis), skin depigmentation (leopard skin), edema and skin atrophy, inflammatory process in the cornea leading to irreversible blindness, growth arrest, and epilepsy. The proportion of depigmentation and blindness is most common in older (>40 years) age groups. The disease may lead to excess mortality.

Diagnostic tests: Microscopy of fresh skin snips to detect microfilariae. Nodule palpation. Rapid card tests based on antibody detection have been produced with promising results (but not yet available commercially). Luciferase immunoprecipitation system with a mixture of four *O. volvulus* antigens. Less-invasive techniques for disease surveillance are diethylcarbamazine patch tests (may become commercially available in near future), which provoke a local Mazzotti skin reaction.

Therapy: Ivermectin, given as a single, oral dose annually or every 6 months. There is a risk of SAEs in patients coinfected with *L. loa*. Doxycycline gives good results by destroying the endosymbiotic *Wolbachia* bacteria and has fewer side effects. Surgical removal of subcutaneous nodules.

Prevention: Insect repellent, protective clothing, and insecticiding of vector-breeding sites. Mass treatment with ivermectin (see 'Therapy'). In case transmission is interrupted with ivermectin, it can recur if ivermectin mass treatment is stopped prematurely.

Epidemiology: It is estimated that 37 million people are infected worldwide, 97% of them in Africa, and remaining in small foci in Central and South America and Yemen. Onchocerciasis was imported into Latin America by the slave trade. Onchocerciasis prevalence is related to the proximity to riverine breeding sites of black flies, with the highest disease burden in communities adjacent to rivers. Prevalence of infection rises with age until around 20 years, after which infection profiles vary between geographical region and sex. Higher rates of morbidity are reported in men. This variation can be explained by heterogeneity in age, gender, and occupational exposure to vectors.

Map sources: The Onchocerciasis map is reproduced with permission from M.G. Basáñez et al. (2006).

Key references

Basáñez MG, et al. (2006) River blindness: a success story under threat? *PLoS Med* **3**(9):e371.

Dadzie Y, et al. (2003) Final report of the conference on the eradicability of Onchocerciasis. *Filaria J* **2**:2.

Taylor MJ, et al. (2010) Lymphatic filariasis and onchocerciasis. *Lancet* **376**:1175–1185.

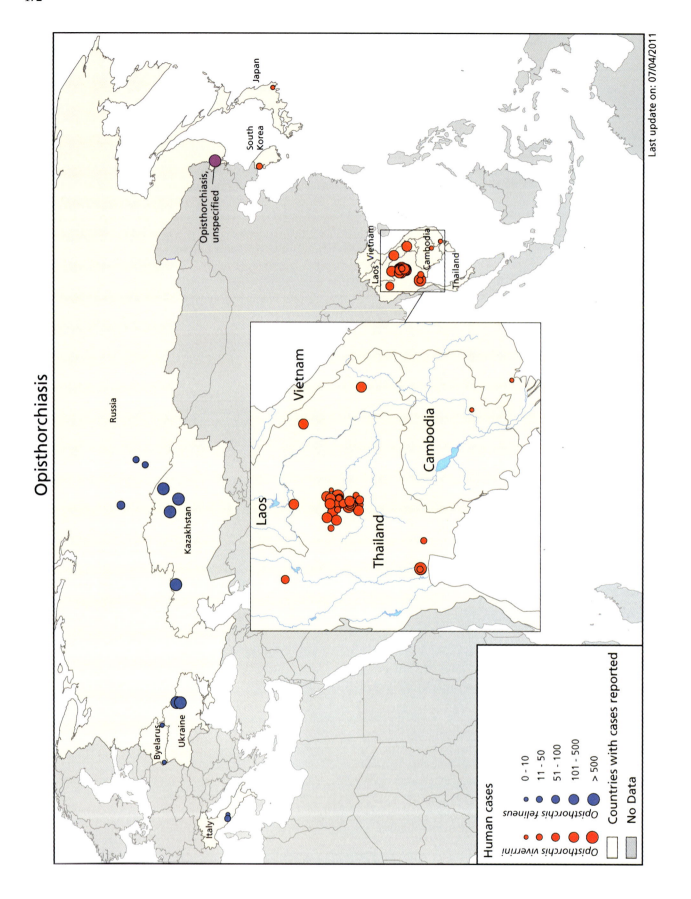

Opisthorchiasis

Last update on: 07/04/2011

Disease: Opisthorchiasis

Classification: ICD-9 121.0; ICD-10 B66.0

Syndromes and synonyms: Cat liver fluke disease, food-borne trematodiasis

Agent: Small (6–18 mm long) trematode liver fluke of dogs, cats, and some other fish-eating mammals: *Opisthorchis felineus* in Europe and northern Asia, *O. viverrini* in Southeast Asia. Both species live in bile ducts.

Reservoir: Humans and fish-eating mammals.

Vector: Freshwater snails (*Bithynia* spp.).

Transmission: Consumption of raw, undercooked, dried, salted, or pickled freshwater fish. There is no direct person-to-person transmission.

Cycle: Eggs excreted by the mammalian host in the feces into freshwater are ingested by the snail vector. They hatch and in 2 months pass through various stages in the snail to produce motile cercariae, which leave the snail and penetrate freshwater fish. In 6 weeks the cercariae encyst, and when the fish is eaten by another mammalian host, they exit the cyst and penetrate the bile duct, where in a month they mature into adult worms and start to produce eggs.

Incubation period: Depends on infecting dose. For acute disease, usually 3 to 4 weeks. For chronic disease, up to several years.

Clinical findings: *O. viverrini*: usually asymptomatic. Occasionally abdominal pain, flatulence, fatigue, mild hepatomegaly, jaundice, and cholangitis. Cholangiocarcinoma is the most serious complication. *O. felineus*: fever and hepatitis-like symptoms in the acute stage (right upper quadrant abdominal pain, nausea, and emesis). Chronic symptoms: biliary tract obstruction, inflammation and fibrosis of the biliary tract, liver abscesses, pancreatitis, and suppurative cholangitis.

Diagnostic tests: Microscopy for eggs in stool smear (Kato–Katz technique) is often inconclusive due to the similarity to eggs of other trematodes. Intradermal test is rapid and sensitive, but not specific. Immunodiagnosis is regarded supportive but not confirmatory. Radiology to demonstrate bile duct pathology. PCR test for *O. viverrini* is available.

Therapy: Praziquantel; the cure rate for *O. viverrini* is over 90%.

Prevention: Sanitation to reduce contamination of vector snail habitat, together with mass treatment with praziquantel and health education.

Epidemiology: Food-borne trematodiasis is focal and occurs in areas where the snail and freshwater fish – that is consumed raw or undercooked – coexist. The disease is the leading cause of cholangiocarcinoma in the world. *O. viverrini* is common in Southeast Asia in the Mekong region with 8 million infected in Thailand and 2 million in Laos. In Thailand about 8.7% of the population is infected and mainly in the northern provinces. Control activities in Thailand were able to reduce the prevalence from 34% to 10% in several areas. No data is available for Cambodia, China, or Vietnam, although opisthorchiasis is likely common there. *O. felineus* is found in Europe and northern Asia with approximately 5 million infected. Infected fish can be shipped and consumed in non-endemic areas.

Map sources: The Opistorchiasis map was made by geocoding reported cases in the medical literature up to 2009.

Key references

Andrews RH, et al. (2008) *Opisthorchis viverrini*: an underestimated parasite in world health. *Trends Parasit* **24**(11):497–501.

Kaewpitoon N, et al. (2008) *Opisthorchis viverrini*: the carcinogenic human liver fluke. *World J Gastroenterol* **14**(5):666–674.

Keiser J, et al. (2009) Food-borne trematodiasis. *Clin Microbiol Rev* **22**(3):466–483.

Marcos LA, et al. (2008) Update on hepatobiliary flukes: fascioliasis, opisthorchiasis and clonorchiasis. *Curr Opin Infect Dis* **21**(5):523–530.

Paragonimiasis

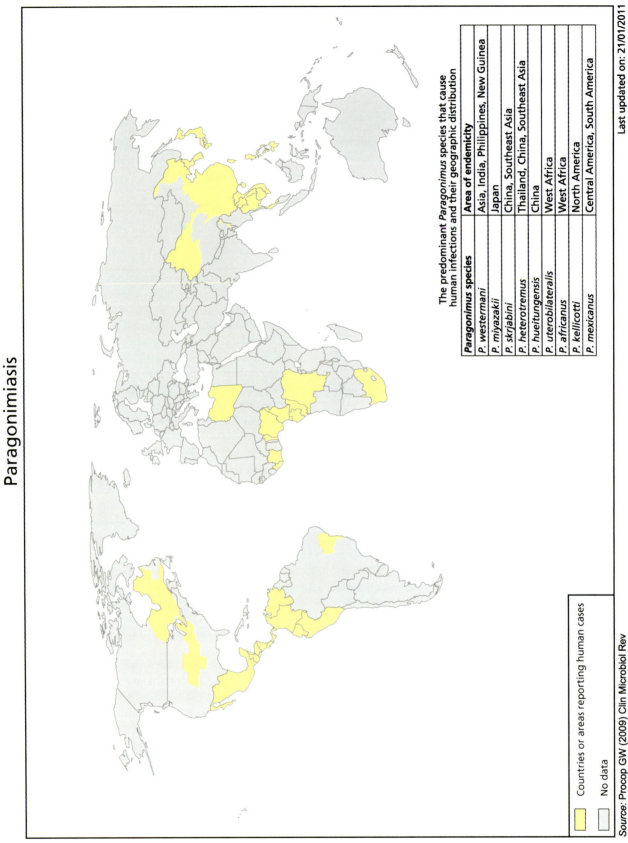

The predominant *Paragonimus* species that cause
human infections and their geographic distribution

Paragonimus species	Area of endemicity
P. westermani	Asia, India, Philippines, New Guinea
P. miyazakii	Japan
P. skrjabini	China, Southeast Asia
P. heterotremus	Thailand, China, Southeast Asia
P. hueitungensis	China
P. uterobilateralis	West Africa
P. africanus	West Africa
P. kellicotti	North America
P. mexicanus	Central America, South America

Last updated on: 21/01/2011

Countries or areas reporting human cases

No data

Source: Procop GW (2009) Clin Microbiol Rev

Disease: **Paragonimiasis**

Classification: ICD-121.2; ICD-10 B66.4

Syndromes and synonyms: Pulmonary distomiasis, lung fluke disease

Agent: Several species of *Paragonimus* trematode flatworms: *P. westermani, P. heterotremus, P. miyazakii, P. skrjabini,* and *P. hueitungensis* (the last two may be the same) in Asia, *P. africanus* and *P. uterobilateralis* in Africa, *P. mexicanus* (*P. peruvianus*) and *P. kellicotti* in the Americas.

Reservoir: Humans, dogs, cats, pigs, and wild carnivores.

Vector: Freshwater snails: *Semisulcospira, Thiara, Aroapyrgus,* and others.

Transmission: By consumption of infected raw, salted, marinated, pickled or undercooked freshwater crabs and crayfish. Infected humans can excrete worm eggs in sputum and feces for up to 20 years. There is no person-to-person transmission.

Cycle: Crustaceans infected with metacercaria larvae are ingested by the reservoir host, excyst in the gut and migrate to the tissues, usually the lungs. There they encapsulate, mature, and lay eggs. Eggs enter the sputum which is coughed up and swallowed, then pass out in the feces into water and hatch in 2–4 weeks into miracidia larvae. These penetrate the body of the vector snail, where they develop in about 2 months into cercaria larvae which enter and encyst in freshwater crabs and crayfish.

Incubation period: Flukes begin to lay eggs 6–10 weeks after ingestion of larvae. In humans, incubation is long and highly variable depending on the number of larvae ingested and organs affected.

Clinical findings: Fever, cough, hemoptysis, and pleuritic chest pain. Flukes may invade the brain and rarely the spinal cord, causing meningitis, intracranial hemorrhage, epilepsy, and paralysis. They may also cause acute and chronic inflammation of the pleura, pericardium, and mediastinum. Chest X-ray findings are similar to tuberculosis. Complications include pleural effusion, pneumothorax, bronchiectasis, and pulmonary fibrosis.

Diagnostic tests: Microscopic examination of sputum for eggs (acid-fast staining destroys eggs), and examination of feces after using concentration techniques; ELISA for serology.

Therapy: Praziquantel and triclabendazole. Bithionol is an alternative treatment but has more side effects. In cerebral paragonimiasis, steroids are added.

Prevention: Thorough cooking of crustaceans, sanitary disposal of sputum and feces and use of molluscicides.

Epidemiology: The major endemic area is China, with an estimated 20 million people infected, followed by India, Laos, and Myanmar. In the Americas, Ecuador has an estimated 1.5 million cases, but up to 2010 only 9 autochthonous cases of paragonimiasis have been reported from North America (excluding 2 outbreaks in 2006 in California from eating raw freshwater crab imported from Japan). In 1992, the Chinese mitten crab from Korean and Chinese waters positive with *Paragonimus* eggs was found in western US waters.

Map Sources: The Paragonimiasis map was made with data from G.W. Procop (2009) and human cases reported in the medical literature up to 2009.

Key references

Aka NA, et al. (2008) Human paragonimiasis in Africa. *Ann African Med* **7**(4):153–162.

Liu Q, et al. (2006) Paragonimiasis: an important food-borne zoonosis in China. *Trends in Parastol* **24**(7):318–323.

Prasad PK, et al. (2009) Phylogenetic reconstruction using secondary structures and sequence motifs of ITS2 rDNA of *Paragonimus westermani* (Kerbert, 1878) Braun, 1899 (Digenea: Paragonimidae) and related species. *BMC Genomics* **10** (Suppl 3):S25.

Procop GW (2009) North American paragonimiasis (caused by *Paragonimus kellicotti*) in the context of global paragonimiasis. *Clin Microbiol Rev* **22**(3):415–446.

Atlas of Human Infectious Diseases, First Edition. Heiman F.L. Wertheim, Peter Horby and John P. Woodall.
© 2012 Blackwell Publishing Ltd. Published 2012 by Blackwell Publishing Ltd.

Schistosomiasis, Africa & Americas

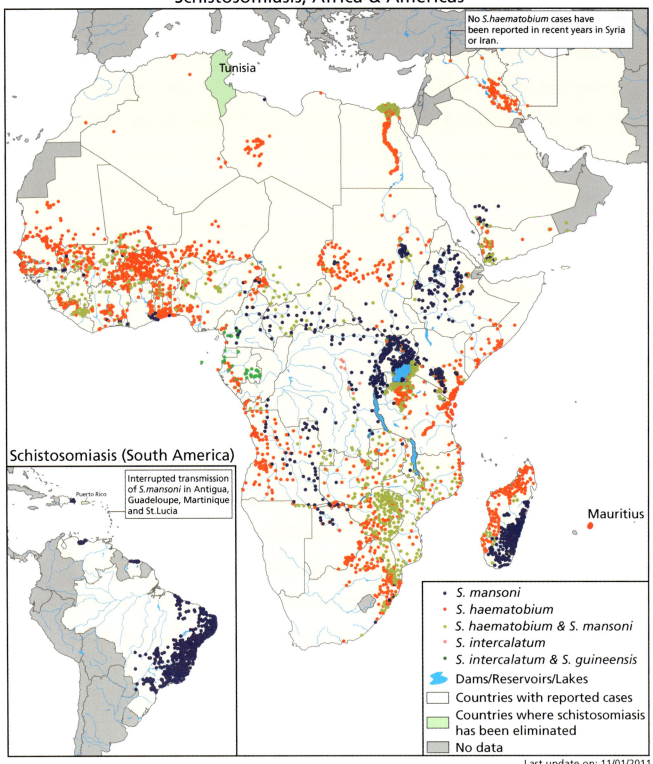

No *S. haematobium* cases have been reported in recent years in Syria or Iran.

Tunisia

Mauritius

Schistosomiasis (South America)

Puerto Rico

Interrupted transmission of *S. mansoni* in Antigua, Guadeloupe, Martinique and St. Lucia

- S. mansoni
- S. haematobium
- S. haematobium & S. mansoni
- S. intercalatum
- S. intercalatum & S. guineensis
- Dams/Reservoirs/Lakes
- Countries with reported cases
- Countries where schistosomiasis has been eliminated
- No data

Last update on: 11/01/2011

Disease: Schistosomiasis, Africa & Americas

Classification: ICD-9 120; ICD-10 B65

Syndromes and synonyms: Bilharziasis, Katayama fever or syndrome, urogenital and intestinal schistosomiasis.

Agent: Trematode worms *Schistosoma mansoni, S. haematobium, S. intercalatum,* and *S. guineensis* (formerly known as *S. intercalatum). S. haematobium* species group contains 8 species, of which not all cause human disease.

Reservoir: Humans are the main reservoir. *S. haematobium* can infect primates, livestock and rodents. *S. mansoni, S. intercalatum,* and *S. guineensis* can infect rodents.

Vector: Freshwater snails: *Biomphalaria* spp. for *S. mansoni, Bulinus* spp. for *S. haematobium, S. intercalatum,* and *S. guineensis.* Technically, humans are the 'vector' as they harbor the parasite's sexual stage. Snails are intermediate hosts.

Transmission: Contact with freshwater bodies containing cercariae that penetrate skin or mucous membranes; drinking contaminated water (uncommon).

Cycle: Snail–human–snail. Infected humans shed eggs into the water, which hatch into larvae (miracidia) that enter snails and develop into motile larvae (cercariae). The cercariae are shed into the water and penetrate the skin of humans in the water, enter the bloodstream and settle in the liver. When matured to adult male and female worms, they migrate to the abdominal veins (*S. mansoni, S. intercalatum, S. guineensis*) or pelvic veins (*S. haematobium*), mate and produce eggs. Snails remain infectious for up to 3 months, humans for more than 10 years.

Incubation period: Usually 14–84 days for acute schistosomiasis (Katayama syndrome); chronic schistosomiasis can be asymptomatic for a long period, months to years.

Clinical findings: Katayama syndrome is an acute form of schistosomiasis, caused by the host immune response to developing larvae and early egg production and presents with nocturnal fever, cough, myalgia, headache, and abdominal pain. Katayama syndrome is more common among infected non-immune individuals (e.g. travelers) and relatively rare among local residents with exposure since childhood. *S. mansoni* causes intestinal schistosomiasis with: diarrhea, abdominal pain, blood in the stool, hepatosplenomegaly. *S. haematobium* causes urogenital schistosomiasis with dysuria, hematuria, hemospermia, and dyspareunia. *S. intercalatum* and *S. guineensis*: granulomas, rectal polyps and ulcers. Chronic infection may lead to liver fibrosis, hepatosplenomegaly, and portal hypertension (*S. mansoni*), obstructive uropathy, bacterial infection, infertility, and bladder cancer (*S. haematobium*); rectitis, salpingitis, infertility and abortion (*S. intercalatum, S. guineensis*); anemia and altered growth and cognitive development in infected children. Rarely, CNS disease may follow *S. haematobium* and *S. guineensis* infection.

Diagnostic tests: Microscopy for eggs in stool (*S. mansoni*) or urine (*S. haematobium*) samples; quantification of eggs in stool by Kato–Katz method and in urine by standardized filtration techniques; PCR.

Therapy: Praziquantel is recommended; alternative: oxamniquine for *S. mansoni*, metrifonate for *S. haematobium*.

Prevention: Access to clean water and sanitation; protective clothing for occupational risk; after accidental exposure, dry the skin and apply 70% alcohol; mollusciciding; avoid contact with contaminated water bodies.

Epidemiology: It is estimated that more than 207 million people are infected world wide, with 85% of them in Africa. Infection does not produce full immunity, so reinfection occurs. Schistosomiasis is a water-based disease that mainly affects rural agricultural and fishing communities. Higher disease prevalence rates in endemic regions are found close to irrigation projects or dams. Man-made water bodies like dams can lead to changes in snail habitat and cause a shift from urogenital to intestinal schistosomiasis (Egypt) and vice versa (Senegal). *S. mansoni* was presumably introduced with the slave trade from west Africa into South America and the Caribbean *S. intercalatum* and *S. guineensis* are geographically restricted to Central Western Africa.

Map sources: The Schistosomiasis map is modified from WHO (1987) Global Schistosomiasis Atlas at: www.who.int/wormcontrol/documents/maps/en/.

Key references

Murinello A, et al. (2006) Liver disease due to *Schistosoma guineensis* – a review. *J Port Gastrenterol* **13**:97–104.

Ross AGP, et al. (2007) Katayama syndrome. *Lancet Infect Dis* **7**:218–224.

Steinman P, et al. (2006) Schistosomiasis and water resources development. *Lancet Infect Dis* **6**:411–425.

World Health Organization (2011) Schistosomiasis. *Factsheet* Nr 115 (www.who.int).

Atlas of Human Infectious Diseases, First Edition. Heiman F.L. Wertheim, Peter Horby and John P. Woodall.
© 2012 Blackwell Publishing Ltd. Published 2012 by Blackwell Publishing Ltd.

Schistosomiasis, Asia

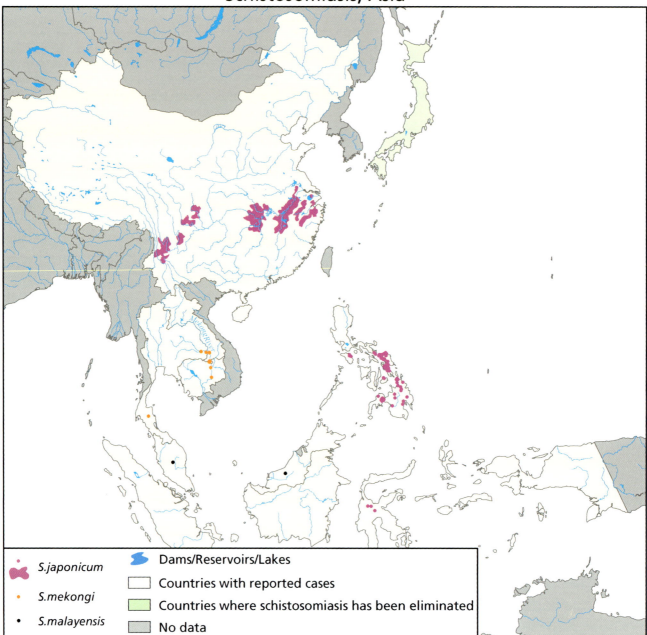

S.japonicum

S.mekongi

S.malayensis

Dams/Reservoirs/Lakes

Countries with reported cases

Countries where schistosomiasis has been eliminated

No data

Last update on: 11/01/2011

Disease: Schistosomiasis, Asia

Classification: ICD-9 120; ICD-10 B65

Synonyms: Bilharziasis, snail fever, Katayama fever or syndrome, intestinal schistosomiasis.

Agent: Trematode worms *Schistosoma japonicum, S. malayensis,* and *S. mekongi.*

Reservoir: Humans, dogs, cats, pigs, cattle, water buffalo and wild rodents for *S. japonicum,* rodents for *S. malayensis,* pigs and dogs for *S. mekongi.*

Vector: Freshwater snails: *Oncomelania* spp. for *S. japonicum, Robertsiella* spp. for *S. malayensis, Neotricula* spp. for *S. mekongi.*

Transmission: Contact with freshwater bodies containing cercariae that penetrate skin or mucous membranes; drinking contaminated water (less common).

Cycle: Snail–human–snail. Infected humans shed eggs into the water, which hatch into larvae (miracidia) that enter snails and develop into motile larvae (cercariae). The cercariae are shed into the water and penetrate the skin of humans with water contact. Cercariae enter the bloodstream and settle in the liver, where they grow into adult male and female worms that migrate to the abdominal veins, mate, and produce eggs. Snails are infectious for up to 3 months, humans for 10 years or more.

Incubation period: Usually 14–84 days for acute schistosomiasis (Katayama syndrome); chronic schistosomiasis can be asymptomatic for a long period, months to years.

Clinical findings: Katayama syndrome is an acute form of schistosomiasis, caused by the host immune response to developing larvae and early egg production and presents with nocturnal fever, cough, myalgia, headache, and abdominal pain. Katayama syndrome is more common among infected non-immune individuals (e.g. travelers) and relatively rare among local residents with exposure since childhood. *S. japonicum* causes intestinal schistosomiasis with: diarrhea, abdominal pain, blood in the stool, hepatosplenomegaly. Chronic infection leads to liver fibrosis and portal hypertension, anemia, and altered growth and cognitive development in infected children; seizures due to egg granulomas in brain or spinal cord. Infection does not produce full immunity, so reinfection occurs.

S. mekongi causes similar, but milder, disease compared to *S. japonicum.*

Diagnostic tests: Microscopy for eggs in stool samples; quantification of eggs by Kato–Katz method; PCR.

Therapy: Praziquantel is the drug of choice for all.

Prevention: Access to clean water and sanitation; protective clothing (rubber boots and gloves) for those with occupational exposure; after accidental exposure, dry the skin and apply 70% alcohol; mollusciciding. Replace water buffaloes by tractors, and livestock management like fencing off water buffaloes.

Epidemiology: Approximately 1 million people are infected with *Schistosoma* spp. in Cambodia, China, Lao PDR, and the Philippines. Schistosomiasis has been eliminated from Japan and the burden has been greatly reduced in China through extensive control efforts. Schistosomiasis is a water-based disease, that mainly affects rural agricultural and fishing communities. Higher disease prevalence rates in endemic regions are found close to large irrigation projects or dams. *S. japonicum* is found in China, Philippines, and Indonesia. In Indonesia, schistosomiasis is confined to two endemic areas in Central Sulawesi. *S. mekongi* is found in the Mekong River area of Cambodia and Laos, and has also been detected in Thailand. *S. malayensis* has only been reported from Malaysia and is a rare cause of human disease.

Map sources: The Schistosomiasis map is modified from WHO (1987) *Global Schistosomiasis Atlas,* at: www.who.int/wormcontrol/documents/maps/en/.

Key references

Chitsulo L, et al. (2000) The global status of schistosomiasis and its control. *Acta Trop* **77**:41–51.

Ross AGP, et al. (2001) Schistosomiasis in the People's Republic of China. *Clin Microbiol Rev* **14**(2):270–295.

Ross AGP, et al. (2007) Katayama syndrome. *Lancet Infect Dis* **7**:218–224.

Steinman P, et al. (2006) Schistosomiasis and water resources development. *Lancet Infect Dis* **6**:411–425.

World Health Organization (2011) Schistosomiasis. *Factsheet Nr 115* (www.who.int).

Atlas of Human Infectious Diseases, First Edition. Heiman F.L. Wertheim, Peter Horby and John P. Woodall.
© 2012 Blackwell Publishing Ltd. Published 2012 by Blackwell Publishing Ltd.

Strongyloidiasis

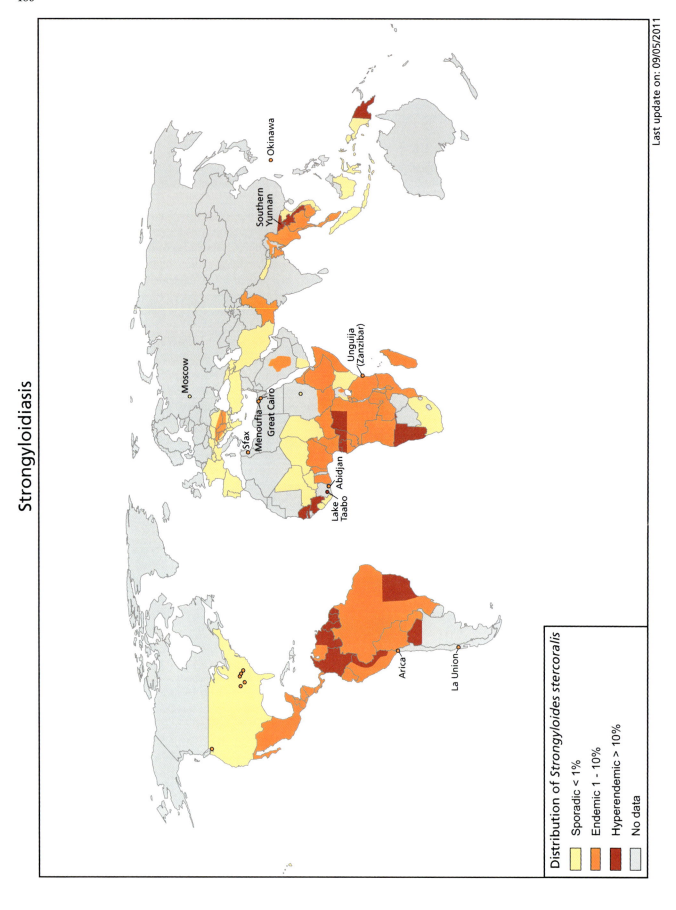

Distribution of *Strongyloides stercoralis*

- Sporadic < 1%
- Endemic 1 - 10%
- Hyperendemic > 10%
- No data

Last update on: 09/05/2011

Okinawa

Southern Yunnan

Moscow

Unguija (Zanzibar)

Sfax
Menoufia
Great Cairo

Abidjan
Lake Taabo

Arica

La Union

Disease: Strongyloidiasis

Classification: ICD-9 127.2; ICD-10 B78

Syndromes and synonyms: Larva currens.

Agent: *Strongyloides stercoralis*, a minute nematode round-worm (up to 2.2 mm long). *S. fuelleborni* (not shown on the map) is a less common agent and can cause human disease in Africa and Papua New Guinea ('swollen belly syndrome' in infants).

Reservoir: For *S. stercoralis*: mainly humans, although infections in non-human primates and dogs have been described. *S. fuelleborni* is mainly found in in monkeys, but human-to-human transmission may occur in some geographical regions.

Transmission: Mainly skin contact with fecally contaminated soil, but oral transmission cannot be excluded.

Cycle: *S. stercoralis* has a free-living (asexual) and parasitic (sexual) lifecycle. Free-living filariform (L3) larvae in the soil penetrate the skin, enter the bloodstream, reach the lungs, travel up to the throat, and are swallowed. In the duododenal wall they mature into adult female worms, produce eggs that hatch immediately, thus only larvae (L1) are excreted. These non-infectious (L1) larvae develop further in the soil into either adult worms or infectious (L3) larvae. Some non-infectious L1 larvae may develop faster into infectious L3 larvae in the human intestine and penetrate the perianal skin or colon wall. This process of auto-infection may lead to hyperinfection in immunocompromised individuals.

Incubation period: Indefinite and variable; from skin penetration to larvae in the stool takes 2–4 weeks.

Clinical findings: Most infections with *S. stercoralis* are asymptomatic. Symptoms may include: upper abdominal pain; cough; diarrhea; a red and painful, creeping urticarial eruption on the skin; and vomiting. Pulmonary symptoms (including Loeffler syndrome) can occur. Disseminated strongyloidiasis occurs in immunocompromised patients and presents with abdominal pain, distension, shock, pulmonary and neurologic complications, and septicemia. High mortality rates (15–87%) have been described in patients with disseminated disease.

Diagnostic tests: Demonstration of *Strongyloides* larvae on repeated stool specimens by microscopy after concentration (coproculture or Baermann). Stool examination has poor sensitivity, particularly in chronic cases. Serological tests vary in sensitivity and specificity, and perform better in chronic cases and are therefore used for screening patients at risk for hyperinfection. PCR has higher sensitivity than microscopy. Hyperinfection: larvae or parasite DNA can be found in sputum and other specimens.

Therapy: Ivermectin; alternative: albendazole or thiabendazole.

Prevention: Access to clean water and sanitation; regular deworming; use of closed footwear. Infection control in immunocompromised patients with hyperinfection. Immunocompromised patients who have been in endemic areas should be screened and treated if positive.

Epidemiology: The estimated prevalence of strongyloidiasis is between 30 and 100 million infections in 70 countries world wide; however, the accuracy of these estimates is uncertain due to poor performance of screening methods. Most cases are found in tropical and subtropical areas (warm, moist). Rarely, it is found in foci in North America and Europe. It is of significance in developed nations as it can cause hyperinfection in immunocompromised patients that have been infected years before in an endemic region. The most important risk factor for hyperinfection is corticosteroid therapy; other risk factors are: hematologic malignancies, malnutrition, alcoholism, HTLV-1 infection, and immunosuppressive medication (e.g. for organ transplantation). Interestingly, hyperinfection is not commonly seen in HIV-infected individuals in endemic countries.

Map sources: The Strongyloidiasis map is modified from M. Farthing et al. (2004) and updated with data from the medical literature.

Key references

Farthing M, et al. (2004) *WGO Practice Guideline; Management of Strongyloidiasis.* World Gastroenterology Organization.

Keiser PB, et al. (2004) *Strongyloides stercoralis* in the immuno-compromised population. *Clin Microb Rev* **17**(1):208–217.

Marcos LA, et al. (2008) Strongyloides hyperinfection syndrome: an emerging global infectious disease. *Trans R Soc Trop Med Hyg* **102**:314–318.

Montesa M, Sawhney C, Barrosa N (2010) *Strongyloides stercoralis*: there but not seen. *Curr Opin Infect Dis* **23**:500–504.

Olsen A, et al. (2009) Strongyloidiasis – the most neglected of the neglected tropical diseases? *Trans R Soc Trop Med Hyg* **103**:967–972.

Atlas of Human Infectious Diseases, First Edition. Heiman F.L. Wertheim, Peter Horby and John P. Woodall.
© 2012 Blackwell Publishing Ltd. Published 2012 by Blackwell Publishing Ltd.

Trypanosomiasis, African

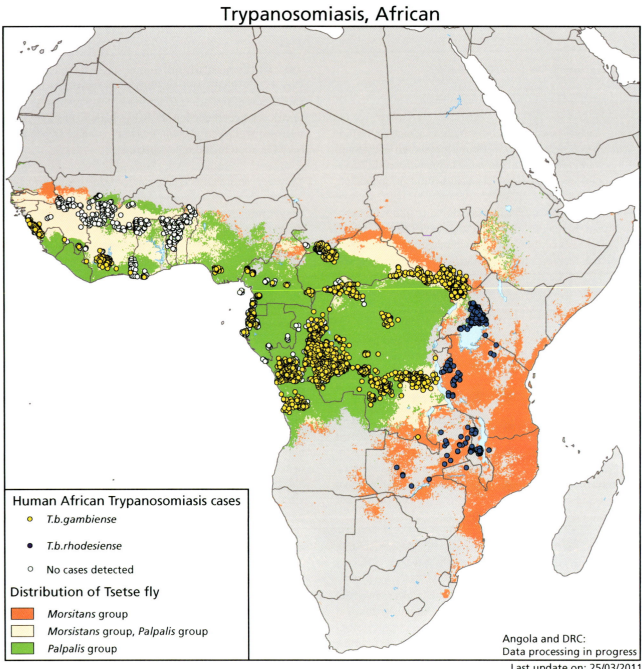

Human African Trypanosomiasis cases

- ○ (yellow) *T.b.gambiense*
- ● (dark blue) *T.b.rhodesiense*
- ○ No cases detected

Distribution of Tsetse fly

- (orange) *Morsitans* group
- (cream) *Morsistans* group, *Palpalis* group
- (green) *Palpalis* group

Angola and DRC:
Data processing in progress

Last update on: 25/03/2011

Disease: Trypanosomiasis, African

Classification: ICD-9 086.3-086.4; ICD-10 B56.0, B56.1

Syndromes and synonyms: Sleeping sickness, Gambian trypanosomiasis, Rhodesian trypanosomiasis, West African sleeping sickness, East African sleeping sickness.

Agent: Extracellular, unicellular hemoflagellate *Trypanosoma brucei*, with two subspecies: *T. b. gambiense* in West and Central Africa (tropical forest), *T. b. rhodesiense* in East and Southern Africa (savannah).

Reservoir: Humans for *T. b. gambiense*; livestock and wildlife for *T. b. rhodesiense*.

Vector: Tsetse fly (*Glossina*). The main human vectors belong to the *palpalis* (riverine flies) and *morsitans* (forest and savannah flies) complex. The palpalis complex (*G. fuscipes, G. palpalis, G. tachinoides*) mainly transmit *T. b. gambiense* and the morsitans complex (*G. morsitans, G. pallidipes, G. swynnertoni*) mainly transmit *T. b. rhodesiense*. *G. fuscipes* and *G. tachinoides* can transmit both subspecies.

Transmission: By tsetse fly bite (day biters); blood transfusion, and congenital.

Cycle: The parasite is ingested by a tsetse fly during feeding on an infected host, and enters the salivary glands after 12–30 days, and can be transmitted to new susceptible hosts during the life of the fly (3 months). There is no vertical transmission in the fly.

Incubation period: 3 days to a few weeks for *T. b. rhodesiense*, several months to years for *T. b. gambiense*.

Clinical findings: A papule at the bite site develops into a painful chancre (mainly *T.b. rhodesiense*), with fever, severe headache, lympadenopathy, insomnia and progresses to variable neurological symptoms including a disrupted sleep cycle, confusion, seizures, and, if left untreated, eventually death.

Diagnostic tests: Detection of trypanosomes in blood, lymph, or CSF after concentration; IgM ELISA, IFA, PCR. A card agglutination trypanosomiasis test (CATT) is available for *T. b. gambiense* but not *T. b. rhodesiense*.

Therapy: Early stage disease: suramin for *T. b. rhodesiense*, pentamidine for *T. b. gambiense*; Late stage disease: melarsoprol for both forms; eflornithine with or without nifurtimox for gambiense. These drugs can cause SAEs.

Prevention: Treat patients to reduce the *T. b. gambiense* reservoir, and cattle to reduce the *T. b. rhodesiense* reservoir; screen blood donations; vector control: fly traps, insecticide-treated screens, ground and aerial spraying, release of sterile male tsetse flies.

Epidemiology: WHO estimates that 50,000 to 70,000 people are infected each year, with about 60 million people at risk in 36 countries. The disease distribution is limited by the range of the tsetse fly vector. Cases outside the tsetse fly distribution are likely imported. The disease distribution is patchy, with discrete foci and little to no disease between these foci. It is a disease of poverty and mainly occurs in remote rural areas. African trypanosomiasis was close to eradication through a variety of control programs, a loosening of these control programs caused the disease to reemerge in the 1980s. However, recent disease control programs are reversing this trend. The chronic *gambiense* form in West and Central Africa accounts for 95% of cases and is seperated from *rhodesiense* by the Great Rift Valley. Uganda is the sole country reporting both forms, with *rhodesiense* in the south and *gambiense* in the northwest.

Map sources: The African Trypanosomiasis map was made with data obtained from P.P. Simarro et al. (2010). The tstetse fly distribution data is based on statistical distribution models produced by the Environmental Research Group Oxford, available at: www.fao.org/ag/againfo/programmes/en/paat/maps.html.

Key references

Aksoy S (2011) Sleeping sickness elimination in sight. *PloS Negl Trop Dis* **5**(2):e1008.

Food and Agriculture Organization (2000) *Consultant's Report; Predicted Distributions of Tsetse Fly in Africa*. Rome, Italy.

Simarro PP, et al. (2008) Eliminating human African trypanosomiasis: where do we start and what comes next? *PLoS Med* **5**(2):e55.

Simarro PP, et al. (2010) The Atlas of Human African Trypanosomiasis. *Int J Health Geogr* **9**:57.

Simarro PP, et al. (2011) The human African trypanosomiasis control and surveillance program of the World Health Organization 2000–2009. *PLoS Negl Trop Dis* **5**(2):e1007.

World Health Organization (2011) African trypanosomiasis (sleeping sickness) fact sheet: www.who.int/trypanosomiasis_african/en/.

Atlas of Human Infectious Diseases, First Edition. Heiman F.L. Wertheim, Peter Horby and John P. Woodall.
© 2012 Blackwell Publishing Ltd. Published 2012 by Blackwell Publishing Ltd.

Trypanosomiasis, American

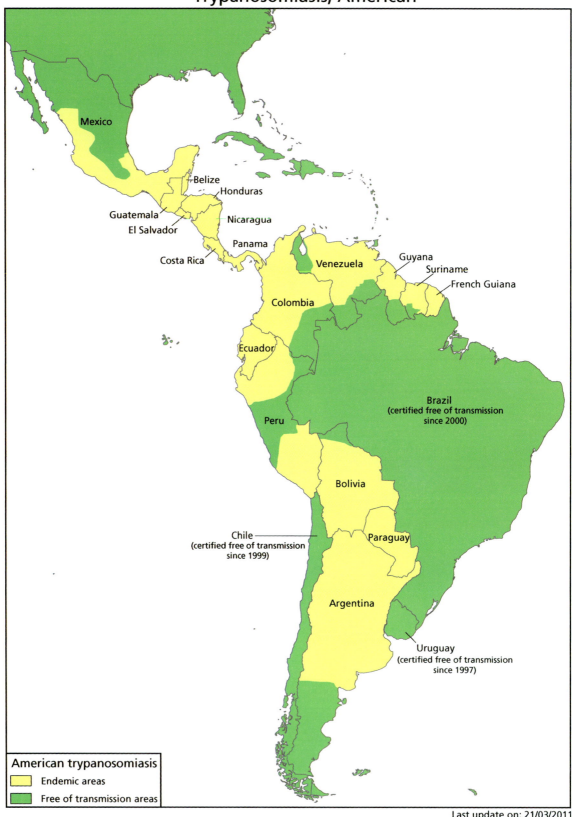

Mexico

Belize
Honduras
Guatemala
Nicaragua
El Salvador
Panama
Costa Rica
Venezuela
Guyana
Suriname
French Guiana
Colombia
Ecuador
Brazil
(certified free of transmission
since 2000)
Peru
Bolivia
Chile
(certified free of transmission
since 1999)
Paraguay
Argentina
Uruguay
(certified free of transmission
since 1997)

American trypanosomiasis
Endemic areas
Free of transmission areas

Last update on: 21/03/2011

Disease: **Trypanosomiasis, American**

Classification: ICD-9 086.2; ICD-10 B57

Synonyms: Chagas disease.

Agent: *Trypanosoma cruzi*, a protozoan, with a flagellate form in the bloodstream and an intracellular form without flagellum.

Reservoir: Humans and a wide variety of domestic and wild mammals, especially dogs, cats, guinea-pigs, rodents, and opossums.

Vector: Blood feeding reduviid bugs of the genera *Triatoma, Rhodnius,* and *Panstrongylus.* The most common vector in south America is *Triatoma infestans.* The vector lives up to 2 years.

Transmission: The vector defecates during feeding, and the infected feces are rubbed into the bite wound or conjunctivae, mucous membranes, or abraded skin; blood transfusion, organ transplant and shared needles. Congenital infection occurs in 2–8% of infected pregnancies. Oral transmission occurs by eating or drinking contaminated food or drink.

Cycle: 10–30 days in the vector after first infected meal, then 5–42 days in the reservoir host.

Incubation period: 5–14 days after infected bite, 30–40 days after infected blood transfusion.

Clinical findings: Most infections produce few or no symptoms. Acute symptoms include variable fever, lymphadenopathy, malaise, and hepatosplenomegaly. The entry site may be inflamed for up to 8 weeks, and a diagnostic unilateral bipalpebral edema (Romana's sign) appears in a few cases. After a latent period which may last 10–30 years, chronic irreversible sequelae occur in 20–30% of cases: myocardial lesions with arrhythmia, often fatal, and lesions of the esophagus, colon, and peripheral nervous system. Variations in clinical presentations can be related to the strain involved. Group I *T. cruzi*, rare north of the Amazon region, produce cardiac but not digestive tract lesions. Group II *T. cruzi* can produce both cardiac and digestive tract lesions. AIDS patients may develop meningoencephalopathy. CFR from encephalomyelitis or cardiac failure among untreated symptomatic patients is 5–10%.

Diagnostic tests: Direct examination of blood smear (low sensitivity), PCR, serology (indirect immunofluorescence, indirect hemagglutination). Serology can give false positive results. Culture takes weeks.

Therapy: Benznidazole, pentamidine, melarsoprol, eflornithine, suramin, and nifurtimox are effective in acute cases; melarprosol and eflornithine can have SAEs. Patients need to be followed up for 1–2 years.

Prevention: Application of residual insecticides or insecticidal paint inside dwellings, use of insecticide-treated bed nets, screening of blood and organ donors from infected areas. Application of these methods has eradicated intradomiciliary transmission from Uruguay (1997), Chile (1999), Guatemala (2005), Brazil (2006), the eastern region of Paraguay, and five of the endemic provinces of Argentina. Honduras and Nicaragua are awaiting certification of eradication. Only the food-borne risk remains in those areas.

Epidemiology: An estimated 7.6 million people are infected with *T. cruzi* and 75 million are at risk in Mexico, Central and South America, determined by the range of the vector. Originally American trypanosomiasis was a disease of agricultural workers (mainly adult men) living in rural areas in poor housing conditions. In urban areas transmission is mainly via blood transfusion, and occasionally via ingestion of contaminated sugarcane juice or palm fruit juice. Control programs between 1990 and 2006 resulted in the estimated annual number of deaths falling from more than 45,000 to 12,500, and the incidence of new cases from an estimated 700,000 to 41,200. Chronic cases are diagnosed in non-endemic countries in immigrants. In the USA ±300,000 immigrants have Chagas disease, and an estimated 30,000 cases of Chagas cardiomyopathy annually.

Map sources: The American Trypanosomiasis map was modified from P.D. Marsden (1997) and updated with data from A. Moncayo et al. (2009) and medical literature.

Key references

Marsden PD (1997) The control of Latin American trypanosomiasis. *Rev Soc Brasil Med Trop* **30**(6):521–527.

Moncayo A, et al. (2009) Current epidemiological trends for Chagas disease in Latin America. *Mem Inst Oswaldo Cruz* **104** (Suppl. I):17–30.

Prata A (2001) Clinical and epidemiological aspects of Chagas disease. *Lancet Inf Dis* **1**(2):92–100.

Atlas of Human Infectious Diseases, First Edition. Heiman F.L. Wertheim, Peter Horby and John P. Woodall.
© 2012 Blackwell Publishing Ltd. Published 2012 by Blackwell Publishing Ltd.

Viral Infections

Avian Influenza A/H5N1

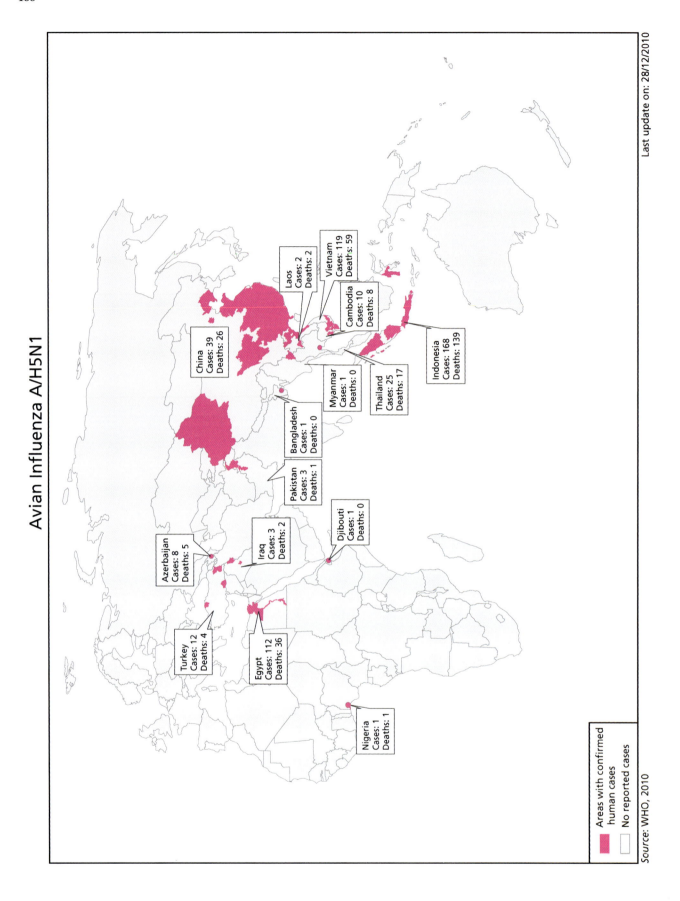

Laos
Cases: 2
Deaths: 2

Vietnam
Cases: 119
Deaths: 59

Cambodia
Cases: 10
Deaths: 8

China
Cases: 39
Deaths: 26

Myanmar
Cases: 1
Deaths: 0

Thailand
Cases: 25
Deaths: 17

Indonesia
Cases: 168
Deaths: 139

Bangladesh
Cases: 1
Deaths: 0

Pakistan
Cases: 3
Deaths: 1

Djibouti
Cases: 1
Deaths: 0

Azerbaijan
Cases: 8
Deaths: 5

Iraq
Cases: 3
Deaths: 2

Turkey
Cases: 12
Deaths: 4

Egypt
Cases: 112
Deaths: 36

Nigeria
Cases: 1
Deaths: 1

Last update on: 28/12/2010

Areas with confirmed human cases

No reported cases

Source: WHO, 2010

Disease: Avian Influenza (A/H5N1)

Classification: ICD-9 488.01; ICD-10 J09.0

Synonyms: Bird flu, avian influenza, highly pathogenic avian influenza, H5N1.

Agent: Influenza A subtype H5N1, a RNA virus, family Orthomyxoviridae. Avian influenza H5N1 occurs in two forms, a virulent form known as highly pathogenic avian influenza H5N1 (HPAI H5N1) and a milder form known as 'low pathogenic' (LPAI H5N1). H5N1 viruses have diverged into geographically distinct strains (genetic clades).

Reservoir: LPAI viruses naturally circulate in wild birds, principally waterfowl and gulls, in which they generally cause no symptoms. LPAI viruses are transmitted to terrestrial poultry (chickens, turkeys). LPAI most likely evolved to HPAI in aquatic birds (ducks and geese). Transmission of HPAI into migratory birds can result in large die-offs.

Transmission: Direct contact with sick or dead poultry (most common) infected with HPAI, and possibly via inhalation of virus-laden particles or contact of contaminated material with the eyes or respiratory mucosa. Other postulated routes: ingestion of water contaminated with the feces of infected birds, consumption of undercooked products from infected birds. Often, however, the route of exposure is not clear. Limited person-to-person transmission of HPAI H5N1 is possible following prolonged close contact with an infected patient.

Incubation period: 3 days (range 2–9 days).

Clinical findings: Sudden onset fever and cough. Other early symptoms include: myalgia, headache, vomiting, diarrhea, nausea, and epigastric pain. The disease rapidly progresses to severe viral pneumonia. Patients may present with encephalitis or gastroenteritis. The CFR is around 60%.

Diagnostic tests: Virus detection by RT-PCR of respiratory specimens is recommended; virus culture requires a BSL-3 facility. Microneutralization assay is recommended to detect antibodies to A/H5N1. Rapid antigen tests are not recommended due to lack of sensitivity.

Therapy: Oseltamivir may improve survival, if given early after onset. Otherwise treatment is supportive.

Prevention: Prevention of exposure to the wild aquatic bird reservoir and domestic poultry (farm biosecurity). Surveillance for infected poultry flocks and culling of infected flocks (stamping out). Poultry workers and cullers must wear protective clothing. Education of poultry farmers and the general public to reduce high-risk exposures. Human cases must be isolated, close contacts monitored, and healthcare workers must wear personal protective equipment.

Epidemiology: Since the end of 2003 the A/H5N1 virus has spread globally, infecting poultry in over 60 countries and causing the loss of over 250 million poultry. In 2010 HPAI H5N1 remained entrenched in poultry in several Asian countries and Egypt. While migratory waterfowl plays a role in the long-distance spread of H5N1 (see Bird Migration map), the intensification of poultry farming and poorly regulated movement and trade in poultry is probably the most important factor in sustaining the current epizootic. HPAI H5N1 is highly contagious between birds and has a high fatality in most poultry species, making it an economically important disease. However, it is the risk to humans that has driven most of the control activities. Over 500 human cases have been detected in 15 countries. The concern remains that H5N1 may evolve or reassort with another influenza A virus to become either more transmissible from poultry to humans or transmissible from person to person.

Map sources: The Avian Influenza map was reproduced from WHO, available at: http://gamapserver.who.int/mapLibrary/ (accessed dec. 2010).

Key references

Abdel-Ghafar AN, et al. (2008) Virus update on avian influenza A (H5N1) virus infection in humans. *N Engl J Med* **358**(3):261–273.

Gambotto A, et al. (2008) Human infection with highly pathogenic H5N1 influenza virus. *Lancet* **371**(9622):1464–1475.

Food and Agriculture Organization (revised in 2007) *The Global Strategy for the Prevention and Control of H5N1 Highly Pathogenic Avian Influenza*. FAO/OIE Strategy document.

Peiris JSM, et al. (2007) Avian influenza vírus (H5N1): a threat to human health. *Clin Microb Rev* **20**:243–267.

Barmah Forest and Ross River Virus Disease

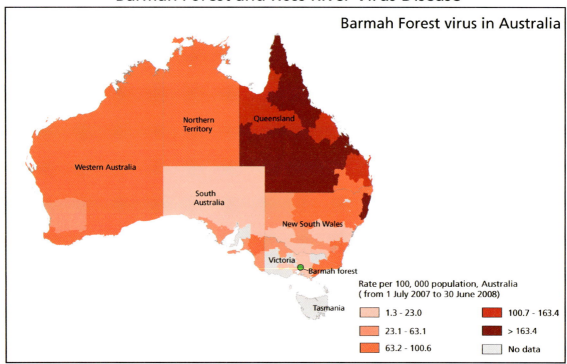

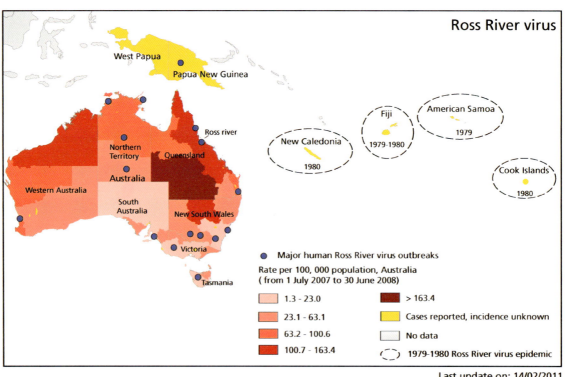

Disease: Barmah Forest & Ross River Virus Disease

Classification: ICD-9 066.3; ICD-10 R50.9 (Barmah Forest) and B33.1 (Ross River)

Syndromes and synonyms: Polyarthritis and rash, epidemic polyarthritis, Barmah Forest virus disease, and Ross River virus disease, Murweh virus disease.

Agent: Barmah Forest virus (BFV) and Ross River virus (RRV), enveloped RNA viruses, genus *Alphavirus* in the family Togaviridae. An early isolate of BF from Queensland was initially named Murweh virus. There are two topotypes of Ross River virus, from eastern and western Australia; a third, in northeastern Australia, has not been found since the mid-1970s.

Reservoir: Large marsupials, particularly kangaroos and wallabies.

Vector: Mainly *Ochlerotatus vigilax* and *Culex annulirostris*. *Aedes camptorhynchus*, *A. normanensis*, *A. notoscriptus*, and *Coquillettidia linealis* are vectors in some circumstances.

Transmission: Mosquito bite; transovarial transmission has been demonstrated in *Aedes vigilax*. There is no direct person-to-person transmission.

Cycle: Viremic reservoir host to mosquito during feeding, then after an extrinsic cycle of a few days, the virus is transmitted to a new reservoir host during feeding.

Incubation period: 3–12 days (usually 7–9).

Clinical findings: Self-limiting disease. Sudden onset of joint pain, fatigue, marked arthralgia and myalgia in more than 40%, stiff and swollen joints in 60–85% of cases; anorexia, headache, back pain, photophobia, sore throat, lethargy, and lymphadenopathy also occur, with fever and a maculopapular rash, usually on the trunk and limbs but also on palms and soles, in 50% of cases. Relapses occur; joint pains and swelling may relapse for as long as 6 years. Patients eventually recover completely.

Diagnostic tests: Viral RNA dection in blood by RT-PCR; serology (IgM ELISA; four-fold increase in IgG); virus isolation is insensitive.

Therapy: Supportive, there is no specific treatment

Prevention: Anti-mosquito measures: light-colored clothing with long sleeves mosquito repellents containing DEET on exposed skin, avoid as much as possible outdoor activities at dawn and dusk, when mosquitoes are most active, and removal of mosquito-breeding sites from around the home.

Epidemiology: There are only about 5,000 cases of RRV and usually only a few hundred cases of BFV annually. Peak incidence is in the 30–40 year age group, the disease is rare in children. RRV disease is the most common arboviral disease in Australia, accounting for about 90% of cases, often occurring in mixed epidemics with BFV disease on mainland Australia (to which BFV is restricted). Most BFV cases occur in Queensland and are only sporadic. RRV cases have been reported from the island of New Guinea and caused epidemics in Pacific islands in 1979–1980. Transmission occurs year-round, especially in coastal northern and northeastern Australia, but is more intense during the mosquito season in most of the country. Birds are presumed to be involved in spread around Australia; a viremic tourist from Australia is believed to have introduced the eastern topotype of RRV to the Pacific islands. Detailed epidemiological data is available on line at: http://www9.health.gov.au/cda/source/cda-index.cfm.

Map sources: The Barmah Forest and Ross River Virus disease map was made with data obtained from the Australian Government, Department of Health and Ageing, available at: www.health.gov.au/internet/main/publishing.nsf/Content/cdi3202.

Key references

Harley D, et al. (2001) Ross River virus transmission, infection, and disease: a cross-disciplinary review. *Clin Microbiol Rev* **14**(4):909–932.

Mackenzie JS (2001) in Service MW (ed.) *The Encyclopedia of Arthropod-Transmitted Infections*. CAB International, pp. 67–69.

Atlas of Human Infectious Diseases, First Edition. Heiman F.L. Wertheim, Peter Horby and John P. Woodall.
© 2012 Blackwell Publishing Ltd. Published 2012 by Blackwell Publishing Ltd.

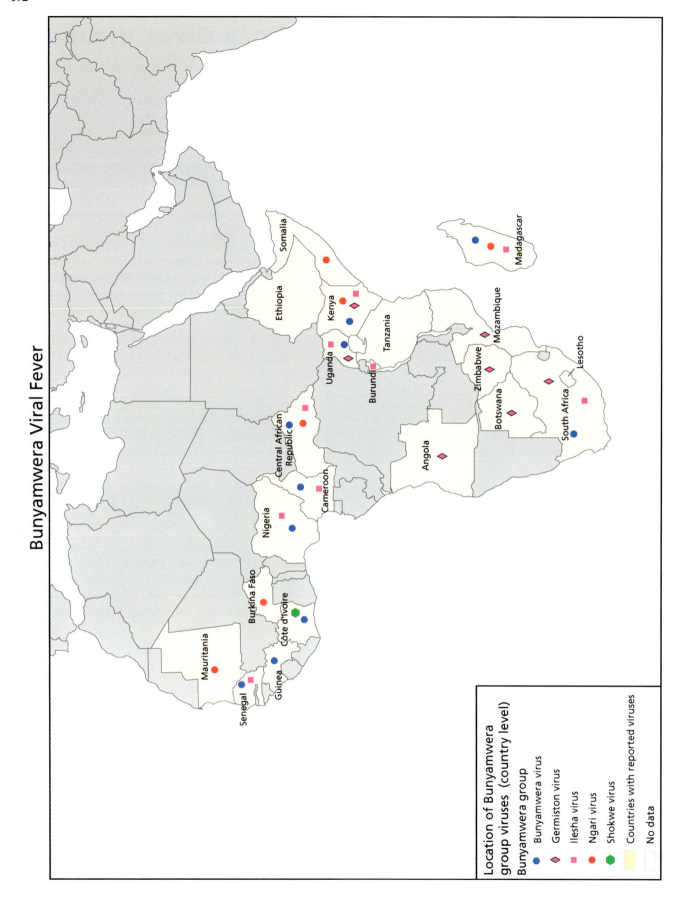

Bunyamwera Viral Fever

Location of Bunyamwera
group viruses (country level)
Bunyamwera group

- Bunyamwera virus
- Germiston virus
- Ilesha virus
- Ngari virus
- Shokwe virus
- Countries with reported viruses
- No data

Disease: **Bunyamwera Viral Fever**

Classification: ICD-9 066.3; ICD-10 A92.8

Syndromes and synonyms: Bunyamwera encephalitis, Bunyamwera viral disease, Cache Valley encephalitis.

Agent: Bunyamwera group viruses are enveloped, single-stranded, RNA viruses genus *Orthobunyavirus* of the family Bunyaviridae (see also Bunyavirus Group C map). Bunyamwera group viruses that can cause human disease in Africa are: Bunyamwera virus (BUNV), Germiston virus (GERV), Ilesha virus (ILEV), Ngari virus (NRIV), and Shokwe virus. Cache Valley complex viruses (CVV) have been isolated from human cases in North America, but are not shown on this map.

Reservoir: Not completely understood; most Bunyamwera viruses are likely maintained in nature involving a transmission cycle with various small mammals (mainly wild rodents) as amplifying hosts and mosquitoes. African rodents replicate BUNV and develop viremia. Livestock (goats, sheep, cattle), horses and rodents are hosts for GERV as shown by seroprevalence studies. Amplifying hosts for CVV are mainly large mammals (caribou, deer, horses, sheep).

Vector: Many species of mosquitoes of the genera *Aedes*, *Mansonia*, *Culex*, and *Anopheles*.

Transmission: By mosquito bite.

Cycle: The mosquito becomes infected when feeding on a viremic vertebrate host. The virus crosses the mosquito gut wall and replicates in the organs of the mosquito. After several days, the virus reaches the salivary glands and is injected into the next host during feeding.

Incubation period: Estimated at less than 2 weeks.

Clinical findings: Sudden onset fever, frontal headache, backache, diarrhea and a rash; usually resolves without sequelae; fatalities are rare and the result of hemorrhage or meningoencephalitis. ILEV and NRIV can cause hemorrhagic fever outbreaks. CVV rarely causes encephalitis, with only one fatal case reported in the USA in 1995.

Diagnostic tests: Several serologic tests are available. Virus can be isolated or RNA detected in acute blood by RT-PCR.

Therapy: Supportive; there is no specific therapy.

Prevention: Anti-mosquito precautions.

Epidemiology: African Bunyamwera viruses known to cause human disease circulate in Sub-Saharan Africa. Virus transmission peaks in the rainy season when mosquitoes are abundant. All age groups can be infected, though BUNV mainly affects children. BUNV is particularly active in the riverine forests in Nigeria and CAR. 100% of adults living in tropical rainforest of the DRC are seropositive. Neutralizing antibody rates of over 50% for ILEV have been found in people in savannah areas of Nigeria. Lower seroprevalences of ILEV are found in rainforests. GERV is endemic in southern African countries. To date, GERV has not been reported to be responsible for any major human disease outbreaks, and is therefore considered of minor public health importance.

Map source: The Bunyamwera Viral Fever map was made by geocoding human cases reported in the medical literature up to 2010 and the CDC Arbovirus Catalog, available at: http://wwwn.cdc.gov/arbocat/index.asp

Key references

Bouloy M (2001) Bunyamwera virus. In Service MW (ed.) *The Encyclopedia of Arthropod-transmitted Infections*. CAB International, pp. 94–97.

Gavrilovskaya I (2001) Issyk-Kul virus disease. In Service MW (ed.) *Encyclopedia of Arthropod-Transmitted Infections*. CAB International, pp. 231–234.

Gerrard SR (2004) Ngari virus is a Bunyamwera virus reassortant that can be associated with large outbreaks of hemorrhagic fever in Africa. *J Virol* **78**(16):8922–8926.

Grimstad PR (2001) Cache Valley virus. In Service MW (ed.) *The Encyclopedia of Arthropod-transmitted Infections*. CAB International, pp. 101–104.

Morvan JM (1994) Ilesha virus: a new aetiological agent of haemorrhagic fever in Madagascar. *Trans R Soc Trop Med Hyg* **88**:205.

Atlas of Human Infectious Diseases, First Edition. Heiman F.L. Wertheim, Peter Horby and John P. Woodall.
© 2012 Blackwell Publishing Ltd. Published 2012 by Blackwell Publishing Ltd.

Bunyavirus Group C Disease

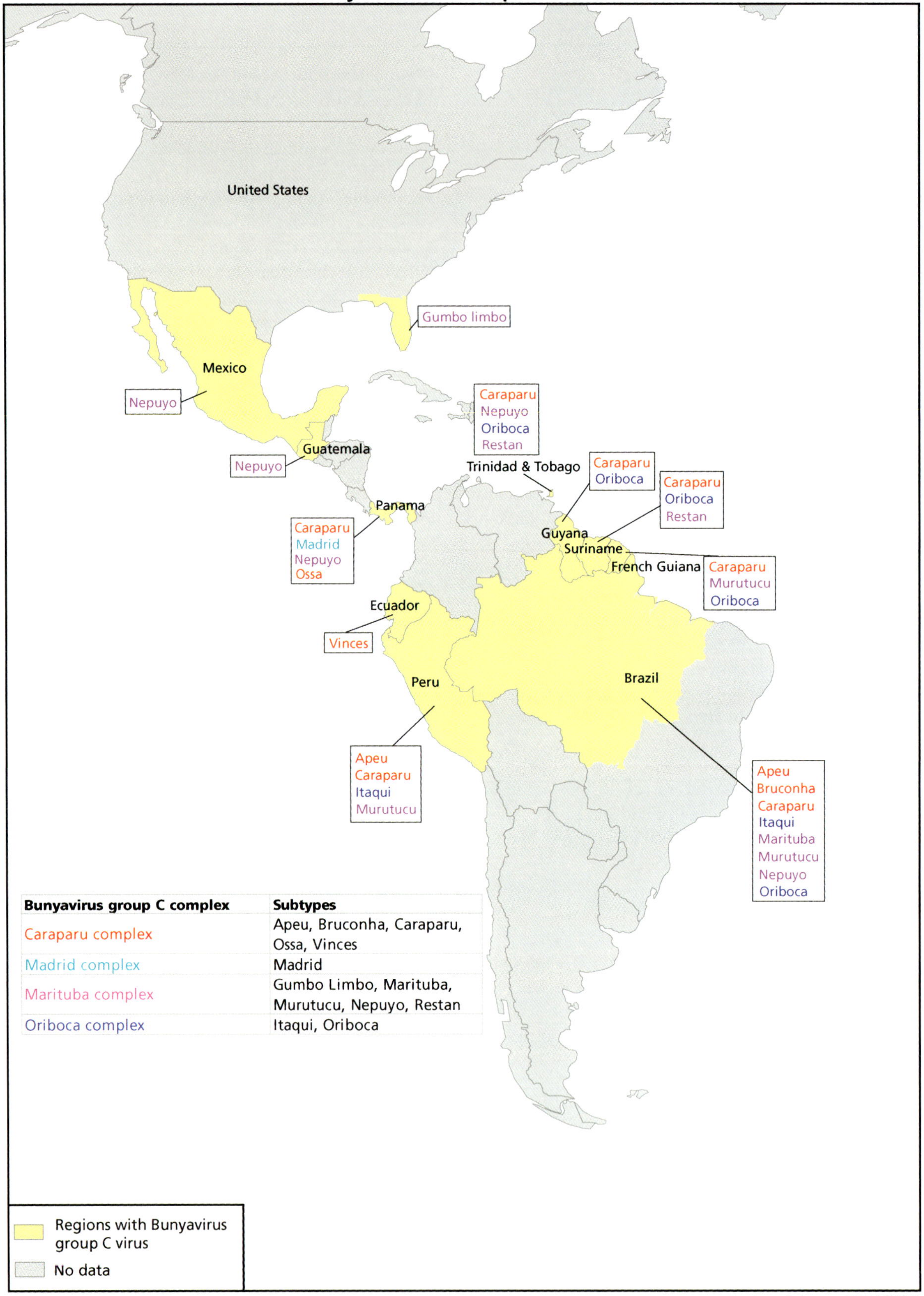

United States

Gumbo limbo

Mexico

Nepuyo

Guatemala

Nepuyo

Caraparu
Nepuyo
Oriboca
Restan

Trinidad & Tobago

Caraparu
Oriboca

Caraparu
Oriboca
Restan

Panama

Caraparu
Madrid
Nepuyo
Ossa

Guyana

Suriname

French Guiana

Caraparu
Murutucu
Oriboca

Ecuador

Vinces

Peru

Brazil

Apeu
Caraparu
Itaqui
Murutucu

Apeu
Bruconha
Caraparu
Itaqui
Marituba
Murutucu
Nepuyo
Oriboca

Bunyavirus group C complex	Subtypes
Caraparu complex	Apeu, Bruconha, Caraparu, Ossa, Vinces
Madrid complex	Madrid
Marituba complex	Gumbo Limbo, Marituba, Murutucu, Nepuyo, Restan
Oriboca complex	Itaqui, Oriboca

Regions with Bunyavirus group C virus

No data

Last update on: 16/11/2010

Disease: Bunyavirus Group C Disease

Classification: ICD-9 066.3; ICD-10 A92.8

Synonyms: None.

Agent: Spherical, enveloped orthobunyaviruses with single-stranded, negative-sense, tripartite RNA genomes, with considerable recognized reassortment. The name derives from the original classification of arthropod-borne viruses in to A, B and C groups. Group C viruses can be divided into four complexes: (1) Caraparu complex [Apeu virus (APEUV), Bruconha virus (BRCV), Caraparu virus (CARV), Ossa virus (OSSAV), and Vinces virus (VINV)]; (2) Madrid virus (MADV); (3) Marituba complex viruses [Gumbo Limbo virus (GLV), Marituba virus (MTBV), Murutucu virus (MURV), Nepuyo virus (NEPV), Restan virus (RESV)], and (4) Oriboca complex viruses [Itaqui (ITQV), Oriboca viruses (ORIV)].

Reservoir: Forest rodents, marsupials, and bats.

Vector: Mosquitoes (*Aedes* and *Culex* spp.).

Transmission: By mosquito bite. There is no direct person-to-person transmission.

Cycle: Mosquito-host-mosquito. The mosquito becomes infected when feeding on a viremic reservoir host. Depending on ambient temperature, the virus reaches the salivary glands and is transmitted by feeding on the next host in several days.

Incubation period: 3–12 days.

Clinical findings: Dengue-like fever with headache, malaise, arthralgia or myalgia for about 2 to 5 days; occasionally nausea and vomiting, lower limb weakness, conjunctivitis, photophobia and a rash. The fever resolves in a few days; the disease is non-fatal.

Diagnostic tests: IgM capture or IgG ELISAs is most commonly used on paired acute and convalescent sera. Virus isolation in suckling mice or cell culture and identified by RT-PCR.

Therapy: Self-limiting disease.

Prevention: Standard anti-mosquito precautions. There is no vaccine available.

Epidemiology: There is little known about the epidemiology of these viruses. Group C viruses are geograpically limited to the tropical and subtropical areas of the Americas, and were first described in the Brazilian Amazon in the 1950s. Studies show that these viruses circulate in a compact ecosystem in which co-infection with more than one virus is possible in reservoir hosts, leading to genetic reassortment. Genetic analysis shows evidence of intense traffic of these viruses in the Americas. Nepuyo virus has the widest distribution reported, from Mexico to Brazil. There is no sex or age preference for infection. Inapparent and mild infections are common, overt disease is mostly seen in children residing in endemic areas.

Map source: The Bunyavirus Group C Disease map was made by showing which bunyavirus group C virus is reported by country, according to the medical literature up to 2010.

Key reference

Nunes MRT, et al. (2005) Molecular epidemiology of group C viruses (Bunyaviridae: *Orthobunyavirus*) isolated in the Americas. *J Virol* **79**(16):10561–10570.

Atlas of Human Infectious Diseases, First Edition. Heiman F.L. Wertheim, Peter Horby and John P. Woodall.
© 2012 Blackwell Publishing Ltd. Published 2012 by Blackwell Publishing Ltd.

196

California Group Virus Disease

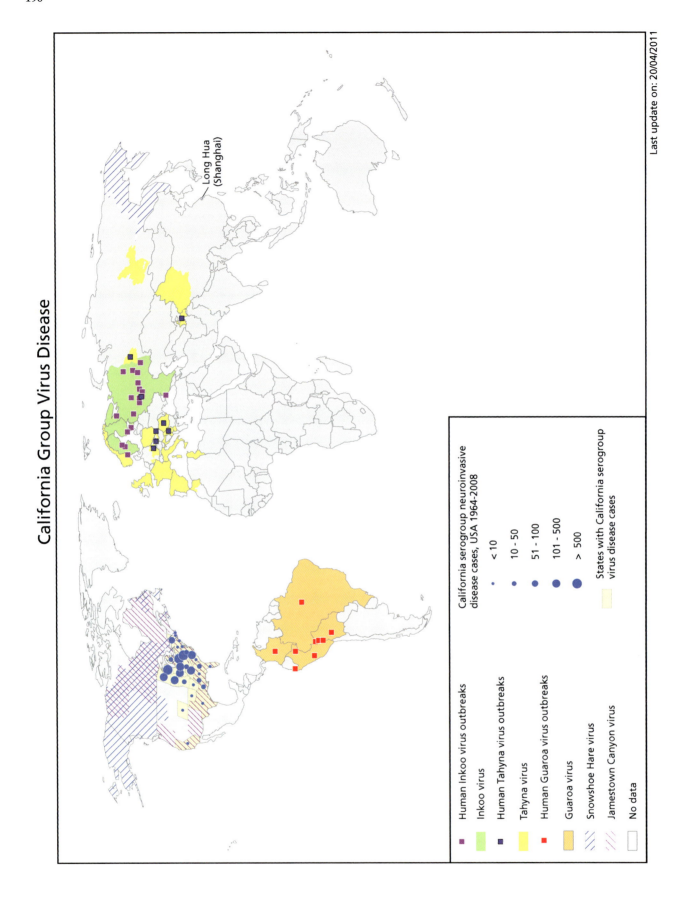

Last update on: 20/04/2011

Disease: California Group Virus Disease

Classification: ICD-9 062.5; ICD-10 A83.5

Syndromes and synonyms: California encephalitis, Jamestown Canyon encephalitis, La Crosse encephalitis.

Agents: Spherical, enveloped, negative sense RNA viruses forming a subgroup of the Bunyaviridae family. In the Americas, human pathogens belonging to the group are Guaroa virus (GROV), Jamestown Canyon virus (JCV), LaCrosse virus (LACV), and snowshoe hare virus (SSHV). Those reported to cause human disease in Europe or Asia are Inkoo virus (INKV), Tahyna virus (TAHV), and SSHV.

Reservoir: Small wild mammals such as rodents, snowshoe hares, deer and vector mosquitoes (venereal and transovarian transmission occur). Dayfeeding chipmunks and squirrels are the principal amplifying hosts of LACV, as the main vector (*Aedes triseriatus*) only bites in daytime. For this reason, night-feeding small mammals are rarely infected with LACV. The white-tailed deer is the main amplifying host for JCV (horses can also be an amplifying host). Snowshoe hares and the arctic ground squirrel are the amplifying hosts of SSHV.

Vector: Mosquitoes, primarily *Aedes* and *Ochlerotatus* spp., secondarily *Anopheles* spp. *Ae. triseriatus* (eastern treehole mosquito) is the most important vector of LACV in the USA. LACV is abundant in forests with oak trees (basal holes are important breeding sites) and hickory hardwoods drained by rapid streams. Different species of cold-tolerant mosquitoes serve as vectors for JCV and SSHV.

Transmission: By mosquito bite.

Cycle: Mosquito–reservoir host–mosquito. The mosquito becomes infected during feeding on a viremic reservoir host; once the virus reaches the salivary glands it can be transmitted during feeding to the next reservoir host.

Incubation period: Usually 5–15 days.

Clinical findings: Fever, headache, vomiting, sometimes progressing to acute CNS and respiratory involvement, with recurrent seizures in 25% of CNS cases. INKV is associated with severe illness and chronic neurologic disease in Russia.

Diagnostic tests: Serology (IgM and IgG ELISA) on acute and convalescent sera; cross-reactivity exists leading to misidentification. RT-PCR has been used to test human brain tissue samples.

Therapy: Supportive, there is no specific treatment. Ribavirin may limit the severity and improve the prognosis of LACV infections. Anticonvulsant medication in those with seizures.

Prevention: As mosquito vectors and wildlife reservoirs are widespread, control is not feasible; personal anti-mosquito measures; eliminating potential breeding sites (e.g. old tires) and filling of basal tree-holes with concrete.

Epidemiology: The California group viruses are widely distributed over all types of terrain. Each has its preferred vector mosquito species and host, for instance snowshoe hare for SSHV. LACV is the primary cause of arboviral encephalitis in children in the USA. Most LACV infections occur in those residing close to woodland breeding sites of *Ae. triseriatus* from July to September. Boys are more often affected with LACV, as they more often play in the woods. JCV is most commonly found around the Great Lakes in USA and Canada. The JCV vectors prefer hilly woodlands where they breed in ponds from April to June. SSHV, has a different ecosystem: (sub)arctic forests and tundras in Canada and Siberia. SSHV has been detected in China. SSHV transmission occurs during the arctic summer from May to August, and mainly affects children (<10 years), especially boys. Lumbo virus is a strain of TAHV isolated from mosquitoes in Mozambique (Africa), but no human cases have been diagnosed there.

Map sources: The California Group Virus Disease map was made by geolocating human outbreaks reported in the medical literature up to 2010. La Crosse virus epidemiology data was obtained from the CDC, available at: www.cdc.gov/lac/tech/epi.html (accessed Dec 2010).

Key references

Beaty BJ (2001) La Crosse virus. In Service MW (ed.) *The Encyclopedia of Arthropod-transmitted Infections*. CAB International, pp. 261–265.

Grimstad PR (2001) Jamestown Canyon virus. In Service MW (ed.) *The Encyclopedia of Arthropod-transmitted Infections*. CAB International, pp. 235–239.

Labuda M (2001) Tahyna virus. In Service MW (ed.) *The Encyclopedia of Arthropod-transmitted Infections*. CAB International, pp. 482–483.

Rust RS, et al. (1999) La Crosse and other forms of California encephalitis. *J Child Neurol* **14**(1):1–14.

Atlas of Human Infectious Diseases, First Edition. Heiman F.L. Wertheim, Peter Horby and John P. Woodall.
© 2012 Blackwell Publishing Ltd. Published 2012 by Blackwell Publishing Ltd.

Chikungunya Fever

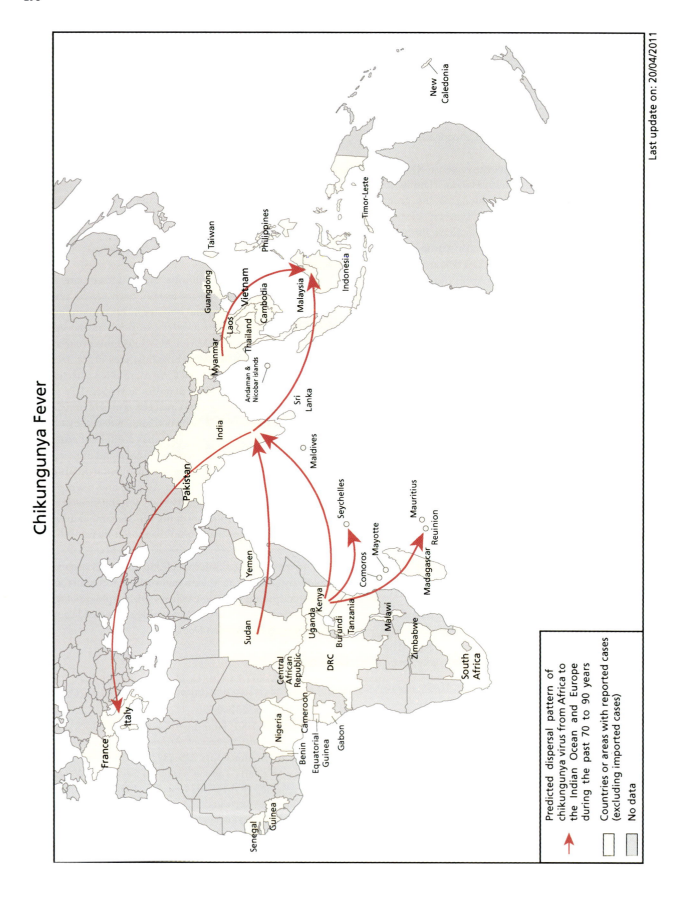

New Caledonia

Taiwan

Guangdong

Vietnam
Laos
Myanmar
Cambodia
Thailand
Malaysia

Philippines

Indonesia

Timor-Leste

Andaman &
Nicobar islands

Sri
Lanka

India

Maldives

Pakistan

Seychelles

Comoros
Mayotte

Mauritius
Reuinion

Yemen

Madagascar

Sudan

Kenya
Uganda
Burundi
Tanzania

Central
African
Republic

DRC

Malawi

Zimbabwe

South
Africa

Nigeria
Cameroon

Benin
Equatorial
Guinea
Gabon

Italy

France

Guinea

Senegal

Last update on: 20/04/2011

Predicted dispersal pattern of
chikungunya virus from Africa to
the Indian Ocean and Europe
during the past 70 to 90 years

Countries or areas with reported cases
(excluding imported cases)

No data

Disease: **Chikungunya Fever**

Classification: ICD-9 066.3; ICD-10 A92.0

Syndromes and synonyms: Chikungunya means 'that which bends up' in Makonde language, to describe the pain.

Agent: Chikungunya virus (CHIKV), an enveloped RNA virus, genus *Alphavirus* in the family Togaviridae. CHIKV belongs to the same antigenic complex as Mayaro, Ross River, and o'nyong-nyong viruses. Phylogenetic analysis suggests an African origin about 500 years ago, with spread to Asia within the last century.

Reservoir: Non-human primates in Africa and humans in Asia; Asian monkeys can be infected, but do not seem to constitute an important reservoir. During intra-epidemic periods, several vertebrates have been implicated as potential reservoirs.

Vector: In Africa, the principal vectors are the sylvan mosquitoes *Ae. furcifer* and *Ae. africanus*, *Ae. luteocephalus*, and *Ae. taylori*; in Asia, urban *Ae. aegypti*, *Ae. albopictus*, and various *Culex* species.

Transmission: By mosquito bite. Transmission from mother to neonate can occur in the intrapartum period; blood-borne transmission is possible.

Cycle: Humans are viremic at a titer high enough to infect mosquitoes for 3 to 7 days post illness onset. The virus travels from the mosquito gut to the salivary glands in 5–7 days, after which it can infect another human by bite.

Incubation period: 3–7 days (range 1–12 days).

Clinical findings: Sudden onset fever, chills, fatigue, transient maculopapular rash constant polyarthralgia/arthritis of small joints (hands, wrists, ankles, feet); leucopenia and mild thrombocytopenia. Neurological, cardiac, and hepatic complications rare . The acute stage in infants and young children can be atypical (epidermolysis, myocarditis, or encephalitis), but is rarely fatal. Infected neonates (mother-to-child transmission) are at a high risk of severe encephalopathy and death. Chronic inflammatory joint symptoms were observed in up to 50% of adult cases, and after 2 years in some outbreaks.

Diagnostic tests: Within 5 days of disease onset: RT-PCR on whole blood, virus isolation; After 5 days: IgM ELISA on serum; serological tests can cross-react.

Therapy: Supportive with pain management.

Prevention: Standard anti-mosquito precautions.

Epidemiology: Before 2004, CHIKV was considered a minor arboviral disease, but since then has spread globally, infecting millions of people. Most cases are symptomatic. CHIKV has been endemic in Africa for centuries, typically causing small epidemics in rural areas. CHIKV spread to Asia within the last 60 years producing urban outbreaks, similar to dengue fever, involving *Ae. egypti*. The global epidemic started since a mutation in the CHIKV E1 glyco-protein gene (*A226V*) occurred, that enhanced its infectivity and transmission by *Ae. albopictus*. The mutated CHIKV is succesful in spreading in tropical and temperate regions where *Ae. albopictus* is present. In 2005–2006 CHIKV spread from East Africa to virgin soil in the Indian Ocean Islands to produce epidemics affecting up to three-quarters of the population. Since 2006, CHIKV outbreaks with are reported from several (sub)tropical countries in the new world. CHIKV virus was imported into several European countries and caused a small outbreak with autochthonous transmission in northern Italy. CHIKV-viremic travelers can cause autochthonous transmission in previous CHIKV-free areas if *Ae. albopictus* or other competent mosquitoes are present.

Map sources: The Chikungunya Virus Disease map is made by showing regions with reported outbreaks reported to WHO, ProMED-mail, and the medical literature up to 2010. Data was also used from the CDC, available at: www.cdc.gov/ncidod/dvbid/Chikungunya/CH_GlobalMap.html, and De Lamballerie et al. (2008).

Key references

De Lamballerie X, et al. (2008) Chikungunya virus adapts to tiger mosquito via evolutionary convergence: a sign of things to come? *Virol J* **5**:33.

Simon F, et al. (2011) Chikungunya virus infection. *Curr Infect Dis Rep.* **13**(3):218–228.

Volk SM, et al. (2010) Genome-scale phylogenetic analyses of chikungunya virus reveal independent emergences of recent epidemics and various evolutionary rates. *J Virol* **84**(13):6497–6504.

Colorado Tick Fever

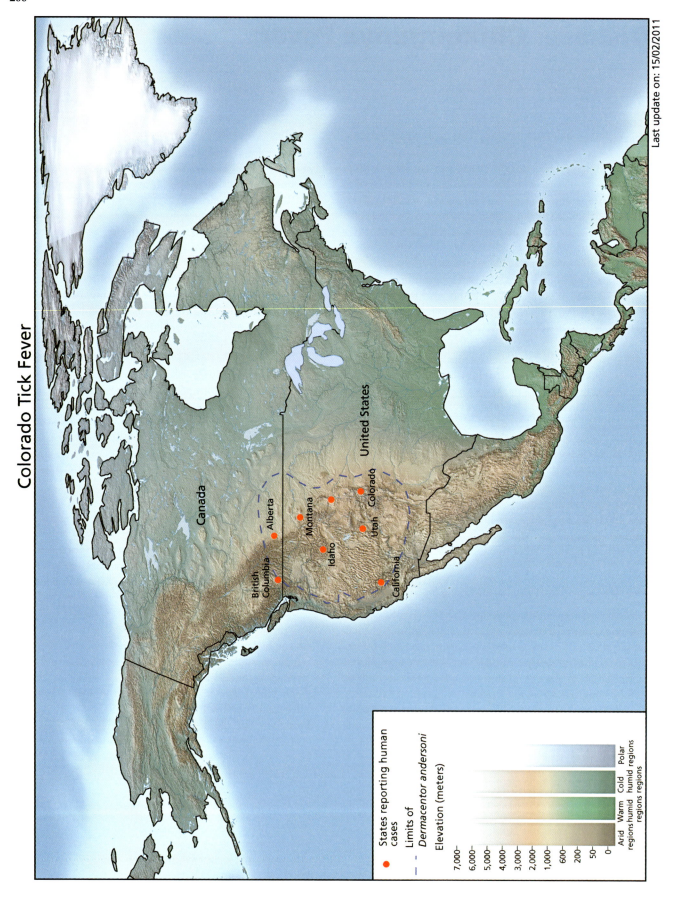

Canada

United States

British Columbia

Alberta

Montana

Idaho

Utah

Colorado

California

States reporting human cases

Limits of *Dermacentor andersoni*

Elevation (meters)

7,000—
6,000—
5,000—
4,000—
3,000—
2,000—
1,000—
600—
200—
50—
0—

Arid regions

Warm humid regions

Cold humid regions

Polar regions

Disease: Colorado Tick Fever

Classification: ICD-9 066.1; ICD-10 A93.2

Syndromes and synonyms: None.

Agent: Colorado Tick Fever Virus (CTFV), a prototype virus of the genus *Coltivirus* of the family Reoviridae; a spherical, enveloped virus with a double-stranded RNA genome of 12 segments.

Reservoir: High altitude rodents, including ground squirrels and porcupines; ticks by trans-stadial transmission; possibly transovarial, but this is considered unlikely.

Vector: Ixodid wood tick (*Dermacentor andersoni*).

Transmission: By tick bite, blood transfusion; bone marrow for transplantation is routinely screened in endemic areas.

Cycle: The tick feeds on an infected host, the virus multiplies in the tick's midgut and spreads to the salivary glands, to be injected into another host at the next feed, where it infects erythrocytes. As the virus infects erythrocytes, it is partially protected from immune clearance, leading to prolonged viremia in both humans (up to 4 months) and rodents, favoring spread.

Incubation period: <1–19 days, average about 3–4 days, depending on the infecting dose. Viremia in humans may last for 4 months or more.

Clinical findings: Sudden onset of high fever (biphasic), chills, myalgia, arthralgia, severe headache, ocular pain, conjunctivitis, anorexia, nausea, and sometimes vomiting. Spleen and liver can be palpable, and pericarditis or myocarditis may be found. A few cases have a petechial or maculopapular rash. Prolonged convalescence may follow. Children may have a more severe syndrome with hemorrhagic manifestations, including a more pronounced rash, DIC, and GI bleeding; or CNS involvement including meningitis and encephalitis. Fatalities are rare.

Diagnostic tests: Serology (IgM ELISA, IFA of erythrocytes). Diagnosis is confirmed by a significant (>=4-fold) change in antibody titer between acute and convalescent sera. Virus isolation or RNA detection by RT-PCR from the blood or CSF.

Therapy: Supportive.

Prevention: Personal anti-tick precautions (appropriate clothing, acaricide, repellent). Vaccine production ceased in the 1970s and there is no possibility of vector control due to the habitat. Screening of bone marrow donors in endemic areas.

Epidemiology: Colorado tick fever is only present in North America (USA and Canada). In the USA, besides the states with human cases shown on the map, the virus has been isolated from ticks within the range of *D. andersoni*. The typical habitat of the tick and its rodent hosts is a south-facing slope above 1,500 meters with Ponderosa pine and shrubs on dry, rocky surfaces. Infection is seasonal, coinciding with the period of greatest tick activity in early summer. Human cases can be detected from March to September in the Rocky Mountain region, USA. Most human cases are males, aged 20–29 years, probably reflecting the frequency of outdoor activity in the mountains.

Map sources: The Colorado Tick Fever map was made with geolocating reported cases in the medical literature up to 2010.

Key references

Attoui H, et al. (2005) Coltiviruses and Seadornaviruses in North America, Europe, and Asia. *Emerg Infect Dis* **11**(11):1673–1679.

Brackney MM, et al. (2010) Epidemiology of Colorado tick fever in Montana, Utah, and Wyoming, 1995–2003. *Vector Borne Zoonotic Dis* **10**(4):381–385.

Calisher CH (1994) Medically important arboviruses of the United States and Canada. *Clin Microbiol Rev* **7**(1):89–116.

Calisher CH (2001) Colorado tick fever. In Service MW (ed.) *The Encyclopedia of Arthropod-Transmitted Infections*. CAB International, pp. 121–126.

Klasco R (2002) Colorado tick fever. *Med Clin North Am* **86**(2):435–440.

Atlas of Human Infectious Diseases, First Edition. Heiman F.L. Wertheim, Peter Horby and John P. Woodall.
© 2012 Blackwell Publishing Ltd. Published 2012 by Blackwell Publishing Ltd.

Crimean-Congo Hemorrhagic Fever

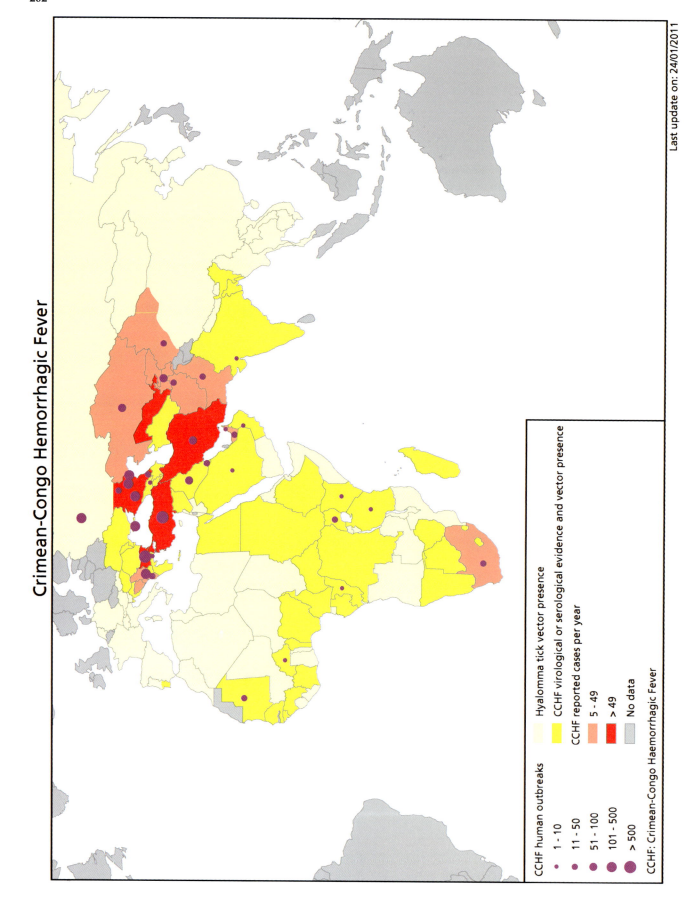

CCHF human outbreaks
- 1 - 10
- 11 - 50
- 51 - 100
- 101 - 500
- > 500

Hyalomma tick vector presence

CCHF virological or serological evidence and vector presence

CCHF reported cases per year
- 5 - 49
- > 49
- No data

CCHF: Crimean-Congo Haemorrhagic Fever

Last update on: 24/01/2011

Disease: Crimean–Congo Hemorrhagic Fever

Classification: ICD-9 065.0; ICD-10 A98.0

Synonyms: Congo fever, Congo–Crimean hemorrhagic fever, Central Asian hemorrhagic fever

Agent: Crimean-Congo hemorrhagic fever virus (CCHFV) is an enveloped, spherical virus with a tripartite, single-stranded, negative sense RNA genome, belonging to the genus *Nairovirus* in the family Bunyaviridae. It has 7 geno-types distinguished by the small (S) segment of the RNA.

Reservoir: Hares, hedgehogs, wild mice, livestock, ostriches. Since hard ticks overwinter and can pass the virus transova-rially, ticks also serve as reservoirs.

Vector: Hard ticks, principally *Hyalomma* spp., also *Boophilus* spp. and *Rhipicephalus* spp.

Transmission: By tick bite; larval ticks are carried on migrat-ing birds, which are refractory to the virus. The virus is also spread among veterinarians, farmers, shepherds, butchers, and slaughter-house workers by contact with the blood of infected livestock. Person-to-person spread is by contact with infectious body fluids of patients.

Cycle: Tick–vertebrate–tick, with humans as incidental hosts.

Incubation period: 1–12 days, usually 3–7.

Clinical findings: Sudden onset of fever (which may be biphasic), malaise, weakness, irritability, headache, severe pain in limbs and loins and marked anorexia; occasionally vomiting, abdominal pain, and diarrhea. Hemorrhage in oropharynx, nose, lungs, uterus, intestines; hematomas, echy-mosis, and petechiae; hematuria and albuminuria. In Russia, estimates are that only 1 in 6 cases is hemorrhagic. The CFR ranges from 2 to 80% in different countries.

Diagnostic tests: Virus isolation in cell culture; RT-PCR; antigen detection; serology by IgM ELISA. The virus is a BSL-4 agent.

Therapy: Supportive; intravenous ribavirin and convalescent human serum are recommended.

Prevention: Personal anti-tick precautions. An inactivated mouse-brain vaccine is in use in Russia and eastern Europe. Healthcare workers caring for CCHF patients are at risk and need to take proper barrier precautions.

Epidemiology: The disease is limited geographically to the range of the vector tick. *Hyalomma* spp. do not occur in the Americas and Oceania. Historically the tick does not appear above 50°N latitude, but possibly due to changes in climate and environment the tick and CCHFV outbreaks have occurred above this latitude. In the northern hemisphere, *H. marginatum* becomes more active by increasing tempera-tures during spring (April–May) and immature stages are active from May to September. The potential roles of migra-tory birds and the movement of livestock carrying ticks in the spread of the virus are unclear. CCHFV outbreaks mainly occur in those working in agricultural areas. About 90% of the cases in a recent outbreak in Turkey were farmers. Cases regularly had skin contact with livestock or other animals. Also outdoor activities (hiking, camping) in endemic areas are a risk factor. Countries on the map marked as having no data (western Sahara, Palestine, parts of the Arabian peninsula, Kashmir) are within the range of the vector tick and likely at risk for CCHFV outbreaks. CCHFV genotypes cluster geo-graphically, with exceptions: the Asia 1 genotype has been found in Madagascar, where it was possibly introduced by migrating birds, and Africa 1 in the Middle East, which may have been introduced with infected livestock.

Map sources: The Crimean–Congo Hemorrhagic Fever map was made with data on CCHF outbreaks between 1943 and 2010 obtained from ProMED mail, the medical literature and WHO, available at: www.who.int/csr/disease/.

Key references

Ergonul O, et al. (2006) Crimean–Congo haemorrhagic fever. *Lancet Infect Dis* **6**:203–214.

Leblebicioglu H, et al. (2010) Crimean–Congo haemorrhagic fever in Eurasia. *Int J Antimicrob Agents* **36**(Suppl. 1): S43–S46.

World Health Organization (2004) *The Vector-Borne Human Infections of Europe, their Distribution and Burden on Public Health.* Publication from the WHO Regional Office for Europe.

Atlas of Human Infectious Diseases, First Edition. Heiman F.L. Wertheim, Peter Horby and John P. Woodall.
© 2012 Blackwell Publishing Ltd. Published 2012 by Blackwell Publishing Ltd.

204

Dengue

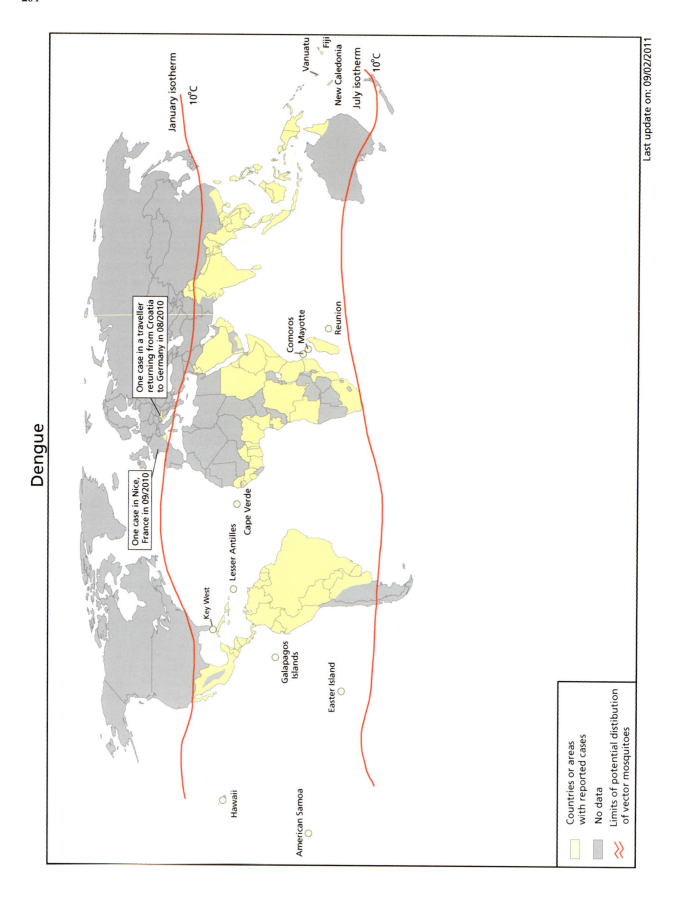

One case in a traveller returning from Croatia to Germany in 08/2010

One case in Nice, France in 09/2010

January isotherm
10°C

July isotherm
10°C

Vanuatu
Fiji
New Caledonia

Comoros
Mayotte
Reunion

Cape Verde

Lesser Antilles

Key West

Galapagos Islands

Easter Island

Hawaii

American Samoa

Countries or areas with reported cases

No data

Limits of potential distibution of vector mosquitoes

Disease: Dengue

Classification: Dengue fever (DF): ICD-9 061, ICD-10 A90; Dengue hemorrhagic fever/Dengue shock syndrome (DHF/DSS): ICD-9 065.4; ICD-10 A91.

Synonyms: Breakbone fever.

Agent: Dengue virus (DENV) is an enveloped RNA virus, genus *Flavivirus* in the family Flaviviridae. There are four antigenically related, but distinct, dengue virus serotypes (DEN-1, DEN-2, DEN-3, and DEN-4), all of which can cause DF/DHF.

Reservoir: Humans; forest monkeys in West Africa and Southeast Asia.

Vector: Most commonly, the urban container-breeding, day-biting mosquitoes *Aedes aegypti* and *Ae. albopictus*; in Polynesia, *Ae. scutellaris* complex spp.; in Malaysia, *Ae. nivaeus* complex spp., in West Africa, *Ae. furcifer-taylori* complex spp., and recently in Europe by *Ae. albopictus* (see *Aedes* map).

Transmission: By mosquito bite.

Cycle: Human–mosquito–human around housing; monkey–mosquito–monkey and monkey–mosquito–human in the forests of West Africa and Malaysia. Human viremia lasts 3–5 days since onset of symptoms; the mosquito can transmit 8–12 days after taking a viremic blood meal, depending on the ambient temperature.

Incubation period: 3–14 days (usually 4–7 days).

Clinical findings: Sudden onset of fever lasting 2–7 days, sometimes biphasic, severe headache, myalgia, arthralgia, retro-orbital pain, anorexia, nausea, vomiting and a maculopapular rash (not easily seen on dark skin). Most cases recover. Minor occurrence of petechiae, epistaxis, or gingival bleeding may be seen. Serious hemorrhagic manifestations, like a severe drop in blood platelets, indicate dengue hemorrhagic fever (DHF), that can progress to dengue shock syndrome (DSS) and death. Infection with any serotype results in lasting homologous immunity, but little cross-immunity to other serotypes. Cross-immunity may exacerbate, rather than diminish, disease severity when infected with a new serotype; DHF leading to DSS can occur as a secondary infection with a different serotype, but DHF/DSS has also been reported in primary infections. CFR for DHF is up to 20%, for untreated DSS up to 50%, and 1–2% if correctly treated.

Diagnostic tests: IgM capture ELISA; NS1 antigen test; RT-PCR of blood or tissue; virus isolation in mosquitoes or mosquito cell culture with identification by IFA.

Therapy: Supportive, including rehydration. Avoid aspirin because of potential hemorrhage.

Prevention: Removal of breeding sites in any type of container that holds water (e.g. vase, tire). Larviciding standing water, adulticiding with non-persistent insecticides. Personal protection with suitable clothing, mosquito repellents, nets, and screens.

Epidemiology: The global dengue distribution follows vector presence and introduction of the virus, and occurs basically between the 10 °C isotherms. Autochthonous dengue fever cases appeared in Europe for the first time in 2010, north of 10 °C isotherm and likely transmitted by *Ae. albopictus* (see *Aedes agypti* and *Aedes albopictus* map). There is strong seasonality, correlated with the rainy season, which produces a marked increase in vectors because more mosquito-breeding sites become available then. Two, 3 or all 4 serotypes may occur concurrently. DHF/DSS in many countries is most often seen in children suffering a secondary infection with a different serotype. Incidence rates of up to 3% have been seen in dengue naïve populations such as are found in some Pacific islands.

Map sources: The Dengue map was made with data obtained from the CDC and WHO websites, available at: http://gamapserver.who.int/ and www.cdc.gov/dengue/. Discrepancies were resolved by cross-checking with the medical literature. Recent autochthonous cases in Europe (north of 10 °C isotherm) were added to the map.

Key references

Guzman A, et al. (2010) Update on the global spread of dengue. *Int J Antimicrob Agents* **36**(Suppl. 1):S40–S42.

Jelinek T (2009) Trends in the epidemiology of dengue fever and their relevance for importation to Europe. *Euro Surveill* **14**(25):19250.

Kyle JL, et al. (2008) Global spread and persistence of dengue. *Ann Rev Microbiol* **62**:71–92.

Atlas of Human Infectious Diseases, First Edition. Heiman F.L. Wertheim, Peter Horby and John P. Woodall.
© 2012 Blackwell Publishing Ltd. Published 2012 by Blackwell Publishing Ltd.

206

Eastern Equine Encephalitis

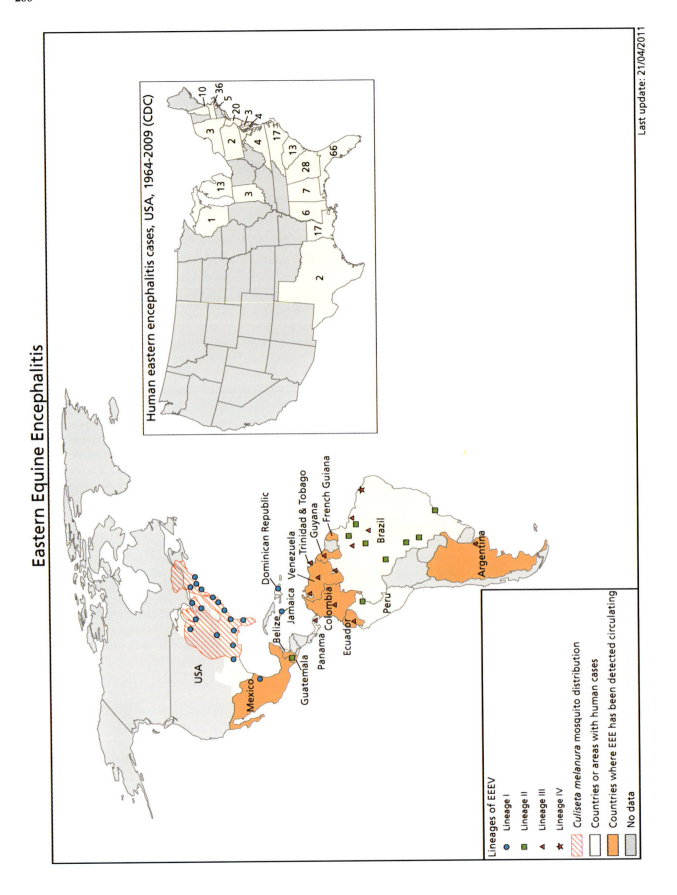

Human eastern encephalitis cases, USA, 1964-2009 (CDC)

Lineages of EEEV
- Lineage I
- Lineage II
- Lineage III
- Lineage IV

Culiseta melanura mosquito distribution

Countries or areas with human cases

Countries where EEE has been detected circulating

No data

Last update: 21/04/2011

Disease: Eastern Equine Encephalitis

Classification: ICD-9 062; ICD-10 A83.2

Synonyms: None.

Agent: Eastern equine encephalitis virus (EEEV) is an enveloped, single-stranded positive-sense RNA alphavirus, genus *Alphavirus* in the family Togaviridae, with four lineages: Group I is endemic in North America and the Caribbean and causes most human disease cases; the other three groups (IIA, IIB, and III) infrequently cause equine or human illness in Central and South America.

Reservoir: Principally wild birds in North America. Wild rodents, bats, reptiles, or amphibians may also be involved. Pheasants may serve as sentinels as they develop fatal disease. Chickens are more typically used as sentinels by detection of seroconversion.

Vector: Mosquitoes. In North America, *Culiseta melanura* bird-to-bird; *Aedes* or *Coquillettidia* spp. from bird to other vertebrates (including horses and humans). In South America, *Culex* spp.

Transmission: By mosquito bite. There is no direct person-to-person transmission.

Cycle: *Culiseta melanura*: bird to bird; *Aedes* or *Coquillettidia* spp.: from bird to other vertebrates (including horses and humans). Viremia lasts 2–5 days in birds, and the extrinsic cycle in mosquitoes lasts 2–3 days. Horses and humans are dead-end hosts because their viremia is generally not high enough to infect mosquitoes.

Incubation period: 4–10 days.

Clinical findings: Sudden onset of high fever, headache, chills, vomiting, myalgias, photophobia and dysthesias; 50–90% of apparent cases develop encephalitis. In the USA, one-third of encephalitis cases die and one-third of the survivors are moderately to severely disabled.

Diagnostic tests: IgM antibody detection in CSF (in serum may not be from the current infection), neutralization test on paired acute and convalescent sera; RT-PCR. Virus isolation takes time. IFA in necropsy brain tissue is definitive.

Therapy: Supportive, there is no specific treatment.

Prevention: Personal anti-mosquito precautions. Adulticide spraying is practiced in areas where horse cases appear. A human vaccine against only the North American strain is available for laboratory personnel.

Epidemiology: In the USA, an average of only 6 neuroinvasive cases of EEE are reported annually. The annual number of cases has declined in recent years. Incidence is similar among different age groups and ethnicities, but it is twice as high among men. Persons aged over 50 and under 15 are at greatest risk for developing severe disease. In North America, outbreaks occur during the mosquito season. In tropical South America transmission to horses is year-round, but human cases are rare. *Culiseta* breeds in swampy areas in woodland, transmitting the virus from marsh-nesting birds to horses kept in such areas; unvaccinated horses often die. Outbreaks in Mexico and islands of the Caribbean have all been due to the North American subtype, indicating spread by migratory birds. South American strains are distinct and of three different lineages, probably determined by the range of different rodent hosts. Only a single human case has been reported from Brazil, and none from Guatemala, Belize, Colombia, Ecuador Peru, Cuba, or Trinidad and Tobago in spite of detection of the virus in mosquitoes or horses in those countries. The virus has also been isolated from horses in eastern Canada.

Map sources: The Eastern Equine Encephalitis map was made with distribution data obtained from the medical literature and CDC (www.cdc.gov/EasternEquineEncephalitis/tech/epi.html). The distribution of the vector *Culiseta melanura* was obtained from CIESIN, available at: www.ciesin.org/docs/001-613/001-613.html.

Key references

Davis LE, et al. (2008) North American encephalitic arboviruses. *Neurol Clin* **26**(3):727–757.

Reimann CA, et al. (2008) Epidemiology of neuroinvasive arboviral disease in the United States, 1999–2007. *Am J Trop Med Hyg* **79**:974–979.

Smith DW (2009) Arbovirus infections. Chapter 40 in *Manson's Tropical Diseases*, 22nd edn.

Weaver SC (2001) Eastern equine encephalitis. In Service MW (ed.) *The Encyclopedia of Arthropod-transmitted Infections*. CAB International, pp. 151–159.

Ebola and Marburg Virus Disease

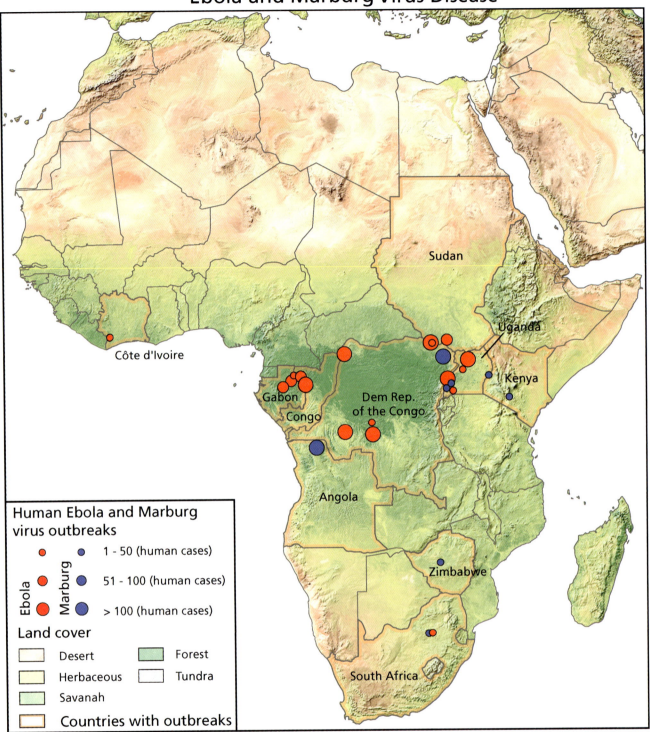

Human Ebola and Marburg
virus outbreaks

Ebola Marburg

● ● 1 - 50 (human cases)

● ● 51 - 100 (human cases)

● ● > 100 (human cases)

Land cover

☐ Desert ☐ Forest

☐ Herbaceous ☐ Tundra

☐ Savanah

☐ Countries with outbreaks

Last update on: 21/04/2011

Disease: Ebola and Marburg Virus Disease

Classification: ICD-9 065.8 and 078.89; ICD-10 A98.4 and A98.3

Syndromes and synonyms: Ebola or Marburg hemorrhagic fever.

Agent: Ebola viruses (genus *Ebolavirus*), marburg viruses (genus *Marburgvirus*), and 'cueva viruses', family Filoviridae, order Mononegavirales; enveloped, single-stranded, negative-sense RNA viruses. There are five ebola viruses: Bundibugyo virus (BDBV), Ebola virus (EBOV), Reston virus (RESTV), Sudan virus (SUDV), and Taï Forest virus (TAFV); two marburg viruses: Marburg virus (MARV) and Ravn virus (RAVV); and one 'cuevavirus': Lloviu virus (LLOV).

Reservoir: Ebola viruses: possibly fruit bats, unknown for BDBV, SUDV, and TAFV; Marburg viruses: infectious MARV and RAVV have been isolated from Egyptian fruit bats; 'Cuevaviruses': Schreiber's long-fingered bats.

Transmission: Ebola viruses: unknown route. Bats have not yet been implicated in the initiation of ebola outbreaks. However, most outbreaks are associated with the consumption or contact with diverse non-human primates, suggesting that transmission could occur from bats to monkeys to humans; exposure to contaminated body fluids; by direct person-to-person contact; via injection with re-used syringes; preparing bodies of cases for burial. Marburg viruses: most outbreaks are associated with index cases visiting caves or working in mines. As Egyptian fruit bats are cave animals, transmission may occur directly from bats to humans or via contact with their excreta and secreta; transmission between humans is similar as for ebola virus. 'Cuevaviruses' are probably apathogenic for humans.

Cycle: Not completely understood (see 'Transmission').

Incubation period: 2–21 days.

Clinical findings: Sudden onset of fever, chills, malaise, myalgia, and headache, followed by pharyngitis, vomiting, diarrhea, and a maculopapular rash. Severe cases have internal and external hemorrhages, CNS involvement and multiorgan failure leading to terminal shock. The case fatality rate (CFR) varies, depending on location, virus involved, and clinical care: 0% for RESTV and TAFV, 34% for BDBV; 78% for EBOV, 53% for SUDV, 82% for MARV. Recovery may be prolonged and accompanied by long term sequelae, particularly hearing loss. Filoviruses can persist for months and disease may recur.

Diagnostic Tests: Must be done in BSL-4 facilities if samples contain infectious virus. IgM ELISA, RT-PCR and virus isolation can be used on acute specimens; in convalescence, antibody tests; on autopsy specimens, electron microscopy and immunohistochemistry.

Therapy: Supportive, there is no specific treatment.

Prevention: Isolation and barrier nursing of cases; discourage butchering of wildlife that died from unknown causes and burial practices of cases involving ritual embalming. Avoid bat-infested caves or mines in endemic areas.

Epidemiology: Ebola viruses, except RESTV, are endemic in the tropical rain forests of equatorial Africa. Most outbreaks started from a single case admitted to a hospital that had inadequate infection control, resulting in rapid nosocomial transmission. Cases have been imported from endemic countries into South Africa and Switzerland, and laboratory infections have occurred in the UK and Russia.

Marburg viruses are endemic in arid woodlands of equatorial Africa. Outbreaks are usually limited to a few cases, with the exception of one outbreak in the DRC and Angola. Cases have been imported into South Africa, the Netherlands, and possibly the USA. A laboratory outbreak in 1967 in Germany and in Yugoslavia, led to the discovery of the disease (not shown on the map).

Map sources: The Ebola and Marburg Virus Disease map was made with data obtained from CDC, available at: www.cdc.gov/ncidod/dvrd/spb/mnpages/disinfo.htm.

Key references

Klenk H-D, Feldmann H (2004) *Ebola and Marburg viruses: Molecular and Cellular Biology*. Wymondham, Norfolk, UK: Horizon Bioscience.

Kuhn JH (2008) *Filo viruses – A Compendium of 40 Years of Epidemiological, Clinical, and Laboratory Studies. Archives of Virology Supplement*, Vol. 20. Vienna, Austria: Springer, Wien, New York.

Kuhn JH, et al. (2010) Proposal for a revised taxonomy of the family Filoviridae. *Arch. Virol* **155**(12):2083–2103.

Atlas of Human Infectious Diseases, First Edition. Heiman F.L. Wertheim, Peter Horby and John P. Woodall.
© 2012 Blackwell Publishing Ltd. Published 2012 by Blackwell Publishing Ltd.

Hantaviral Disease, New World

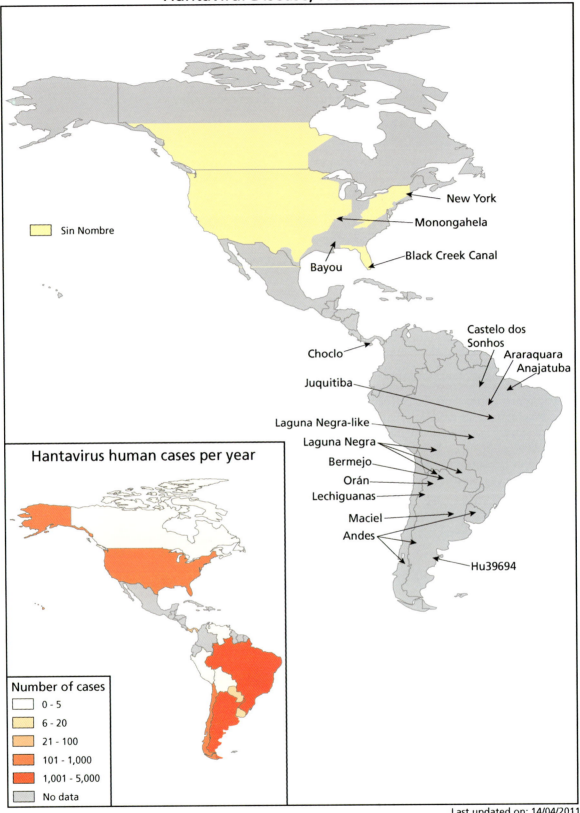

Sin Nombre

New York
Monongahela
Black Creek Canal
Bayou

Choclo

Castelo dos
Sonhos
Araraquara
Anajatuba

Juquitiba

Laguna Negra-like
Laguna Negra
Bermejo
Orán
Lechiguanas
Maciel
Andes
Hu39694

Hantavirus human cases per year

Number of cases
- 0 - 5
- 6 - 20
- 21 - 100
- 101 - 1,000
- 1,001 - 5,000
- No data

Last updated on: 14/04/2011

Disease: Hantaviral Disease, New World

Classification: ICD-9 480.8; ICD-10 B33.4

Syndromes and synonyms: Hantavirus pulmonary syndrome (HPS), Hantavirus cardiopulmonary syndrome, Four Corners disease.

Agents: Hantaviruses, a large group of different, enveloped, single-stranded, negative-sense viruses with a tripartite RNA genome, that belong to the Bunyaviridae family. Hantaviruses that cause HPS were discovered in 1993; more than 30 new hantaviruses have been detected since then, but not all cause HPS. There at least 14 hantaviruses that cause HPS in the Americas: Sin Nombre virus (SNV), Monongahela virus (MGLV), New York virus (NYV), Bayou virus (BAYV), Black Creek Canal virus (BCCV), Choclo virus, Andes virus (ANDV), Bermejo virus (BMJV), Lechiguanas virus (LECV), Maciel virus (MCLV), Oran virus (ORNV), Laguna Negra virus (LANV), Araraquara virus, Hu39694, and Juquitiba virus. Old World and New World hantaviruses share high similarity in their genome and have comparable lifecycles. Currently, there is no consensus on the classification of hantaviruses.

Reservoir: Each hantavirus has its specific rodent host. HPS is generally caused by the sigmodontine borne hantaviruses. Phylogenetic analysis reveals that hantaviruses have a long co-evolutionary history with their host.

Transmission: By inhalation of aerosols from dried rodent excreta (this is unlike other *Bunyaviruses* that are generally arthropod-borne). Person-to-person transmission has been reported for ANDV.

Cycle: Rodent-to-rodent though saliva, excreta and bite, with humans as an accidental, dead-end host.

Incubation period: Typically 2 weeks (days to 6 weeks).

Clinical findings: Typically a cardiopulmonary infection as opposed to the primarily renal infection produced by Old World hantaviruses; renal involvement and hemorrhage are rare in New World cases. Symptoms are fever, myalgia, and GI pain, followed by sudden onset of respiratory distress and hypotension, with rapid progression to respiratory failure and shock. Convalescence is prolonged. CFR is 35–60%.

Diagnostic tests: Serology (IgM ELISA, Western blot, strip immunoblot, IFA); RT-PCR of biopsy material.

Therapy: Supportive, there is no specific treatment.

Prevention: Domestic and peridomestic rodent control, disinfection of rodent-contaminated areas.

Epidemiology: The first hantavirus found in the New World was Sin Nombre virus in the 'Four Corners' area (USA) in 1993, where an outbreak occurred of severe pulmonary disease in previously healthy adults. Since then, sporadic outbreaks have been detected throughout the Americas, with new strains and reservoir hosts. Approximately 200 cases of HPS per year are reported in the Americas. There is no HPS in the Caribbean, probably because the rodent host *Sigmodontinae* is infrequent there. The number of cases is much smaller than that of HFRS in the Old World, but the CFR is higher. Cases confirmed by serology have been reported in Colombia and Venezuela but the identity of the hantavirus unknown. Seoul virus (see Hantavirus Disease, Old World map) seropositives in humans and *Rattus norvegicus* are found in many port cities in the Americas, spread by shipping, but without evidence of disease. Risk of exposure to hantavirus is correlated with outdoor occupations such as agriculture, in which a person might encounter rodents or their excreta; the greatest risk is entering rodent-infested closed buildings. Epidemiology differs by country and virus. In household contacts of index patients with HPS in Chile, the risk of secondary cases was 17.6% among sex partners and 1.2% among other household members. Infection is more common in males, with most cases occurring within the 20–40 age group.

Map sources: The New World Hantavirus map was made with various sources:

CDC (www.cdc.gov/ncidod/diseases/hanta/hps/), and C.B. Jonsson et al. (2010).

Key references

Bi Z, et al. (2008) Hantavirus infection: a review and global update. *J Infect Dev Ctries* 2(1):3–23.

Jonsson CB, et al. (2010) A global perspective on hantavirus ecology, epidemiology, and disease. *Clin Microbiol Rev* 23(2):412–441.

Padula PJ, et al. (2000) Genetic diversity, distribution, and serological features of hantavirus infection in five countries in South America. *J Clin Microbiol* 38:3029–3035.

Atlas of Human Infectious Diseases, First Edition. Heiman F.L. Wertheim, Peter Horby and John P. Woodall.
© 2012 Blackwell Publishing Ltd. Published 2012 by Blackwell Publishing Ltd.

Hantaviral Disease, Old World

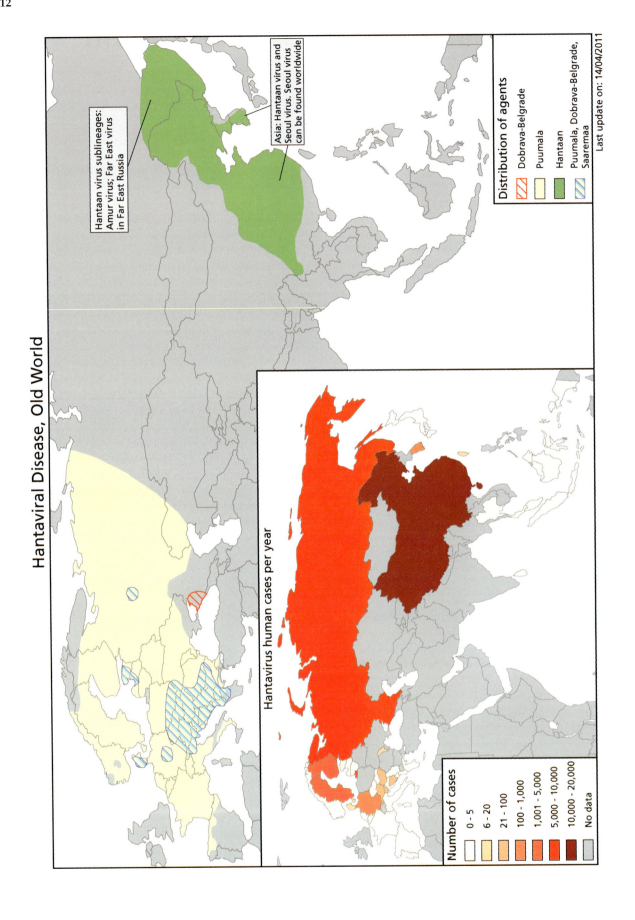

Hantaan virus sublineages:
Amur virus; Far East virus
in Far East Russia

Asia: Hantaan virus and
Seoul virus. Seoul virus
can be found worldwide

Distribution of agents

- Dobrava-Belgrade
- Puumala
- Hantaan
- Puumala, Dobrava-Belgrade, Saaremaa

Last update on: 14/04/2011

Hantavirus human cases per year

Number of cases

- 0 - 5
- 6 - 20
- 21 - 100
- 100 - 1,000
- 1,001 - 5,000
- 5,000 - 10,000
- 10,000 - 20,000
- No data

Disease: Hantaviral Disease, Old World

Classification: ICD-9 078.6; ICD-10 A98.5

Syndromes and synonyms: Hemorrhagic fever with renal syndrome (HFRS), Korean Hemorrhagic Fever, Hemorrhagic Nephrosonephritis, Nephropathia epidemica

Agent: Hantaviruses, a large group of different, enveloped, single-stranded, negative-sense viruses with a tripartite RNA genome, that belong to the Bunyaviridae family. Hantaviruses are named after the Hantan River area in South Korea, where the first hantavirus (Hantaan) was isolated in the 1970s. Old World and New World hantaviruses share high similarity in their genome and have comparable life cycles. Currently, there is no consensus on the classification of hantaviruses. Old World hantaviruses shown on the map are: Dobrava–Belgrade virus (DOBV), Hantaan virus (HTNV), Puumula virus (PUUV), and Saaremaa virus (SAAV). Seoul virus (SEOV) is not shown, it is world wide in major port cities.

Reservoir: HFRS is caused by *Myodes-*, *Rattus-*, and *Apodemus*-borne hantaviruses. Each virus has its particular host: *Apodemus* spp. (striped field mouse) for HTNV, DOBV and SAAV and *Myodes* (= *Clethrionomys*) for PUUV. SEOV infects *Rattus norvegicus* and can therefore be found world wide.

Transmission: By inhalation of aerosols from dried rodent excreta. Person-to-person transmission has not been reported.

Cycle: Rodent-to-rodent though saliva, excreta and bite, with humans as an accidental, dead-end host.

Incubation period: Usually 2–4 weeks (days to 2 months).

Clinical findings: Sudden onset fever, headache, malaise, anorexia, severe abdominal or lower back pain, often with nausea and vomiting, followed by hypotension which may progress to shock, hemorrhages and renal involvement, and death. Convalescence is prolonged. PUUV virus causes less severe disease. The CFR is 5–15% for HFRS; for PUUV and SAAV infection the CFR is 1%; for DOBV the CFR is 9–12%. The differential diagnosis is leptospirosis or rickettsioses.

Diagnostic tests: Serology (IgM ELISA, IFA); RT-PCR. Virus isolation is difficult.

Therapy: Supportive; ribavirin is effective if given within the first 6 days; dialysis if indicated.

Prevention: Domestic and peridomestic rodent control; disinfection of rodent-contaminated areas; formalin-inactivated HTNV vaccines are used in Russia, China and Korea.

Epidemiology: Approximately 150,000 to 200,000 patients with HFRS are hospitalized each year throughout the world, more than half of them in China. The main agent of HFRS in Asia is HTNV. SEOV is also an important cause, but has a wider distribution. The most prevalent hantaviral disease in western and central Europe is caused by PUUV, with >9,000 cases per year. DOBV is restricted to the Balkans. Hantaviral disease is seasonal, linked to the activity of the rodent host. HFRS epidemics are associated with rodent abundance, caused by various seasonal factors. During the agricultural season, infection is linked to outdoor activities, and during the winter, rodents seek shelter in and around buildings and infection is contracted indoors. There have been reports of clinical hantaviral infections in the UK and there is serological evidence of human infection in Israel, Kuwait, Laos, Malaysia, Philippines, Thailand, and Vietnam and in several African nations.

Map sources: The Old World Hantavirus map is made with various sources from the medical literature and ProMED-mail.

Key references

Bi Z, et al. (2008) Hantavirus infection: a review and global update. *J Infect Dev Ctries* 2(1):3–23.

Heyman P, et al. (2009) Hantavirus infections in Europe. *Exp Rev Anti Infec Ther* 7(2):205–217.

Jonsson CB, et al. (2010) A global perspective on hantavirus ecology, epidemiology, and disease. *Clin Microbiol Rev* 23(2):412–441.

Makary P, et al. (2010) Disease burden of Puumala virus infections, 1995–2008. *Epidemiol Infect* 138(10):1484–1492.

Tersago K, et al. (2010) Hantavirus outbreak in Western Europe. *Epidemiol Infect* 139(3):381–390.

Vapalahti O, et al. (2003) Hantavirus infections in Europe. *Lancet Infect Dis* 3(10):653–661.

Atlas of Human Infectious Diseases, First Edition. Heiman F.L. Wertheim, Peter Horby and John P. Woodall.
© 2012 Blackwell Publishing Ltd. Published 2012 by Blackwell Publishing Ltd.

214

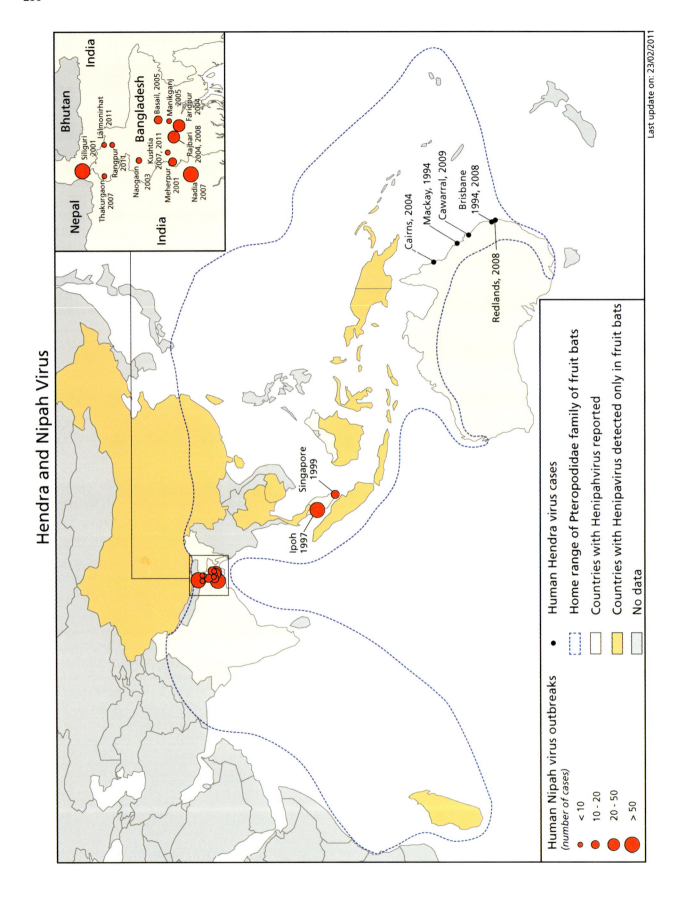

Hendra and Nipah Virus

India · **Bhutan** · **Nepal** · **India**

Bangladesh

Siliguri 2001
Thakurgaon 2007
Lalmonirhat 2011
Rangpur 2011
Naogaon 2003
Kushtia 2007, 2011
Meherpur 2001
Nadia 2007
Rajbari 2004, 2008
Faridpur 2004
Manikganj 2005
Basail, 2005

Cairns, 2004
Mackay, 1994
Cawarral, 2009
Brisbane 1994, 2008
Redlands, 2008

Singapore 1999

Ipoh 1997

Human Nipah virus outbreaks
(number of cases)
- < 10
- 10 - 20
- 20 - 50
- > 50

- Human Hendra virus cases
- - - Home range of Pteropodidae family of fruit bats
- Countries with Henipahvirus reported
- Countries with Henipavirus detected only in fruit bats
- No data

Last update on: 23/02/2011

Disease: Hendra and Nipah Virus

Classification: ICD-9 078.8; ICD-10 B33.8

Synonyms: Hendra virus disease, Nipah virus disease.

Agent: Hendra virus and Nipah virus are negative-stranded RNA viruses, and comprise the *Henipavirus* genus within the family Paramyxoviridae. Hendra virus was discovered in horses and stable staff in Australia in 1994, Nipah virus in pigs and pig farmers in the town Nipah, Malaysia, in 1999.

Reservoir: Primarily Old World fruit-eating bats, mainly in the family Pteropodidae.

Transmission: Hendra virus: through contact with infectious body fluids, including urine, saliva, and nasal discharge, or during autopsy of infected horses. Nipah virus: through contact with infectious body fluids, including bat saliva (on fallen fruit and in date palm sap), or droplets from coughing infected pigs. In Bangladesh, half of reported cases between 2001 and 2008 were due to human-to-human transmission.

Cycle: Bat to bat via unknown route. Humans and domestic animals are incidental hosts.

Incubation period: Varying from 4 to 45 days.

Clinical findings: Hendra virus: encephalitis and pneumonia, with a rapid progression to death (few survive). One case recovered from encephalitis but relapsed 14 months later and died with neurologic signs, suggesting latency and recrudescence. Nipah virus: encephalitis and pneumonia. There has been a case of relapse encephalitis more than 4 years after infection. The CFR can vary from 10 to 75%, but is generally high.

Diagnostic tests: Virus isolation, RT-PCR, serology. Both viruses are BSL-4 agents.

Therapy: Supportive measures such as mechanical ventilation. There is no specific treatment, but ribavirin may have some effect. Monoclonal antibodies as post-exposure prophylaxis before onset of clinical signs.

Prevention: Hendra virus: manage contact between fruit bats and horse by basic husbandry measures such as placing food and water points under cover, regulate movement of horses from areas where the disease is occurring, regulate import of horses from Australia during outbreaks. Nipah virus: avoid contact with fruit bats and their discharges; wash and peel fruit, and wash hands before and after preparing fruit; regulate importation of pigs from outbreak areas.

Epidemiology: Hendra virus: pteropid bats are the primary reservoir of Hendra virus and are asymptomatic. The viruses can be isolated from their reproductive tracts and urine. The epidemiological reasons for the emergence of Hendra virus infection in horses are not clear. All human cases had close contact with infected horses.

Nipah virus outbreaks have occurred only in South Asia and may be associated with the bat-breeding season. In Malaysia, it was hypothesized that the bats fed on fruit trees in pig farms, and that fallen fruit contaminated with bat saliva containing Nipah virus was eaten by pigs, who became infected. Nipah viruses have been isolated from bats in Cambodia and Thailand, and a high seroprevalence has been found in fruit bats in NW India, in the absence of reported pig or human disease. In Bangladesh, there is epidemiologic evidence of bat–human transmission without an intermediate livestock host, and of human–human transmission. Young boys who gather fruit from the trees are at higher risk of disease. Also drinking palm sap from trees is a potential risk factor. Antibodies to henipaviruses have been found in fruit bats in Madagascar (*Pteropus* and *Eidolon* sp.) and in Ghana (*Eidolon* sp.), but in the absence of virus isolation or RNA detection, it is not possible to know which virus is involved. No human or animal cases have been reported in Madagascar or in Africa.

Map sources: The Hendra and Nipah Virus map was made by geocoding reported human cases or outbreaks in the medical literature or reported to WHO up to 2011. The fruit bat distribution was obtained from WHO, available at: http://www.who.int/csr/disease/nipah/en/index.html.

Key references

Field H, et al. (2001) The natural history of Hendra and Nipah viruses. *Microbes Infect* **3**(4):307–314.

Hayman D, et al. (2008) Evidence of henipavirus infection in West African fruit bats. *PLoS ONE* **3**(7):e2739.

Montgomery JM, et al. (2008) Risk factors for Nipah virus encephalitis in Bangladesh. *Emerg Infect Dis* doi 10.3201/eid1410.060507.

Hepatitis A

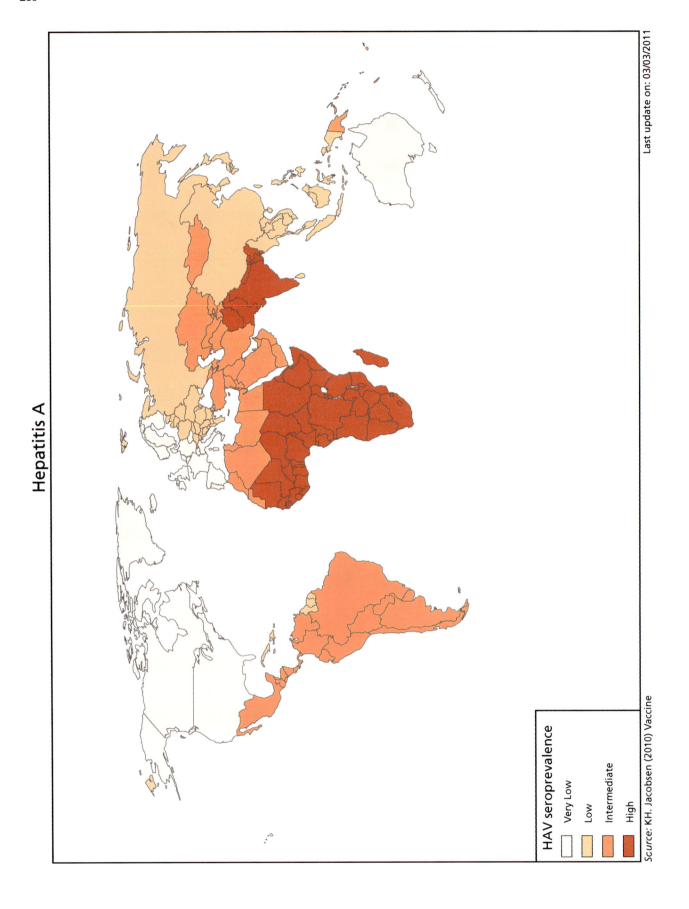

HAV seroprevalence

Very Low
Low
Intermediate
High

Source: KH. Jacobsen (2010) Vaccine

Last update on: 03/03/2011

Disease: Hepatitis A

Classification: ICD-9 070.1; ICD-10 B15.

Synonyms: Epidemic hepatitis, infectious hepatitis, infectious jaundice, catarrhal jaundice.

Agent: Hepatitis A virus (HAV), a single stranded RNA virus, genus *Hepatovirus* in the family Picornaviridae.

Reservoir: Humans are the main reservoir; non-human primates can be infected, rarely.

Transmission: Person-to-person transmission via fecal–oral route (hands, food, water, sexual contact).

Cycle: After ingestion, the virus infects hepatocytes, resulting in periportal necrosis. The virus is shed via bile into the stool and contaminates the environment, leading to new infections in susceptible exposed individuals.

Incubation period: Commonly 28–30 days, ranging from 15 to 50 days.

Clinical findings: Fever, fatigue, anorexia, abdominal discomfort, nausea, vomiting, myalgia, jaundice, dark urine, and light stools. Arthritis and rash may occur. Disease may be mild and short-lived (several weeks) to severe and prolonged (months), with a CFR <0.3%.

Diagnostic tests: Serology to detect specific IgM antibodies; RT-PCR to detect viral RNA in blood or stool.

Therapy: Supportive.

Prevention: Hygiene, access to clean water, and sanitation. An effective vaccine is available; vaccination should be offered to high-risk groups (MSM, liver disease, travelers to endemic areas, IVDUs, outbreaks); passive immunization with immunoglobulins can be given as PEP within 2 weeks of the exposure. The virus remains viable for weeks at room temperature.

Epidemiology: Globally, there exist four patterns of HAV infection, based on age-specific HAV seroprevalence rates. High-endemic areas generally have low disease rates as most infections occur in young children, who are usually asymptomatic. Adults are immune and epidemics in these high-endemic areas are uncommon. High-endemic areas is defined as a region where >90% of the children <10 years are already infected and most cases are asymptomatic. The high-endemic areas are generally in poor regions with poor sanitation and lack of access to clean water (see Human Development Index map and Sanitation map). Improving living conditions leads to intermediate endemicity, which causes high disease rates because more infections now occur in older people (as disease averted in children), who are symptomatic. HAV epidemiology in high-endemic areas is shifting to intermediate endemicity, which results in an increase in disease burden. Large variations exist within countries in HAV incidence. In (very) low-endemic areas, children will not acquire the disease and the adult population will remain susceptible, leading to localized outbreaks. In areas of low endemicity, the overall prevalence is <25%. In developed countries with low endemicity, outbreaks are often caused by contaminated food products, like shellfish, which can concentrate virus, and other food products that are contaminated by an infected food handler.

Map sources: The Hepatitis A map is modified from K.H. Jacobsen et al. (2010).

Key references

Beth BP (2002) Global epidemiology of hepatitis A: implications for control. *Proc. 10th International Symposium on Viral Hepatitis and Liver Disease.*

Jacobsen KH, et al. (2010) Hepatitis A virus seroprevalence by age and world region, 1990 and 2005. *Vaccine* **28**:6653–6657.

Melnick JL (1995) History and epidemiology of hepatitis A virus. *J Infect Dis* **171**:S2–S8.

Atlas of Human Infectious Diseases, First Edition. Heiman F.L. Wertheim, Peter Horby and John P. Woodall.
© 2012 Blackwell Publishing Ltd. Published 2012 by Blackwell Publishing Ltd.

218

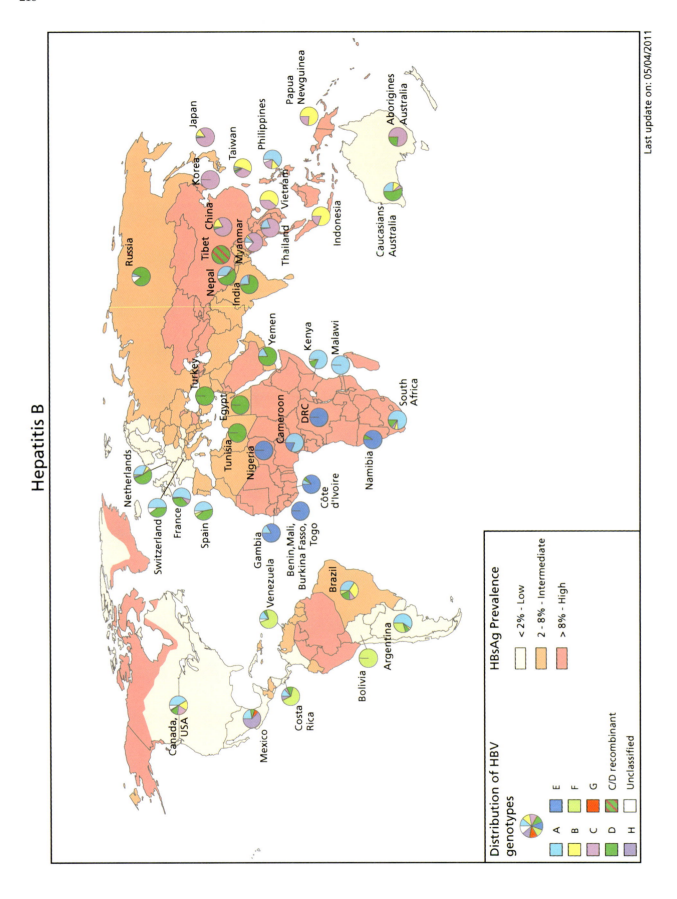

Hepatitis B

Last update on: 05/04/2011

Distribution of HBV genotypes

A	E
B	F
C	G
D	C/D recombinant
H	Unclassified

HBsAg Prevalence

< 2% - Low
2 - 8% - Intermediate
> 8% - High

Disease: Hepatitis B

Classification: ICD-9 070.3; ICD-10 B16 and B18.

Syndromes and synonyms: Type B hepatitis, serum hepatitis, homologous serum jaundice, long-incubation hepatitis.

Agent: Hepatitis B virus (HBV), a DNA virus belonging to the family of Hepadnaviridae. There are 8 genotypes (A to H) with marked differences in disease severity. Genotypes are classified by comparing complete HBV genomes. The map illustrates the distribution of chronic HBV infection. Co-infection with hepatitis D virus (HDV) may occur resulting in severe chronic liver disease. HDV is a defective RNA virus that requires HBV for replication.

Reservoir: Humans.

Transmission: Percutaneous or mucosal exposure to blood or body fluids (e.g. semen, vaginal fluid, saliva) of an infected individual. Person-to-person transmission via sexual contact, needle sharing in IVDUs, sharing toothbrushes or razors, and blood transfusion. Transmission does not occur via kissing, coughing, or sneezing. Mother to child transmission occurs mainly during birth or transplacentally (not via breastfeeding).

Incubation period: 2–3 months.

Clinical findings: HBV disease has an acute and chronic form. 10% of children and 30–50% of adults present with symptoms of acute HBV infection similar to hepatitis A and last several weeks: fatigue, abdominal pain, nausea, vomiting, myalgia, jaundice, dark urine, and light stools. Fever is often absent and arthritis and rash may be present. Chronic disease evolves to cirrhosis or hepatocellular carcinoma and eventually death. 90% of infants who are infected in their first year develop chronic infection. Only 10% of adults who acquire infection develop chronic disease, as the majority is able to clear HBV within 6 months. Differences in disease severity, risk of liver cirrhosis and development of hepatocellular carcinoma are seen by age of infection, level of viral replication, level of inflammation, region and HBV genotype. Also co-infection with HDV leads to more severe chronic liver disease.

Diagnostic tests: Serologic tests to assess active infection: HBsAg, HBeAg; HBV DNA can be detected in blood by PCR; quantitative PCR to monitor treatment.

Therapy: Supportive for acute hepatitis B. Interferon-alpha and reverse transcriptase inhibitors for chronic hepatitis B. Treatment response, particularly interferon treatment, differs by HBV genotype. Treatment is expensive and often not available in developing countries. In Southeast Asia, medicinal herbs are widely used to treat chronic HBV disease, of which the efficacy is yet unclear. Liver transplant is possible for decompensated cirrhosis.

Prevention: WHO recommends vaccination of all newborns. In countries where prevalence is low: HBV vaccination of risk groups and those living in endemic communities; safe sexual practices; screening of blood products; universal precautions when caring for patients; infection control. Vaccine and immunoglobulins as PEP within 24 hours of exposure.

Epidemiology: Hepatitis B is a common disease world wide, despite the existence of a vaccine. The WHO estimates that globally 2 billion individuals have been infected, of which about 360 million have chronic disease. Yearly, it is estimated that there are 500,000 to 700,000 HBV associated deaths world wide. In high-endemic regions like Southeast Asia, Africa, and the Amazon basin, most individuals become infected during childhood (mother-to-child, or child-to-child). In developed regions, the prevalence is low and important routes of transmission are different, consisting mostly of unsafe sexual practices, IVDU, and occupational transmission in healthcare workers. Chronic HBV associated liver cirrhosis is more common in developed nations than in Southeast Asia, but the incidence of hepatocellular carcinoma is lower compared to Southeast Asia. It is not yet fully clear whether this is due to differences in HBV genotype or age of infection.

Map sources: The Hepatitis B Virus map is redrawn from World Health Organization report (2001) and A. Kramvis et al (2005).

Key references

Kramvis A, et al. (2005) Hepatitis B virus genotypes. *Vaccine* **23**:2409–2423.

Liaw YF, et al. (2010) The natural history of chronic HBV infection and geographical differences. *Antivir Ther* **15**(S3):25–33.

Palumbo E (2007) Hepatitis B genotypes and response to antiviral therapy: a review. *Am J Therap* **14**:306–309.

World Health Organization (2001) *Introduction of Hepatitis B Vaccine into Childhood Immunization Services*. Report WHO/V&B/01.31. Geneva.

Atlas of Human Infectious Diseases, First Edition. Heiman F.L. Wertheim, Peter Horby and John P. Woodall.
© 2012 Blackwell Publishing Ltd. Published 2012 by Blackwell Publishing Ltd.

Hepatitis C

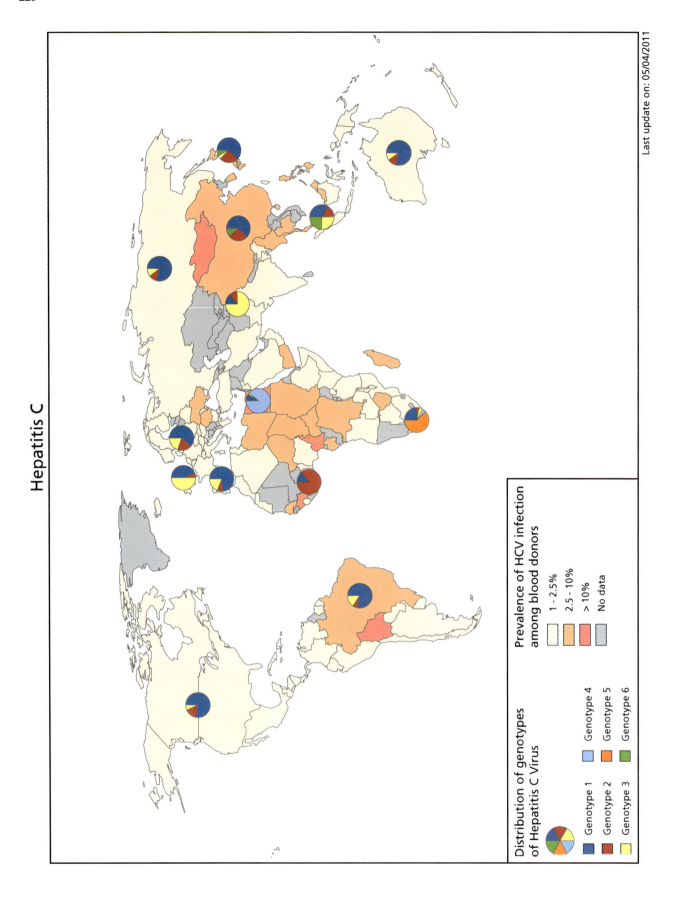

Last update on: 05/04/2011

Distribution of genotypes of Hepatitis C Virus		Prevalence of HCV infection among blood donors	
Genotype 1	Genotype 4		1 - 2.5%
Genotype 2	Genotype 5		2.5 - 10%
Genotype 3	Genotype 6		> 10%
			No data

Disease: **Hepatitis C**

Classification: ICD-9 070.5; ICD-10 B17.1 and B18.2.

Syndromes and synonyms: Non-A non-B hepatitis, HCV infection.

Agent: Hepatitis C virus (HCV) is an enveloped RNA virus (*hepacavirus*) and belongs to the flaviviruses. The HCV genome is highly mutable. There are at least six HCV genotypes and several subtypes with differences in clinical presentation, geographic distribution and treatment response. HCV was discovered in 1989 as another cause of transfusion associated hepatitis (non-A non-B hepatitis).

Reservoir: Humans.

Transmission: Person-to-person transmission occurs parentally (blood to blood). Mother to child transmission or transmission via sexual contact is rare. Mother to child transmission increases if the mother is co-infected with HIV.

Incubation period: Usually 6 to 9 weeks; range from 2 weeks to 6 months.

Clinical findings: Majority will be asymptomatic in the acute phase, but approximately 80% develops chronic HCV disease. Acute disease: insidious onset with right upper quadrant pain, fatigue, nausea, malaise and vomiting; some progress to jaundice and dark urine. Most infected cases (approx. 80%) develop chronic disease with fatigue as main symptom; 20–30% eventually develop severe liver disease: cirrhosis and liver cancer (may take 20 years and is dependent on the presence of other risk factors). HCV infection is an important cause for liver transplantation in developed countries. There is accelerated progression of hepatic fibrosis and increased risk of hepatocellular carcinoma in men, elderly, obese, alcoholics, those infected with HIV or hepatitis B virus.

Diagnostic tests: Serology (EIA, recombinant immunoblot assay (RIBA)); RT-PCR on plasma; quanitiative RT-PCR to monitor treatment; genotyping; liver biopsy for histology to assess disease stage and activity.

Therapy: Ribavirin in combination with peg-interferon. Response to interferon differs by HCV genotype: there is a more sustained virological response in HCV genotype 2 and 3 infections, as compared to HCV genotype1 and 4. The peg-interferon and ribavarin response can be improved by the combination with oral DNA-polymerase and protease inhibitors.

Prevention: Infection control hospitals; safe injection practices by healthcare providers; screening of blood products; clean needle programs. HCV immunoglobulin is not effective. There is no vaccine.

Epidemiology: HCV infection has a worldwide prevalence of 2% and an estimated 130 to 170 million chronic cases globally. The highest prevalences are found in Africa and Asia. Egypt has the highest HCV prevalence rate (22%), likely due to a national schistosomiasis treatment campaign since the 1960s that re-used needles. In developing countries the high prevalence is likely due to poor infection control practices in the healthcare system (therapeutic injections, blood transfusion, surgery). Also local practices in the community, like acupuncture and cutting of the skin with unsterile knives, are other important routes of transmission. In Asia it is common to receive injections for various illnesses outside the hospital setting. In developed countries HCV is mainly transmitted by IVDU, accounting for 70–80% of HCV infections.

Map sources: The Hepatitis C Virus map was made with data obtained from WHO: the prevalence map was redrawn from a map by the World Health Organization (2002); and the genotype data was obtained from WHO (2009) (www.who.int/vaccine_research/documents/ViralCancer7.pdf)

Key references

Khattab MA, et al. (2010) Management of hepatitis C virus genotype 4: Recommendations of an international expert panel. *J Hepatol* **54**(6):1250–1262.

Munir S, et al. (2010) Hepatitis C treatment: current and future perspectives. *Virol J* **7**:296.

Shepard CW, et al. (2005) Global epidemiology of Hepatitis C virus infection. *Lancet Infect Dis* **5**:558–567.

World Health Organization (2002) Hepatitis C. *Guide WHO/CDS/CSR/LYO/2003*. Geneva.

World Health Organization (2002) Map: Hepatitis C, 2001. *Weekly Epid Rep* **6**(77):47.

Atlas of Human Infectious Diseases, First Edition. Heiman F.L. Wertheim, Peter Horby and John P. Woodall.
© 2012 Blackwell Publishing Ltd. Published 2012 by Blackwell Publishing Ltd.

Hepatitis E

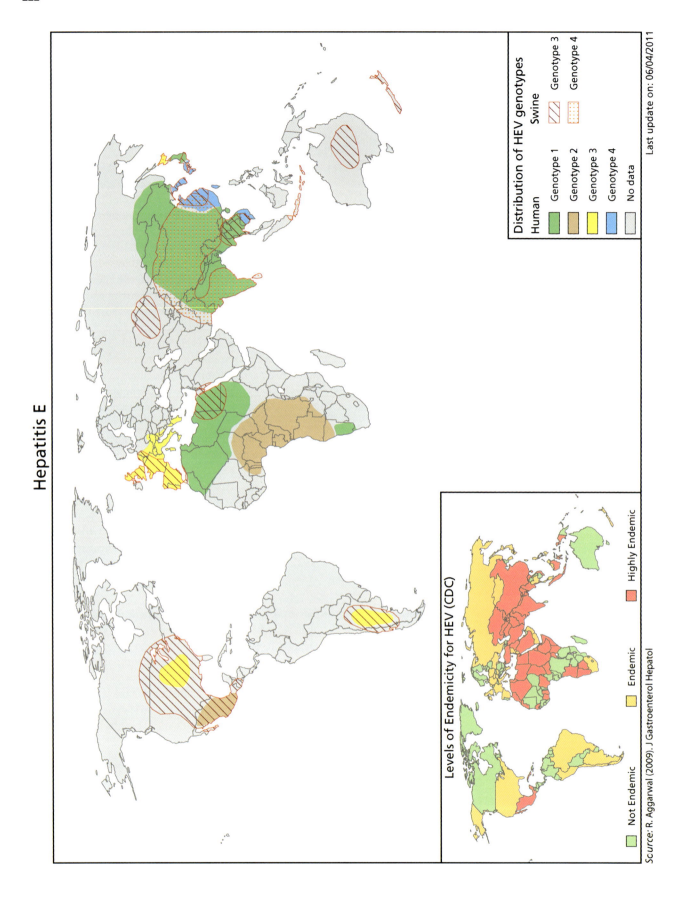

Distribution of HEV genotypes

Human

- Genotype 1
- Genotype 2
- Genotype 3
- Genotype 4
- No data

Swine

- Genotype 3
- Genotype 4

Last update on: 06/04/2011

Levels of Endemicity for HEV (CDC)

- Not Endemic
- Endemic
- Highly Endemic

Source: R. Aggarwal (2009). J Gastroenterol Hepatol

Disease: **Hepatitis E**

Classification: ICD-9 070.5; ICD-10 B17.2.

Syndromes and synonyms: Epidemic non-A non-B hepatitis, fecal–oral non-A non-B hepatitis, enterically transmitted non-A non-B hepatitis.

Agent: Hepatitis E virus (HEV), a non-enveloped single-stranded RNA virus, genus *Hepevirus*, the single member in the Hepeviridae family. The virus can be classified into four genotypes (genotype HEV-1 to HEV-4), and >24 sub-genotypes (1a–1e, 2a–2b, 3a–3j, and 4a–4g). Avian isolates of HEV are now considered to be a separate genus. HEV was discovered in the 1980s as a result of a large water-borne non-A non-B hepatitis outbreak in India between 1978 and 1979.

Reservoir: Humans are the natural host. Numerous mammals have serologic evidence of HEV disease, including but not limited to: pigs, cattle, sheep, goats, horses, macaques, cats, dogs, rabbits, mongoose, deer, wild boar, rats, and mice. HEV in pigs is asymptomatic, but there is transient viremia and excretion of virus into the environment.

Transmission: Fecal–oral route, mainly via fecally contaminated water, but also via: food, materno-fetal, and transfusion of blood products. Direct person to person transmission is uncommon.

Cycle: Human to human and occasionally animal to human. HEV is excreted from the liver into the stool via the bile and eventually into the environment. The amount of infectious virus in the stool is relatively low and explains a lower rate of transmission as compared to hepatitis A (see Hepatitis A map).

Incubation period: On average 40 days (range: 2 to 10 weeks).

Clinical findings: The disease is self-limiting and acute symptoms are similar to acute hepatitis A disease. Children are generally asymptomatic or have mild disease. Clinical evident disease is more common in age group 15–44 years, with following symptoms: fatigue, fever, nausea, vomiting, abdominal pain, jaundice, dark urine, and light stool. Pregnant women are at risk for severe disease, including fulminant hepatitis and death. In immunocompromised persons (e.g. transplant recipients or users of immune-modulating therapy) chronic infection has been reported.

Diagnostic tests: Serology (HEV IgM, IgG); HEV RNA detection in blood and stool by RT-PCR.

Therapy: Supportive.

Prevention: Hygiene; access to clean water; sanitation (see Water and Sanitation map). A vaccine has been developed and proven effective, but is not yet available.

Epidemiology: HEV is more prevalent in areas with hot climates and poor sanitation. Outbreaks are more common during heavy rainfall and flooding, which leads to fecal contamination of the drinking water. Food-borne outbreaks also occur, especially with contaminated shellfish. HEV genotypes have their own geographic distribution. HEV-1 is common in high endemic areas of Asia and Africa. HEV-2 can be found in Mexico and West Africa. HEV-3 has been found in rare cases in the USA and several developed countries in Europe, Japan, Australia, New Zealand, Korea, and Argentina. HEV-4 causes sporadic human cases in Southeast Asia and Japan. HEV-3 and HEV-4 are also reported in pigs on all continents, causing sporadic disease in humans.

Map sources: The Hepatitis E map is redrawn from R. Aggarwal et al. (2009). The data on levels of HEV endemicity was obtained from CDC (2009), available at: www.cdc.gov/hepatitis/HEV.

Key references

Aggarwal R, et al. (2009) Epidemiology of Hepatitis E: current status. *J Gastroenterol Hepatol* **24**(9):1484–1493.

Aggarwal R (2011) Hepatitis E: Historical, contemporary and future perspective. *J Gastroenterol Hepatol* **26** (Suppl. 1): 72–82.

Mushahwar IK (2008) Hepatitis E virus: molecular virology, clinical features, diagnosis, transmission, epidemiology, and prevention. *J Med Virol* **80**(4):646–658.

World Health Organization (2001) Hepatitis E. *Guide WHO/CDSCSR/EDC/2001.12*. Geneva.

Atlas of Human Infectious Diseases, First Edition. Heiman F.L. Wertheim, Peter Horby and John P. Woodall.
© 2012 Blackwell Publishing Ltd. Published 2012 by Blackwell Publishing Ltd.

Human Immunodeficiency Virus
HIV Prevalence

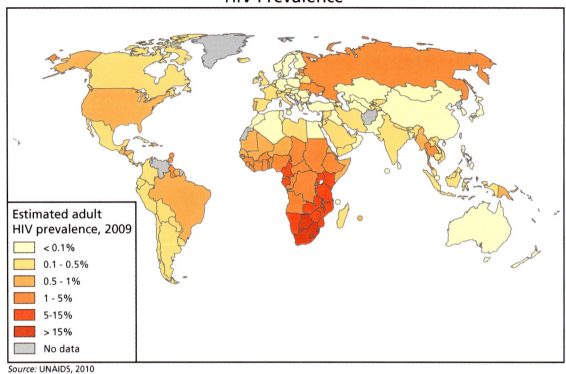

Estimated adult HIV prevalence, 2009

- < 0.1%
- 0.1 - 0.5%
- 0.5 - 1%
- 1 - 5%
- 5-15%
- > 15%
- No data

Source: UNAIDS, 2010

HIV-1 Group M - Subtypes and Recombinants

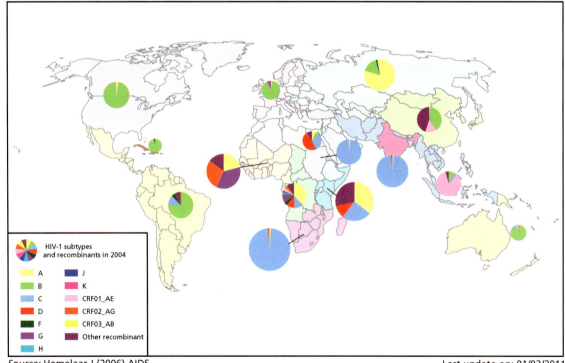

HIV-1 subtypes and recombinants in 2004

- A
- B
- C
- D
- F
- G
- H
- J
- K
- CRF01_AE
- CRF02_AG
- CRF03_AB
- Other recombinant

Source: Hemelaar J (2006) AIDS

Last update on: 01/03/2011

Disease: Human Immunodeficiency Virus

Classification: ICD-9 042-044; ICD-10 B20-24

Syndromes and synonyms: VIH, SIDA, slim disease, acquired immune deficiency syndrome (AIDS).

Agent: Human Immunodeficiency Virus (HIV), an enveloped single-stranded RNA virus of the *Lentivirus* genus and Retroviridae family, is divided into two main species HIV-1 and HIV-2. HIV-1 is more infectious and more virulent than HIV-2 and predominates globally, with HIV-2 transmission restricted to parts of Western and Central Africa.

Reservoir: Humans.

Transmission: HIV is transmitted through contact with HIV-infected body fluids (blood, semen, and vaginal secretions) and is predominantly a sexually transmitted infection. Other routes are: sharing contaminated needles; mother-to-child transmission during pregnancy, childbirth and breastfeeding; blood or blood product transfusion; and organ or tissue transplantation.

Incubation period: Around 50–70% of infected individuals develop a self-limiting 'primary' HIV illness 1–12 weeks after infection. Time from infection to development of clinically apparent immunodeficiency ranges from less than 1 year to over 15 years.

Clinical findings: Primary HIV infection is usually a non-specific illness with fever, headache, myalgia, fatigue, and a sore throat. Generalized lymphadenopathy and a maculopapular rash may occur. Following primary infection there is a prolonged asymptomatic period before the appearance of the clinical manifestations of a loss of immune control over infectious pathogens and cancers. Common presenting AIDS-defining illnesses are tuberculosis, atypical mycobacterial infections, recurrent bacterial infections, *Pneumocystis jirovecii* pneumonia, candidiasis, Kaposi sarcoma, lymphoma, cryptococcal meningitis, and CMV disease.

Diagnostic tests: Enzyme immunoassay to detect anti-HIV antibodies with confirmation by Western blot. Fourth-generation HIV serology tests that consist of antibody detection and p24 antigen detection in combination are now commonly used. Also rapid tests are available for field testing. Viral load and HIV-1 p24 antigen may be used in some circumstances. CD4 cell counts and HIV viral load are used to monitor progression of infection. Genotypic and phenotypic tests are used for HIVdrug-resistance testing.

Therapy: A combination of several ARVs is recommended, known as Highly Active Antiretroviral Therapy (HAART). Additional strategies include prophylaxis and vaccination against opportunistic infections, general measures to maintain nutrition and health, and treatment of specific infections or HIV-associated disorders.

Prevention: Reducing sexual transmission through the promotion of monogamy, condom use, male circumcision, and the detection and treatment of STIs; raising awareness of individual HIV status through voluntary counseling and testing; protecting IVDUs through needle/syringe exchange and methadone replacement programs; reducing mother to child transmission through voluntary counseling and testing and the provision of ARVs.

Epidemiology: HIV was first recognized clinically in 1981. As of 2009, over 25 million people are estimated to have died from HIV and around 33 million people are living with HIV.

HIV epidemics are categorized into 'low-level' (HIV prevalence <1% in the general population and <5% in vulnerable group such as MSM, injecting drug users, sex workers); 'concentrated' (HIV prevalence <1% in the general population but >5% in at least one vulnerable group); and 'generalized' (HIV prevalence >1% in the general population). The greatest burden of HIV continues to fall on Sub-Saharan Africa, with 68% of all people living with HIV and 72% of all HIV-related deaths in 2009. The epidemic in Africa is, however, heterogeneous, with high-prevalence generalized epidemics in Southern African countries; generalized but moderate prevalence epidemics in Central, East and West Africa, and low-level epidemics in North Africa. No countries in Asia have a generalized epidemic.

HIV-1 can be divided in four groups (M, O, N, and P). Over 90% of HIV-1 infections are group M and the map opposite shows the distribution of the 9 subtypes (clades) and recombinants of the M group HIV-1 viruses.

Map sources: The Human Immunodeficiency Virus prevalence map was made with UNAIDS (2009) data. The HIV-1 subtypes and recombinants map is reproduced from J. Hemelaar et al. (2006).

Key references

Joint United Nations Programme on HIV/AIDS (UNAIDS). (2010) *UNAIDS Report on the Global AIDS Epidemic 2010*. ISBN 978-92-9173-871-7.

Hemelaar J, et al. (2006) Global and regional distribution of HIV-1 genetic subtypes and recombinants in 2004. *AIDS* **20**(16):W13–W23.

Human T-Lymphotropic Virus 1

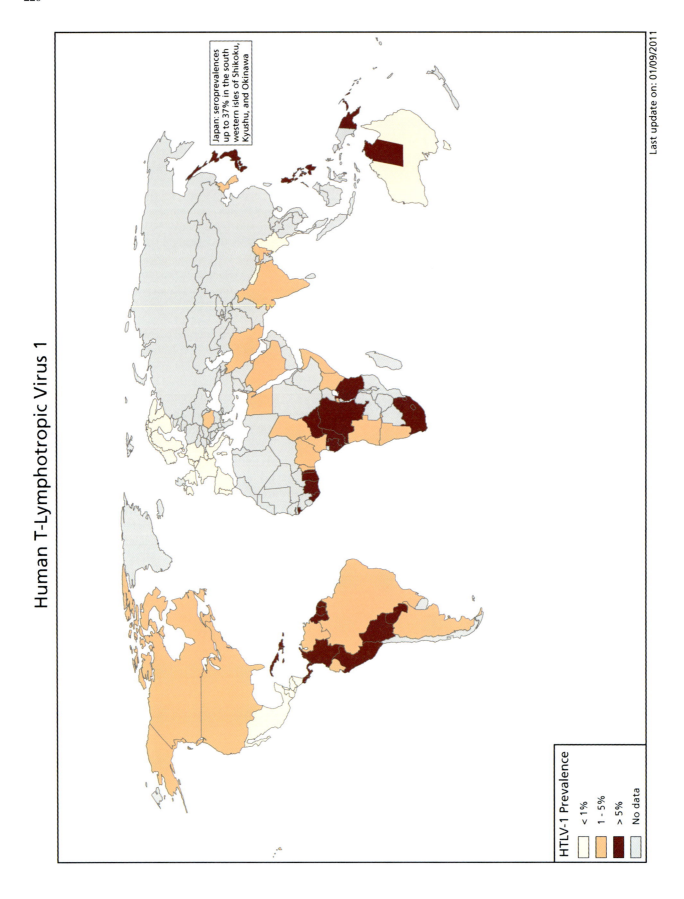

Japan: seroprevalences up to 37% in the south western isles of Shikoku, Kyushu, and Okinawa

HTLV-1 Prevalence

< 1%

1 - 5%

> 5%

No data

Disease: Human T-Lymphotropic Virus 1

Classification: ICD-9 202; ICD-10 B97.33 (virus), C84.1 Sézary disease, C84.5 Other and unspecified T-cell lymphomas, C91.4 Hairy cell leukemia, C91.5 ATL.

Syndromes and synonyms: Adult T-cell leukemia/lymphoma (ATL), T-cell lymphosarcoma, peripheral T-cell lymphoma (Sézary disease), hairy cell leukemia, HTLV-associated myelopathy/tropical spastic paraparesis (HAM/TSP), HTLV-associated uveitis and infective dermatitis.

Agent: Human T-lymphotropic virus 1 (HTLV-1), a type C retrovirus with at least 6 subtypes. The virus was isolated for the first time in the USA in 1980, before HIV-1 (also a retrovirus) was discovered in 1983. Genomically, simian T-lymphotropic virus (STLV) isolates cluster closely with HTLV-1 in the same region, suggesting simian-to-human transmission at multiple occasions.

Reservoir: Human.

Transmission: The virus can be transmitted from mother to child through breast-milk; also through sexual contact, contaminated blood products, organ transplants, and shared syringes during iv drug use.

Incubation period: 20–30 years.

Clinical findings: The most prevalent HTLV-1 clinical manifestations can be divided into those associated with ATL (immunosuppression) or associated with HAM/TSP (immunoactivation). The HTLV-1-infected individual who immunologically tends to immunosuppression can develop opportunistic infections such as *Strongyloides stercoralis* hyperinfection, recurrent skin infections and ATL. The HTLV-1-infected individual who tends to immunoactivation can develop HTLV-associated uveitis, polymyositis, inclusion body myositis, arthritis, pulmonary infiltrative pneumonitis, Sjögren syndrome and HAM/TSP.

Diagnostic tests: Serological tests cross-react with HTLV-2, requiring positive ELISA to be confirmed by Western blot, IFA, or radioimmunoprecipitation (RIPA); RT-PCR.

Therapy: Chemotherapy is ineffective for treating aggressive forms of ATL. There is no satisfactory treatment for HAM/TSP. Access to adequate counseling and correct information about HTLV is of fundamental importance for HTLV-1 seropositive individuals.

Prevention: Screening blood and blood products before use, bottle-feeding (20% of breast-fed infants of infected mothers become infected), using condoms. Counseling and education of IVDUs to implement harm reduction practices.

Epidemiology: Approximately 15 to 20 million people worldwide are believed to be infected. In Africa all HTLV and STLV subtypes are found, and phylogenetic research suggest that HTLV-1 originated in Africa about 27,000 years ago. HTLV-1 infection is more common in women and the prevalence increases with age, with a peak incidence around age 50. Among HTLV-1 carriers, the lifetime risk of developing HAM/TSP ranges from between 0.3% and 4%. For ATL, this risk is estimated to be 1% to 5% and for HTLV-1-associated diseases in general, including ATL, HAM/TSP, uveitis, polymyositis and arthropathy, the lifetime risk may be close to 10%. Japan, Africa, Caribbean islands and South America are the areas of highest prevalence, but the reasons for this are unknown. Most infections world wide are due to subtype HTLV-1a. Distribution of the infection is focal, e.g. Brazil, Japan, and Iran, where HTLV-1 is limited to certain areas of each country. On several Japanese islands the prevalence can reach 37%. Socioeconomic or genetic factors may contribute to the development of HTLV-associated infective dermatitis, since the disease has not been reported in HTLV-1 epidemic Japan. For non-endemic areas such as Europe and North America, HTLV-1 infection is mainly found in immigrants from endemic areas, their offspring and sexual contacts, among sex workers and IVDUs.

Map source(s): The HTLV-1 map was made with data from D.U. Goncalves et al. (2010), S.A. Cooper et al. (2009), and F.A. Proietti et al. (2005).

Key references

Cooper SA, et al. (2009) The neurology of HTLV-1 infection. *Pract Neurol* **9**:16–26.

Goncalves DU, et al. (2010) Epidemiology, treatment, and prevention of human T-cell leukemia virus type 1-associated diseases. *Clin Microbiol Rev* **23**(3):577–589.

Proietti FA, et al. (2005) Global epidemiology of HTLV-I infection and associated diseases. *Oncogene* **24**:6058–6068.

Verdonck K, et al. (2007) Human T-lymphotropic virus 1: recent knowledge about an ancient infection. *Lancet Inf Dis* **7**:266–281.

Atlas of Human Infectious Diseases, First Edition. Heiman F.L. Wertheim, Peter Horby and John P. Woodall.
© 2012 Blackwell Publishing Ltd. Published 2012 by Blackwell Publishing Ltd.

Japanese Encephalitis

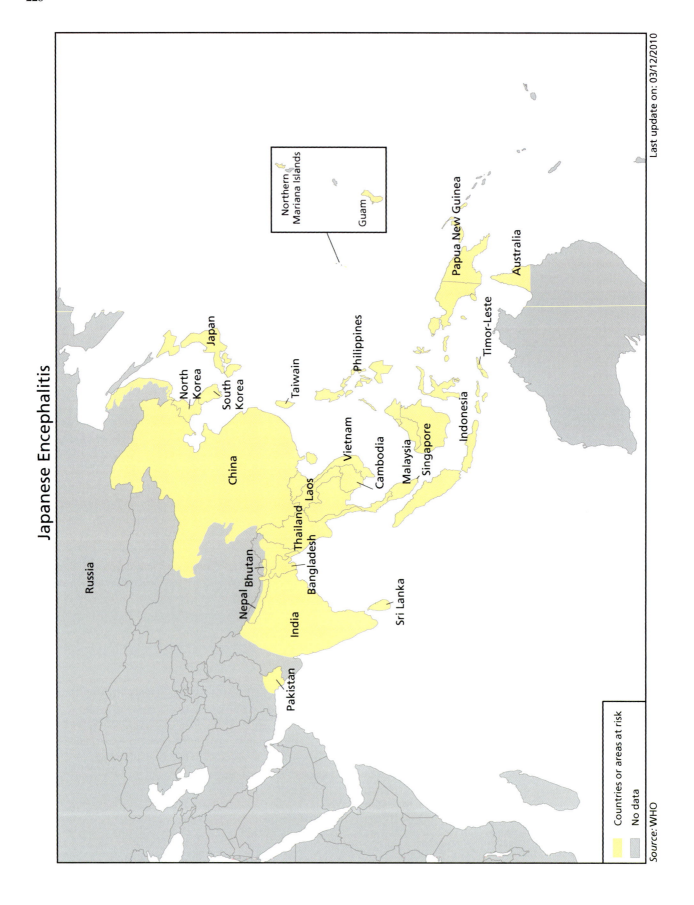

Russia

China

Japan

North Korea

South Korea

Taiwain

Vietnam

Cambodia

Laos

Thailand

Malaysia

Singapore

Indonesia

Philippines

Nepal

Bhutan

Bangladesh

India

Sri Lanka

Pakistan

Papua New Guinea

Australia

Timor-Leste

Northern Mariana Islands

Guam

Countries or areas at risk

No data

Source: WHO

Last update on: 03/12/2010

Disease: Japanese Encephalitis

Classification: ICD-9 062.0; ICD-10 A83.0

Syndromes and synonyms: Japanese B encephalitis.

Agent: Japanese encephalitis virus (JEV), an enveloped, single-stranded, positive sense RNA flavivirus. It is divided into five antigenic groups and four genotypes, which may be linked to differences in virulence.

Reservoir: Wading birds (Ardeidae) and domestic pigs which amplify the virus asymptomatically; mosquitoes by transovarial transmission and possibly overwintering adults.

Vector: Mosquito species that breed in rice fields and marshes, principally *Culex tritaenorhynchus* group; also *C. gelidus* and *C. vishnui*.

Transmission: By mosquito bite.

Cycle: Only ardeid birds and pigs have a sufficient viremia to infect mosquitoes. The mosquito picks up the virus from the blood of a viremic host. After a few days, the virus reaches the salivary glands and is injected into the next host when bitten. Humans are incidental and dead-end hosts as viremia does not reach sufficient levels to infect mosquitoes.

Incubation period: 6–16 days.

Clinical findings: High fever with headache, chills, neck stiffness, anorexia, nausea, and vomiting developing into aseptic meningitis or encephalitis with disorientation, coma, seizures, spastic paralysis, drowsiness, and stupor. Death occurs from respiratory complications or seizures. The case fatality rate is around 20%, but can be as high as 60%; 30% of those who survive suffer lasting damage to the central nervous system.

Diagnostic tests: Serology: IgM capture ELISA on serum or CSF; antibodies can be detected in CSF after 4 days of disease onset, and in serum after 7 days. Virus isolation or viral RNA detection by RT-PCR are insensitive.

Therapy: Supportive, there is no specific treatment.

Prevention: Various vaccines are available; personal anti-mosquito precautions; intermittent irrigation of rice fields disrupts vector breeding; vaccination of pigs reduces amplification.

Epidemiology: JEV is the leading cause of viral encephalitis in Asia: 35,000 to 50,000 cases are reported annually but this believed to be a significant underestimate of the true disease burden. 20–30% die and 30–50% of survivors have neurologic or psychiatric sequelae. It is epidemic in temperate parts of Asia, linked to the seasonal occurrence of mosquitoes, and endemic in tropical regions of Asia due to the year-round mosquito activity. Intensification and expansion of irrigated rice production systems in South and Southeast Asia over the past 20 years have had an important impact on the disease burden caused by Japanese encephalitis, since the vectors breed in rice fields. The vectors prefer non-human hosts, but do feed on humans in periods of peak activity. The disease is mainly seen in children under the age of 15 and the elderly, since most adults are immune from earlier infection; peak age is 3–5 years. The range of JE virus has recently expanded into the Torres Strait of northern Australia, but the disease is rare in western Pacific islands.

Map sources: The Japanese Encephalitis map was made with the following sources:

- CDC Approximate geographic range of Japanese encephalitis, at http://www.cdc.gov/mmwr/preview/mmwrhtml/rr5901a1.htm#fig2 (accessed on 30/10/2010).
- CDC (2010) Risk of Japanese Encephalitis by country, region and season, at http://www.cdc.gov/ncidod/dvbid/jencephalitis/risk-table.htm (accessed on 02/1/2010).
- WHO at http://gamapserver.who.int/mapLibrary/Files/Maps/Global_JE_ITHRiskMap.png (accessed on 26/08/2010).

Key references

Barrett ADT (2001) Japanese encephalitis. In Service MW (ed.), *The Encyclopedia of Arthropod-transmitted Infections*, CAB International, pp. 239–246.

Center for Disease Control and Prevention (2012) *Japanese Encephalitis. Yellow Book.* http://wwwnc.cdc.gov/travel/yellowbook/2012/

Mackenzie JS, et al. (2004) Emerging flaviviruses: the spread and resurgence of Japanese encephalitis, West Nile and dengue viruses. *Nat Med* **10**:S98–S109.

Atlas of Human Infectious Diseases, First Edition. Heiman F.L. Wertheim, Peter Horby and John P. Woodall.
© 2012 Blackwell Publishing Ltd. Published 2012 by Blackwell Publishing Ltd.

Lassa Fever

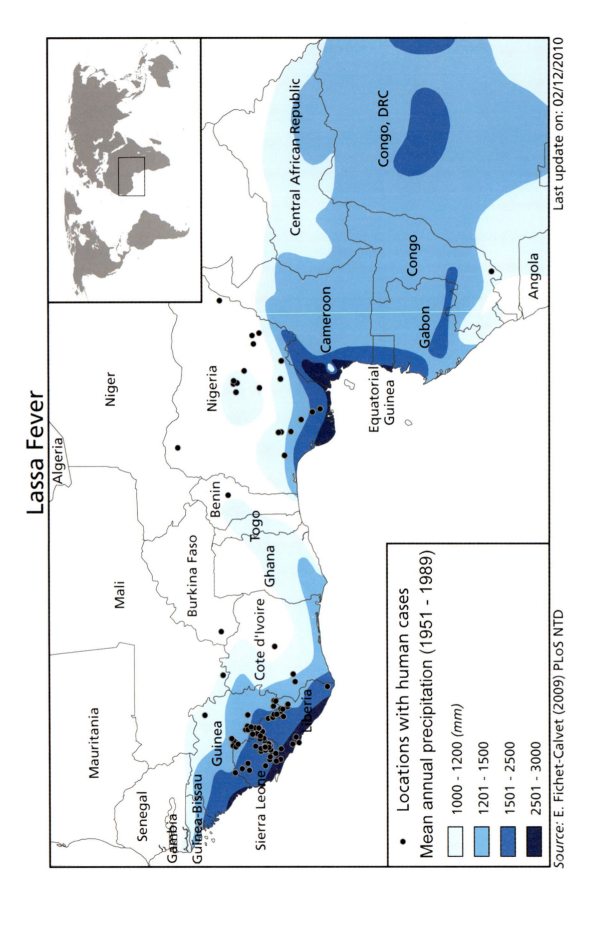

Locations with human cases

Mean annual precipitation (1951 - 1989)

- 1000 - 1200 (*mm*)
- 1201 - 1500
- 1501 - 2500
- 2501 - 3000

Source: E. Fichet-Calvet (2009) PLoS NTD

Last update on: 02/12/2010

Disease: Lassa Fever

Classification: ICD-9 078.8; ICD-10 A96.2

Synonyms: None.

Agent: Lassa fever virus (LFV), a spherical, enveloped, bi-segmented negative strand RNA virus of the genus *Arenavirus* in the family Arenaviridae.

Reservoir: The multi-mammate rat *(Mastomys natalensis)*, which lives in houses and surrounding fields. Previous studies that identified *M. erythroleucus* and *M. huberti* as reservoirs may have confused the species. *M. natalensis* is generally absent in coastal West Africa.

Vector: None.

Transmission: By inhalation of aerosolized excreta of the rodent host, or contact with food or household items contaminated with rodent excreta. Nosocomial transmission is regular in resource-constrained settings.

Cycle: Rodent–rodent, with humans as accidental dead-end hosts. Infected reservoir hosts are asymptomatic and excrete infectious virus in the urine.

Incubation period: 6–21 days, usually 7–12 days.

Clinical findings: Gradual onset, malaise, fever, headache, sore throat, cough, nausea, vomiting, diarrhea, myalgia, chest, and abdominal pain; inflammation and exudation of the pharynx and conjunctivae are common. Progression to multisystem disease occurs in 20% of infections, with hypotension or shock, hemorrhage, pleural effusion, seizures, encephalopathy and edema of the face and neck. Transient alopecia, ataxia, and eighth cranial nerve deafness may follow; deafness may be permanent. In third-trimester pregnant patients, 80% have a fatal outcome and 95% of the fetuses abort. The overall CFR is 1%, but 15–20% in more severe, hospitalized patients.

Diagnostic tests: IgM ELISA, RT-PCR, virus isolation from blood, urine, or throat washing, seroconversion to IgG positive.

Therapy: Supportive care; ribavirin iv is effective if given within the first 6 days after infection. There is no vaccine.

Prevention: Rodent control in and around dwellings; infection control in hospitals, with barrier nursing and precautions to avoid contact with body fluids.

Epidemiology: LFV was isolated from a missionary nurse living in Lassa, Nigeria, in 1969. It is estimated there are 200,000 to 300,000 symptomatic Lassa fever cases in West Africa each year, with an associated mortality of 5,000 to 10,000. Lassa fever occurs in two geographically distinct regions: the Mano River region (Guinea, Sierra Leone, Liberia) in the West, and Nigeria in the East. In the dry season, the multi-mammate rat gathers in houses, and in the rainy season, the rat forages in the surrounding fields. Villages with Lassa fever are all located in rain forest areas or transition zones of rainforest to savannah, where the mean annual rainfall is above 1,500 mm and below 3,000 mm. LFV can be transmitted from rodents to humans both in the rainy and the dry season. However, in the dry season there may be an increased risk for humans due to aggregation of the rats in their houses.

Map Source: The Lassa Fever map is modified from Fichet-Calvet and Rogers (2009), with permission. Positive localities recorded from 1965 to 2007, corresponds to confirmed Lassa cases or studies demonstrating a seroprevalence superior to 10%.

Key references

Fichet-Calvet E, et al. (2007) Fluctuation of abundance and Lassa virus prevalence in *Mastomys natalensis* in Guinea, West Africa. *Vector Borne Zoonotic Dis* **7**(2):119–128.

Fichet-Calvet E and Rogers D (2009) Risk maps of Lassa fever in West Africa. *PLoS Negl Trop Dis* **3**(3):e388.

Frame JD, et al. (1970) Lassa fever, a new virus disease of man from West Africa. *Am J Trop Med Hyg* **19**:670–676.

Gunther S, et al. (2004) Lassa virus. *Crit Rev Clin Lab Sci* **41**:339–390.

Lecompte E, et al. (2006) *Mastomys natalensis* and Lassa fever, West Africa. *Emerg Infect Dis* **12**(12):1971–1974.

McCormick JB (1999) Lassa fever. In Saluzzo JF and Dodet B (eds.), *Emergence and Control of Rodent-Borne Viral Diseases*. Elsevier, pp. 177–195.

Monath TP, et al. (1974) Lassa virus isolation from *Mastomys natalensis* rodents during an epidemic in Sierra Leone. *Science* **185**:263–265.

Atlas of Human Infectious Diseases, First Edition. Heiman F.L. Wertheim, Peter Horby and John P. Woodall.
© 2012 Blackwell Publishing Ltd. Published 2012 by Blackwell Publishing Ltd.

Mayaro Fever

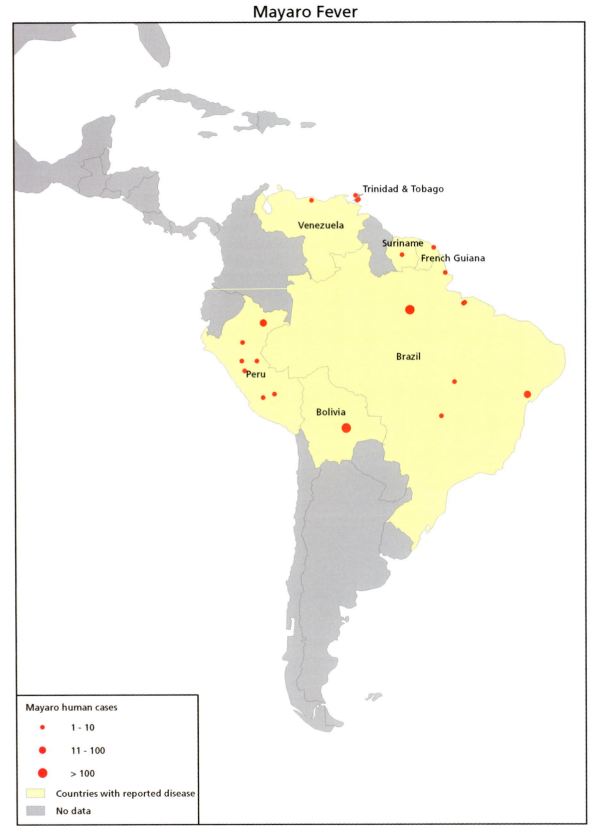

Trinidad & Tobago

Venezuela

Suriname

French Guiana

Brazil

Peru

Bolivia

Mayaro human cases

- 1 - 10
- 11 - 100
- > 100

Countries with reported disease

No data

Last update on: 08/11/2010

Disease: **Mayaro Fever**

Classification: ICD-9 066.3; ICD-10 A92.8

Syndromes and synonyms: Uruma fever.

Agent: Mayaro virus (MAYV), an enveloped, single-stranded, positive sense RNA virus, genus *Alphavirus* in the family Togaviridae, belonging to the Semliki Forest virus complex.

Reservoir: Probably non-human primates; the virus has been isolated from monkeys in Panama and French Guiana, also in the USA from a north-bound migratory bird. Antibody has been found in domestic animals and other vertebrates.

Vector: Mosquitoes, principally canopy-dwelling *Haemagogus* and *Sabethes* spp. The virus has also been isolated from *Psorophora*, *Mansonia* and *Culex* spp.

Transmission: By mosquito bite. Airborne transmission has been reported among laboratory personnel.

Cycle: The mosquito becomes infected with MAYV during feeding on a viremic host. The virus crosses the gut wall and multiplies in the organs of the mosquito. After a few days, depending on the ambient temperature, the virus reaches the salivary glands and is injected into the next host during feeding.

Incubation period: Approx. 1 week.

Clinical findings: Dengue-like acute febrile illness with chills, headache, retro-orbital pain, myalgia and severe arthralgia of the small joints of the hands and feet, sometimes nausea, vomiting and diarrhea, painful lymphadenopathies and often a maculopapular rash. Arthralgias may persist for months, but no fatalities have been recorded.

Diagnostic tests: IgM ELISA; IgG cross-reacts with other alphaviruses. Confirmation needed by neutralization test, virus isolation, or a significant rise in specific antibody between acute and convalescent serum samples; RT-PCR.

Therapy: Supportive.

Prevention: Since the virus has a jungle cycle, environmental insecticide spraying is not feasible; routine personal anti-mosquito measures are indicated.

Epidemiology: MAYV is enzootic in the humid tropical rainforests of South America. Infections peak in the rainy season when the mosquito vectors are most abundant. Most human cases occur sporadically and involve persons who work or reside in humid tropical forest; several small outbreaks of Mayaro fever have been described in residents of rural communities of the Amazon region of Brazil, Bolivia, and Peru. Travelers have imported MAYV from Surinam to the Netherlands and from Brazil into France. The virus has been detected in migratory birds.

Map sources: The Mayaro Fever map was made with multiple sources mentioned under key references.

Key references

Tesh RB, et al. (1999) Mayaro virus disease: an emerging mosquito-borne zoonosis in tropical South America. *Clin Infect Dis* **28**(1):67–73.

Powers AM (2006) Genetic relationships among Mayaro and Una viruses suggest distinct patterns of transmission. *Am J Trop Med Hyg* **75**(3):461–469.

Torres JR (2004) Family cluster of Mayaro fever, Venezuela. *Emerg Infect Dis* **10**(7):1304–1306.

Calisher CH (2001) Mayaro virus. In Service MW (ed.) *The Encyclopedia of Arthropod-transmitted Infections*, CAB International, pp. 335–339.

Atlas of Human Infectious Diseases, First Edition. Heiman F.L. Wertheim, Peter Horby and John P. Woodall.
© 2012 Blackwell Publishing Ltd. Published 2012 by Blackwell Publishing Ltd.

Measles

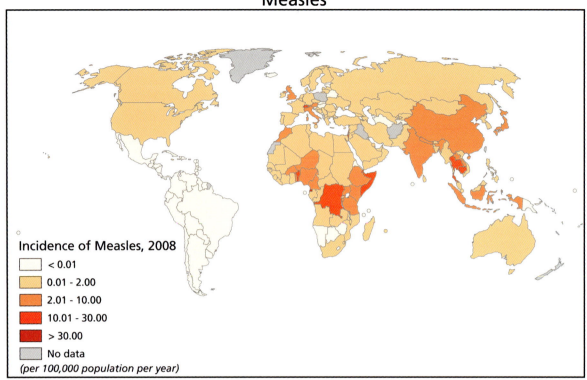

Incidence of Measles, 2008
- [ ] < 0.01
- [ ] 0.01 - 2.00
- [ ] 2.01 - 10.00
- [ ] 10.01 - 30.00
- [ ] > 30.00
- [ ] No data

(per 100,000 population per year)

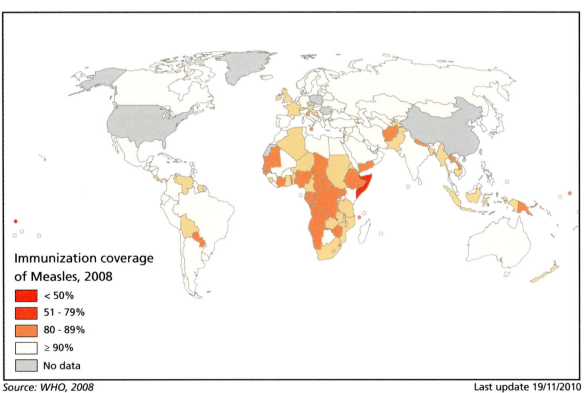

Immunization coverage
of Measles, 2008
- [ ] < 50%
- [ ] 51 - 79%
- [ ] 80 - 89%
- [ ] ≥ 90%
- [ ] No data

Source: WHO, 2008

Last update 19/11/2010

Disease: Measles

Classification: ICD-9 9055.0; ICD-10 B05

Synonyms: Rubeola, morbilli.

Agent: Measles virus, a single-stranded RNA negative-sense morbillivirus, family Paramyxoviridae.

Reservoir: Humans.

Transmission: By airborne droplets from or contact with nose and throat secretions of infected persons, very high from 4 days before to 4 days after rash appears, or with fomites contaminated with those secretions. Droplets remain infectious for several hours, longer under conditions of low humidity. Measles virus is highly contagious.

Incubation period: Median 12.5 days, range 1–3 weeks.

Clinical findings: High fever, conjunctivitis, coryza, cough, maculopapular rash beginning on the face, spreading downwards to reach the hands and feet. Characteristic small white spots (Koplik spots) on the buccal mucosa. Complications may consist of otitis media, pneumonia, laryngotracheal bronchitis (croup), blindness, severe skin infections, severe diarrhea and encephalitis, sometimes fatal. Complications are more common and more severe in people with malnutrition, vitamin A deficiency, and chronic diseases. Very rarely, subacute sclerosing panencephalitis may appear years later.

Diagnostic tests: Detection by RT-PCR on blood or swabs of nasopharyngeal mucosa; virus isolation from swabs, blood, or urine; detection of measles specific IgM or significant rise in antibody titer in paired samples.

Therapy: Supportive; vitamin A supplementation is important to avoid the complications of vitamin A deficiency resulting from the infection. Efficacy of ribavirin is unproven.

Prevention: Vaccination with live attenuated virus vaccine should be routine for children (minimum age: 12 months), preferably with the combined measles, mumps, and rubella vaccine (MMR), with a booster at age 4 to 6 years. Infected children should be kept out of school and away from other child contacts. Displaced persons (e.g. refugees) should be vaccinated within a week of their arrival in a camp. For post-exposure prophylaxis, vaccination is recommended within 72 hours of exposure, with a booster in 5–6 weeks; human immunoglobulin for immunocompromised persons and those for whom vaccine is contraindicated.

Epidemiology: Measles has a worldwide distribution, but is eliminated from the western hemisphere through vaccination. Measles deaths world wide fell by 78% from an estimated 733,000 in 2000 to 164,000 in 2008; all regions but one have achieved the United Nations goal of reducing measles mortality by 90%, however, it remains the leading cause of vaccine-preventable deaths in children and there are fears of a resurgence if vaccination falters for lack of resources. WHO figures for 2008 were 282,000 reported cases, with many thousands more unreported. Some 58% of countries have 90% or more vaccine coverage, adequate to stop transmission, but endemic countries have case fatality rates of up to 30% in places. Most measles deaths (>95%) occur in countries with a per capita income of <US$ 1,000. Measles-free countries still have imported cases and limited outbreaks in subpopulations with low or no vaccination coverage (e.g. religious communities). Measles is being considered for global elimination or even eradication.

Map sources: The Measles map was made with data obtained from WHO, available at: www.who.int/immunization_monitoring/en/.

Key references

De Quadros CA (2004) Can measles be eradicated globally? *Bull World Health Organ* **82**(2):134–138.

Kelly H, et al. (2009) WHO criteria for measles elimination: a critique with reference to criteria for polio elimination. *Euro Surveill* **14**(50):19445.

Strebel P, et al. (2003) The unfinished measles immunization agenda. *J Infect Dis* **187**(Suppl. 1):S1–S7.

World Health Organization (2009) *State of the World's Vaccines and Immunization*, 3rd edn. WHO, UNICEF, World Bank. Geneva.

Atlas of Human Infectious Diseases, First Edition. Heiman F.L. Wertheim, Peter Horby and John P. Woodall.
© 2012 Blackwell Publishing Ltd. Published 2012 by Blackwell Publishing Ltd.

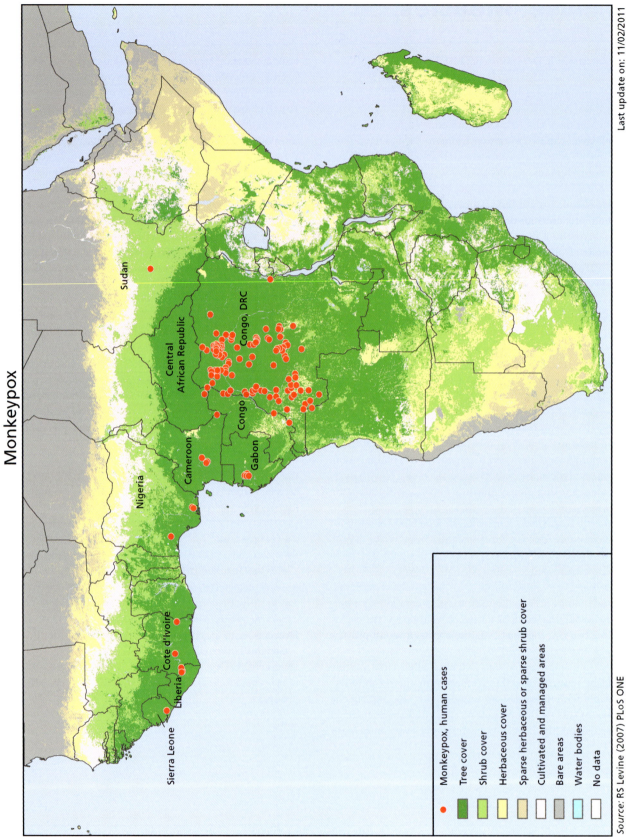

Monkeypox

Sudan

Central
African Republic

Congo, DRC

Congo

Cameroon

Gabon

Nigeria

Cote d'Ivoire

Liberia

Sierra Leone

Monkeypox, human cases
Tree cover
Shrub cover
Herbaceous cover
Sparse herbaceous or sparse shrub cover
Cultivated and managed areas
Bare areas
Water bodies
No data

Last update on: 11/02/2011

Source: RS Levine (2007) PLoS ONE

Disease: **Monkeypox**

Classification: ICD-9 051.9; ICD-10 B04

Syndromes and synonyms: Simian variola.

Agent: Monkeypox virus (MPV), a double-stranded DNA virus of the genus *Orthopoxvirus*, family Poxviridae. Two clades of monkeypox viruses are known: the West African virus and the Congo Basin virus. The Congo Basin strain is more virulent than the West African strain. The MPV genome is > 96% identical to the variola virus genome. However, MPV is not a direct ancestor or descendent of variola virus.

Reservoir: Undetermined. Thought to be forest rodents (squirrels, rats, mice, dormice), shrews and monkeys in the rainforests of West and Central Africa.

Vector: None.

Transmission: By bite or direct percutaneous contact, mucosal or respiratory exposure to blood, tissues, fluids or lesions of infected animals. In Africa, transmission mainly occurs through butchering infected wildlife for food. Person-to-person transmission probably occurs through direct contact with infected tissue/fluid, respiratory droplet spread, and indirect via contaminated objects.

Cycle: Animal to animal, with occasional spill over to humans. Sustained human-to-human transmission has not been documented.

Incubation period: 7–21 days (mean 12 days).

Clinical findings: Symptoms are similar to smallpox, but milder: fever, headache, myalgia, backache, lymphadenopathy (not seen in smallpox), malaise, sore throat, cough, shortness of breath, followed by a vesicular-pustular rash on the face and body; the lesions eventually crust and fall off. The outcome can be fatal (CFR: 1–10%).

Diagnostic tests: The detection of virus by culture or PCR in characteristic skin lesions. Histopathology and immunohistochemistry also support the diagnosis. Laboratory testing should be performed in specialized laboratories.

Therapy: Supportive. Cidofovir has proven anti-monkeypox viral activity *in vitro* and in animal studies, but its efficacy in patients is unknown, neither is any benefit from treatment with vaccinia immune globulin known.

Prevention: Smallpox vaccine is protective, but not a feasible solution in the remote forest habitat where monkeypox is endemic. Hospital personnel should isolate patients and take infection control precautions.

Epidemiology: MPV is endemic in heavily forested areas of Africa, primarily of low altitude and high humidity. The outlier in shrub country in the Sudan is anomalous ecologically and might have been initiated by an infected traveler from the Congo Basin region. Males and females are equally affected, children under 15 more than adults. Comparison of active surveillance data in one health zone in the Democratic Republic of the Congo from the 1980s (0.72 per 10,000) and 2006–2007 (14.5 per 10,000) suggests a 20-fold increase in human monkeypox incidence 30 years after mass smallpox vaccination ceased in that country.

In 2003, multiple cases of monkeypox occurred across the USA among persons who had contact with the excretions of sick prairie dogs (native ground squirrels) either at a child-care center or from pet stores. The animals had been exposed to imported, infected West African rodents on the premises of a distributor of exotic pets. There were more than 70 cases but no fatalities.

Map sources: The Monkeypox map is modified with permission from R.S. Levine et al. (2007) with updates from the medical literature up to 2010.

Key references

Center for Food Security and Public Health (2009) Monkeypox. *Factsheet MNKY_2009*.

Damon IK, et al. (2006) Discovery of monkeypox in Sudan. *N Engl J Med* **355**(9):962–963.

Hutson CL, et al. (2010) Comparison of West African and Congo Basin monkeypox viruses in BALB/c and C57BL/6 mice. *PLoS ONE* **5**(1):e8912.

Levine RS, et al. (2007). Ecological niche and geographic distribution of human monkeypox in Africa. *PloS ONE* **2**(1):e176.

Rimoina AW, et al. (2010) Major increase in human monkeypox incidence 30 years after smallpox vaccination campaigns cease in the Democratic Republic of Congo. *Proc Natl Acad Sci* **107**(37):16262–16267.

Atlas of Human Infectious Diseases, First Edition. Heiman F.L. Wertheim, Peter Horby and John P. Woodall.
© 2012 Blackwell Publishing Ltd. Published 2012 by Blackwell Publishing Ltd.

Mumps

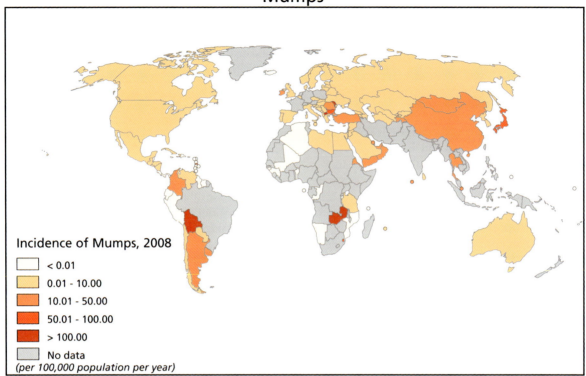

Incidence of Mumps, 2008

- ☐ < 0.01
- ☐ 0.01 - 10.00
- ☐ 10.01 - 50.00
- ☐ 50.01 - 100.00
- ☐ > 100.00
- ☐ No data

(per 100,000 population per year)

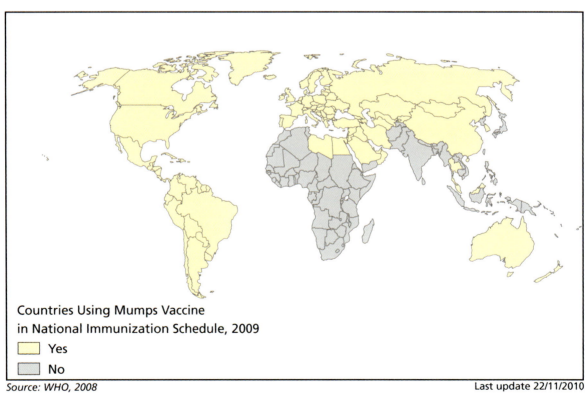

Countries Using Mumps Vaccine
in National Immunization Schedule, 2009

- ☐ Yes
- ☐ No

Source: WHO, 2008   *Last update 22/11/2010*

Disease: **Mumps**

Classification: ICD-9 072; ICD-10 B26

Syndromes and synonyms: Infectious parotitis

Agent: Mumps virus, an enveloped RNA virus of the family Paromyxoviridae. Twelve genotypes are currently recognized.

Reservoir: Humans

Vector: None

Transmission: Through contact with infectious respiratory droplets or saliva.

Incubation period: Median 19 days, range 15–24 days.

Clinical findings: Up to one-third of cases are subclinical. The illness begins with a prodrome of fever, malaise, and headache followed by unilateral or, more commonly, bilateral tender swelling of the parotid (parotitis) or other salivary glands. Parotitis is present in 95% of clinical cases. Infection and inflammation of the testicles (orchitis) occurs in up to 30% of adult males but is rare before puberty. Orchitis results in testicular atrophy in 50% of cases but rarely causes sterility Adult women may rarely suffer inflammation of the ovaries (oophoritis). The commonest nervous system manifestation of mumps infection is meningitis, which is seen in up to 10% of cases but is self-limiting and does not result in death of disability. Other rarer clinical complications include hearing loss, encephalitis, and pancreatitis. Mumps infection in early pregnancy may be associated with an increased risk of spontaneous abortion.

Diagnostic tests: The detection of virus in saliva, cerebrospinal fluid, urine, or seminal fluid by culture or RT-PCR. Detection of mumps specific IgM or significant rise in antibody titer in paired samples.

Therapy: No specific treatment is available.

Prevention: Mumps is preventable by the use of live attenuated mumps virus vaccines. Various vaccine strains are available and may vary in immunogenicity and the incidence of adverse effects, such as fever, rash, parotitis, or meningitis.

Epidemiology: Studies of unvaccinated populations in some western countries indicate that almost everyone will be infected with mumps by adulthood; however the epidemiology of mumps is less well characterized in developing countries. The true number of mumps cases is not known, since it is often a mild disease and reported cases probably represent fewer than 10% of all infections. There is geographic variation in circulating mumps virus genotypes, and there can be several genotypes circulating simultaneously in one area and shifts over time in predominant genotypes. Mumps vaccination is recommended at age 12–18 months and is included in the standard immunization program of most developed countries, usually in a trivalent vaccine with measles and rubella (MMR vaccine). A booster dose in later childhood is also recommended for countries with a good immunization program. Several developed countries with a well-established mumps vaccination program have experienced significant outbreaks in young adults, who were too old to be included in the childhood immunization schedule and had not been exposed to natural infection due to an overall reduction in the transmission of mumps in the population. Other possible reasons for mumps outbreaks in vaccinated populations include a waning of vaccine-induced immunity and genotype mismatch between the vaccine strain and the wild virus. Since the complications of mumps are more common in affected adults compared to affected children, a shift in the average age of infection can lead to an increase in the number of observed complications. However, despite these issues, it must be remembered that comprehensive mumps vaccination programs are associated with a massive overall decrease in the burden of mumps morbidity.

Map sources: The Mumps map was made with data obtained from WHO, available at: www.who.int/immunization_monitoring/en/.

Key references

Galazka AM, et al. (1999) Mumps and mumps vaccine: a global review. *Bull World Health Org* **77**:3–14.

Hiivd A, et al. (2008) Mumps. *Lancet* **371**:932–944.

World Health Organization (2009) *State of the World's Vaccines and Immunization*, 3rd edn. WHO, UNICEF, World Bank. Geneva.

Atlas of Human Infectious Diseases, First Edition. Heiman F.L. Wertheim, Peter Horby and John P. Woodall.
© 2012 Blackwell Publishing Ltd. Published 2012 by Blackwell Publishing Ltd.

O'nyong-nyong Virus Disease

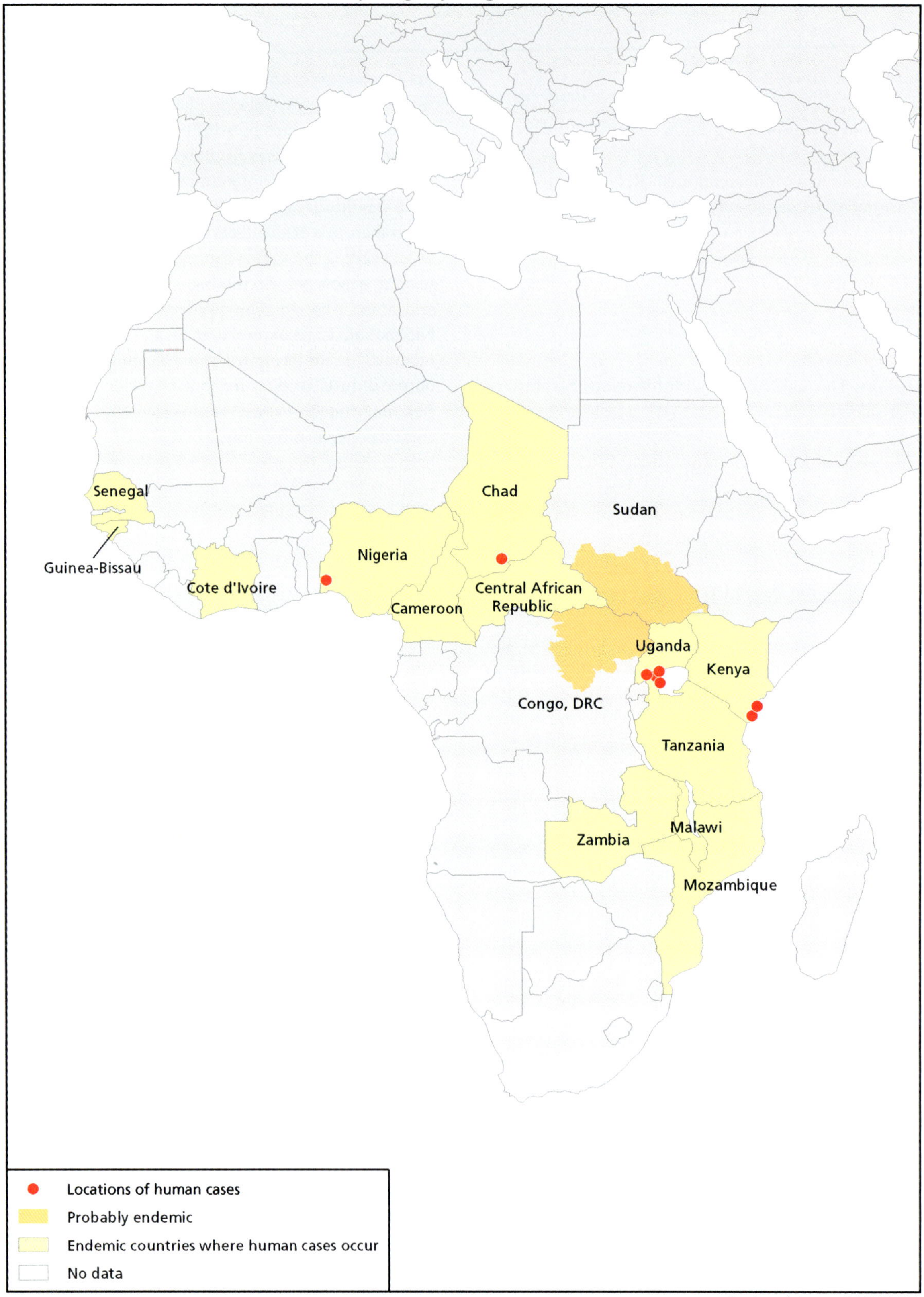

Senegal

Guinea-Bissau

Cote d'Ivoire

Nigeria

Chad

Sudan

Cameroon

Central African
Republic

Uganda

Kenya

Congo, DRC

Tanzania

Zambia

Malawi

Mozambique

● Locations of human cases

Probably endemic

Endemic countries where human cases occur

No data

Last update on: 19/08/2010

Disease: O'nyong-nyong Virus Disease

Classification: ICD-9 066.3; ICD-10 A92.1

Syndromes and synonyms: The name means 'joint-breaker' in the Acholi language of Africa.

Agent: O'nyong-nyong virus (ONNV), an enveloped RNA virus, genus *Alphavirus* in the family Togaviridae, closely related to chikungunya virus (CHIKV, see Chikungunya Fever map). Strains bear the names Gulu, Igbo-Ora, and SG650 viruses.

Reservoir: Unknown.

Vector: ONNV is transmitted by the African malaria vectors *Anopheles funestus* and *An. gambiae*, and probably other members of the complex.

Transmission: By mosquito bite. There is no direct person-to-person transmission documented, and no evidence of congenital transmission.

Cycle: Humans are viremic at a titer high enough to infect mosquitoes for up to 5 days after infection. The virus travels from the mosquito gut to the salivary glands in 5–7 days, depending on the ambient temperature (extrinsic incubation period), after which it can infect another human during feeding.

Incubation period: Estimated to be at least 8 days.

Clinical findings: Dengue-like acute febrile illness with sudden onset fever, severe chills, severe headache, eye pain, symmetrical polyarthralgia of all joints (as opposed to dengue, which attacks mainly elbows and knees), generalized myalgia, sometimes dry cough and coryza, leucopenia and often an itching, descending morbilliform rash. Marked cervical lymphadenitis distinguishes it from chikungunya infection. Hemorrhagic signs have not been seen. Recovery is complete, without sequelae.

Diagnostic tests: RT-PCR on whole blood or serum; virus isolation; plaque reduction neutralization test (there is cross-reactivity with related viruses, including CHIKV).

Therapy: Supportive, there is no specific treatment.

Prevention: Standard anti-mosquito and anti-malarial precautions. There is no vaccine.

Epidemiology: ONNV is a mutant of CHIKV that appeared in 1959 in Uganda and was spread by anopheline mosquitoes across the malaria belt of Africa, leading to a large mosquito-borne virus epidemic. This large epidemic was remarkable because, in spite of the occurrence of millions of cases, no deaths were reported. It ended without a trace in 1962, reappearing as sporadic cases in Africa at rare intervals. In Nigeria in 1966 and 1969, cases were described as a new virus, Igbo-Ora, later recognized as ONNV. There was a small outbreak in Côte d'Ivoire in 1984–1985 and again in 2003, also described as Igbo-Ora virus and a small recurrence in Uganda in 1996. Serological evidence suggested its presence in humans in Kenya in 1994–1995 and in horses in Nigeria, but serological tests are subject to cross-reactions with CHIKV antibody. It is not known how or where the virus survives between outbreaks, but sequence data show very little variation between ONNV strains isolated in Uganda in 1959 and 1996–1997, suggesting that the virus persists, rather than undergoing repeated mutations from CHIKV (which has a non-human primate reservoir).

Map sources: The O'nyong-nyong Virus Disease map was made by visualizing countries with reported human cases reported in the medical literature up to 2010. In case the location of human cases is known, this is shown (red dot).

Key references

Lanciotti RS, et al. (1998) Emergence of epidemic O'nyong-nyong fever in Uganda after a 35-year absence: genetic characterization of the virus. *Virology* **252**:258–226.

Moore DL, et al. (1975) Arthropod-borne viral infections of man in Nigeria, 1964–1970. *Ann Trop Med Parasitol* **69**:49–64.

Powers AM, et al. (2000) Re-emergence of Chikungunya and O'nyong-nyong viruses: evidence for distinct geographical lineages and distant evolutionary relationships. *J Gen Virol* **81**:471–479.

Woodall J (2001) O'nyong-nyong virus. In Service M (ed.) *The Encyclopedia of Arthropod-transmitted Infections*. CAB International, pp. 388–390.

Oropouche Virus Disease

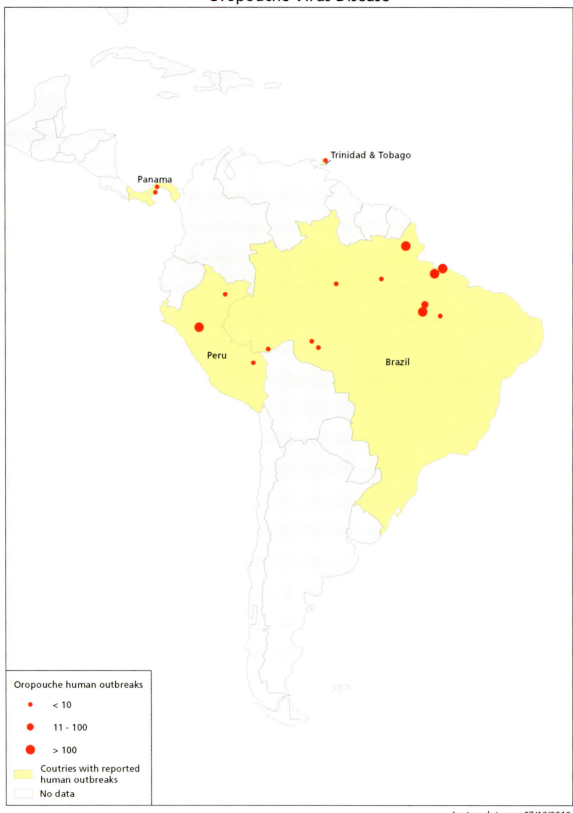

Oropouche human outbreaks

- •   < 10
- ●   11 - 100
- ●   > 100

Coutries with reported human outbreaks

No data

Last update on: 07/12/2010

Disease: Oropouche Virus Disease

Classification: ICD-9 065; ICD-10 A93.0

Syndromes and synonyms: Oropouche fever, fevre de Mojui.

Agent: Oropouche virus (OROV), a spherical enveloped, single-stranded, negative-sense RNA virus, belonging to the Orthobunyavirus group of the Bunyaviridae family, with 3 genotypes.

Reservoir: Monkeys, three-toed sloths (*Bradypus tridactylus*), marsupials, and forest birds.

Vector: During urban epidemics, biting midges (*Culicoides paraensis*); also mosquitoes of *Aedes* and *Culex* genera.

Transmission: By insect bite.

Cycle: The vector becomes infected with OROV by feeding on a viremic host. The virus crosses the gut wall and multiplies in the organs of the insect. After a few days, depending on the ambient temperature, the virus reaches the salivary glands and is injected into the next host during feeding. Jungle cycle: OROV is transmitted among sloths, marsupials, primates, and birds by the mosquitoes *Aedes serratus* and *Culex quinquefasciatus*. Urban cycle: OROV is transmitted to humans by midges (*Culicoides paraensis*).

Incubation period: 2–14 days.

Clinical findings: Sudden onset fever (may be diphasic), headache, myalgia, arthralgia, anorexia, dizziness, chills, and photophobia. Also nausea, vomiting, diarrhea, epigastric and eye pain, conjunctivitis, and meningitis have been reported. Recently, spontaneous hemorrhagic phenomena were reported in human cases. The disease is self-limiting, there are no reports of OROV related deaths.

Diagnostic tests: Serology (IgM ELISA, IFA) or by detection of OROV RNA in blood by RT-PCR.

Therapy: Supportive, there is no specific treatment.

Prevention: Personal anti-insect measures; there is no vaccine. Removal of culicoides breeding sites in cacao husks and felled banana trunks.

Epidemiology: OROV was first isolated in Trinidiad in 1955. In South America, cases are limited to Trinidad, Panama, and the Amazon basin. Oropouche fever is, after dengue fever, the most common arboviral infection in Brazil. The virus has periodically caused large urban epidemics in Brazil and Peru, during which up to 60% of the population has been affected. There also outbreaks in villages and sporadic cases. Approximately 500,000 cases have occurred in Brazil since the 1960s. There are three OROV genotypes circulating in Brazil: genotypes I and II in the Amazon Basin and genotype III in the Southeast Region. Genotype III has been isolated from a marmoset (*Callithrix* species) in southeastern Brazil, and also occurs in Panama. Outbreaks coincide with periods of highest rainfall, when biting midge density is greatest. OROV infections are likely underdiagnosed in South America as was seen during a concurrent outbreak of dengue virus and OROV in Manus (Brazil), where OROV infections were missed by physicians and the Public Health Authority.

Map sources: The Oropouche Virus Disease map was made by geocoding human outbreaks that were reported between 1955 and 2010 in the medical literature and ProMED mail.

Key references
Azevedo RSS, et al. (2007) Reemergence of Oropouche Fever, Northern Brazil. *Emerg Infect Dis* **13**(6):912–915.
Bernardes-Terzian AC, et al. (2009) Sporadic oropouche virus infection, acre, Brazil. *Emerg Infect Dis* **15**(2):348–350.
Mellor PS. (2001) Oropouche virus. In Service MW (ed.) *The Encyclopedia of Arthropod-transmitted Infections*, CAB International, pp. 391–399.
Mourão MPG, et al. (2009) Oropouche fever outbreak, Manaus, Brazil, 2007–2008. *Emerg Infect Dis*. Available from: http://www.cdc.gov/EID/content/15/12/2063.htm.
Nunes MR, et al. (2005) Oropouche virus isolation, southeast Brazil. *Emerg Infect Dis* **11**(10):1610–1613.
Saeed MF (2000) Nucleotide sequences and phylogeny of the nucleocapsid gene of Oropouche virus. *J Gen Virol* **81**:473–478.
Vasconcelos HB (2009) Oropouche fever epidemic in Northern Brazil: Epidemiology and molecular characterization of isolates. *J Clin Virol* **44**:129–133.

Atlas of Human Infectious Diseases, First Edition. Heiman F.L. Wertheim, Peter Horby and John P. Woodall.
© 2012 Blackwell Publishing Ltd. Published 2012 by Blackwell Publishing Ltd.

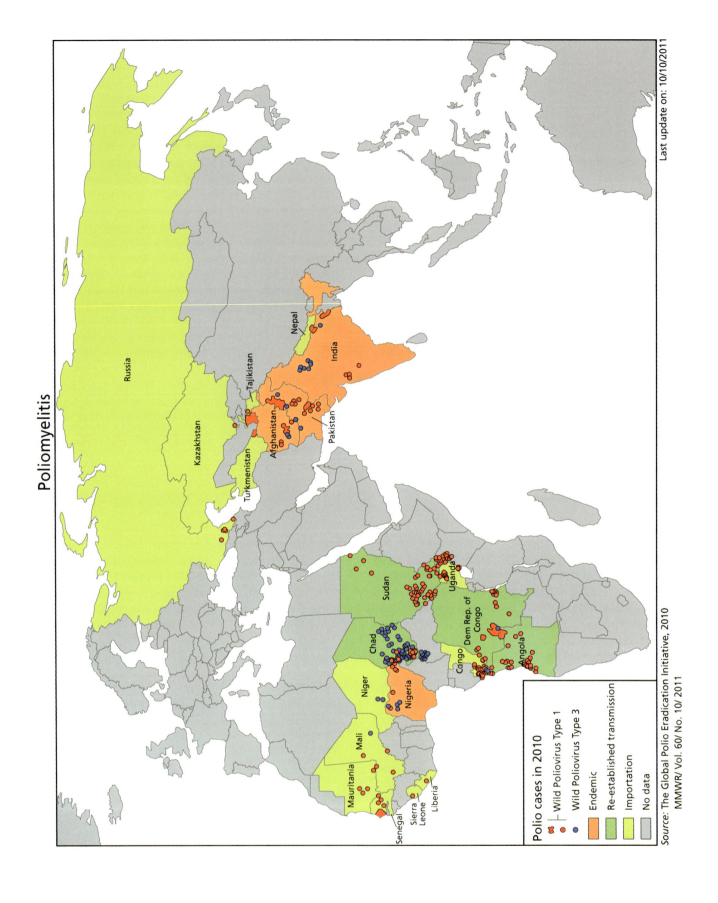

Poliomyelitis

Russia

Kazakhstan

Turkmenistan

Tajikistan

Afghanistan

Pakistan

Nepal

India

Mauritania

Mali

Niger

Nigeria

Chad

Sudan

Uganda

Congo

Dem Rep. of Congo

Angola

Senegal

Sierra Leone

Liberia

Polio cases in 2010

| | Wild Poliovirus Type 1 |
| | Wild Poliovirus Type 3 |

Endemic

Re-established transmission

Importation

No data

Disease: Poliomyelitis

Classification: ICD-9 045; ICD-10 A80

Syndromes and synonyms: Polioviral fever, infantile paralysis, acute flaccid paralysis (AFP), bulbar polio.

Agent: Poliovirus, an RNA enterovirus with three types; type 1 cases are most common, followed by type 3; wild type 2 disappeared in 1999. Rare cases of all three types occur in unimmunized contacts of children vaccinated with the Sabin live attenuated vaccine.

Reservoir: Humans, generally children with inapparent infections.

Transmission: Oro-fecal. 100% of susceptible contacts become infected. Virus appears in the throat < 36 hours after infection, for a week, and in the feces after 72 hours for 3–6 weeks. Transmission through contaminated water and food has been reported rarely.

Incubation period: 3–35 days; 6–20 for paralytic cases.

Clinical findings: Less than 1% of infections result in acute flaccid paralysis, with around 90% of infections being subclinical. In 10% symptoms may include fever, malaise, headache, neck stiffness, pain in the limbs, nausea, and vomiting. Paralysis persists in 0.1–1.0% depending on the virulence of the strain. The flaccid paralysis is usually asymmetric and in one leg. The risk of paralysis is increased by intramuscular injections, immune-compromised state, trauma or surgery (tonsillectomy), and intense physical activity during the incubation period. Also adults are at greater risk of developing paralysis than young children. Aseptic meningitis occurs in around 1% of infections. More severe paralysis with quadriplegia and breathing problems (bulbar polio) may occur.

Diagnostic tests: Virus isolation from stool, CSF or oropharyngeal secretion, followed by typing (to determine if the virus is 'wild type' or a vaccine strain). Alternatively, the diagnosis can be established by serological testing.

Therapy: Supportive, there is no specific polio treatment.

Prevention: In 1988, the WHO launched the Global Polio Eradication Initiative (GPEI). The Americas were certified polio-free in 1994, the WHO Western Pacific Region in 2000 and Europe in 2002 (in 2010, there was importation of polio into Europe). The GPEI has four main strategies to stop transmission of the wild poliovirus: (1) high infant immunization coverage with four doses of oral poliovirus vaccine (OPV) in the first year of life; (2) supplementary doses of OPV to all children under 5 years of age during SIAs; (3) surveillance for wild poliovirus through reporting and laboratory testing of all acute flaccid paralysis (AFP) cases among children under 15 years of age; (4) targeted campaigns once wild poliovirus transmission is limited to a specific focal area. To be certified polio-free, three conditions must be met: (1) there are at least 3 years of zero polio cases due to wild poliovirus; (2) disease surveillance efforts in countries meet international standards; and (3) each country must illustrate the capacity to detect, report, and respond to 'imported' polio cases. Oral live attenuated polio vaccines can give rise to circulation of vaccine-derived polioviruses and rare cases of vaccine-associated paralytic poliomyelitis. For this reason, efforts are underway to develop affordable options for inactivated polio vaccination.

Epidemiology: Since the Global Polio Eradication Initiative, cases have decreased significantly. There were 1,292 reported cases in 2010, of which only 232 were in the endemic countries Afghanistan, India, Nigeria, and Pakistan. In endemic countries most cases are children aged <3 years. In 2009–2010, 23 previously polio-free countries were re-infected due to importation of the virus, notably hundreds of cases in Tajikistan. Most reported polio cases in 2010 ($n = 1,060$) were in non-endemic countries. Polio transmission seems to have been re-established in Chad, Angola, Sudan, and the DRC. This illustrates the difficulties of the global polio eradication program. Risk is seasonal in the temperate climates, with highest risks during the warmer months.

Map sources: The Poliomyelitis map was made with data obtained from the Global Polio Eradication Initiative, available at: www.polioeradication.org.

Key references

World Health Organization (2010) Poliomyelitis. *Factsheet* Nr 114 (www.who.int).

Dutta A (2008) Epidemiology of poliomyelitis – options and update. *Vaccine* **26**(45):5767–5773.

Nathanson N, et al. (2010) From emergence to eradication: the epidemiology of poliomyelitis deconstructed. *Am J Epidemiol* **172**(11):1213–1229.

246

Rabies

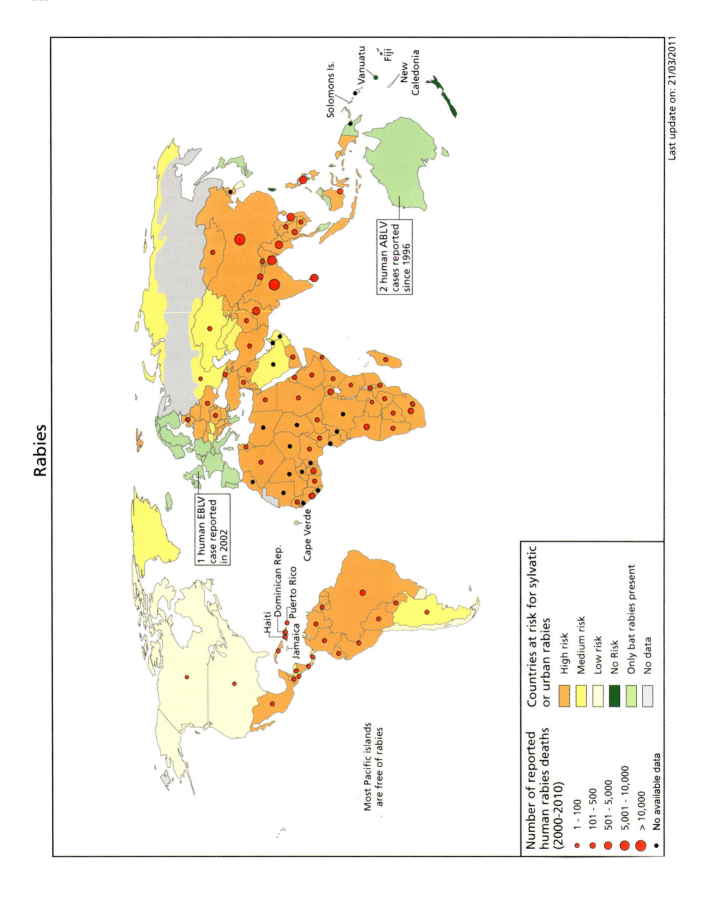

Last update on: 21/03/2011

Disease: Rabies

Classification: ICD-9 071; ICD-10 A82

Syndromes and synonyms: Hydrophobia, furious rabies, paralytic (dumb) rabies, classic rabies, non-classic rabies

Agent: Rabies virus, a rhabdovirus of the genus *Lyssavirus*, with a nonsegmented, negative-stranded RNA genome. At least 11 different genotypes exist, with genotype 1, rabies virus (RABV) causing classic rabies world wide. Genotypes 2–11 have a more limited host-range and geographic distribution: Lagos bat virus (LBV), Mokola virus (MOKV), Duvenhage virus (DUVV), European bat lyssa virus 1 and 2 (EBLV-1/2), Australian bat lyssa virus (ABLV), Aravan virus (ARAV), Irkut virus (IRKV), Khujand virus (KHUV), and West Caucasian bat virus (WCBV).

Reservoir: Wild and domestic canines, also skunks, raccoons, mongooses; vampire, frugivorous and insectivorous bats.

Vector: None.

Transmission: By animal bite through saliva commonly or scratch (rarely). Infected livestock do not bite typically, but may infect a person through their saliva. Very rare: licks upon mucosal surfaces; aerosols in bat-infested caves; person-to-person transmission via organ/tissue transplantation. Rabies can be transmitted via slaughtering of infected reservoir species, for instance dogs in countries where dogs are consumed.

Incubation period: Usually 1–3 months (rarely <1 week and >1 year) depending on virus variant, dose, wound severity and distance of wound from the brain.

Clinical findings: Rabies can manifest itself in two general forms: classic encephalitic (furious) rabies and paralytic (dumb) rabies. Both forms are progressive and generally lead to death. The majority of the cases present as encephalitic rabies, with hydrophobia and hyperexcitability. Paralytic rabies presents with flaccid muscle weakness or as febrile encephalopathy. In some papers, a third form, non-classic atypical rabies, is described.

Diagnostic tests: FA staining of frozen skin sections taken from the nape of the neck, or postmortem brain tissue; RT-PCR on saliva, skin or brain biopsy or buccal swab; serology; cell culture or mouse inoculation from saliva, skin, or brain.

Therapy: Supportive and palliative as rabies is almost invariably fatal. Heavy sedation with supportive management needs further study (Milwaukee protocol). Vaccination after onset of rabies confers no benefit.

Prevention: Thorough cleansing of wounds and postexposure prophylaxis (PEP): rabies-immune globulin and a series of rabies vaccinations. Vaccination of people at high risk (veterinarians, animal rescue personnel, laboratory staff, etc.), avoid contact with stray dogs or cats, sick or dead wildlife; vaccinate all dogs and cats; distribute baits containing oral vaccine in wildlife habitat; quarantine dogs arriving from infected countries. Culling of stray dogs is ineffective; sterilization prevents replacement breeding.

Epidemiology: Rabies occurs in more than 150 countries and territories; world wide, more than 55,000 people die of rabies every year; 40% of people who are bitten by suspect rabid animals are children under 15 years of age. Dogs are the source of 99% of human rabies deaths, which is largely due to low rabies vaccination coverage of dogs in developing countries. Most cases of rabies in North America and Australia have been acquired from bats, often with no documented record of a bite. The USA was declared free of canine rabies transmission in 2007. In the Americas, dog rabies control reduced human cases to 16 by 2009. Every year, more than 15 million people world wide receive a preventive PEP regimen to avert the disease – this is estimated to prevent more than 327,000 rabies deaths annually.

Map sources: The Rabies map is made with data obtained from WHO RabNet, available at: www.who.int/rabies.

Key references

Hemachudha T, et al. (2006) Rabies. *Curr Neurol Neurosci Rep* **6**(6):460–468.

Jackson AC. (2002) Update on rabies. *Curr Opin Neurol* **15**(3):327–331. Milwaukee protocol, available at: www.mcw.edu/rabies

Rupprecht CE, et al. (2006) Current and future trends in the prevention, treatment and controlof rabies. *Expert Rev Anti Infect Ther* **4**(6):1021–1038.

Wertheim HF, et al. (2009) Furious rabies after an atypical exposure. *PloS Med* **6**(3):e44.

WHO (2005) *Expert Consultation on Rabies*. WHO Technical Report 931. (www.who.int).

Atlas of Human Infectious Diseases, First Edition. Heiman F.L. Wertheim, Peter Horby and John P. Woodall.
© 2012 Blackwell Publishing Ltd. Published 2012 by Blackwell Publishing Ltd.

Rift Valley Fever

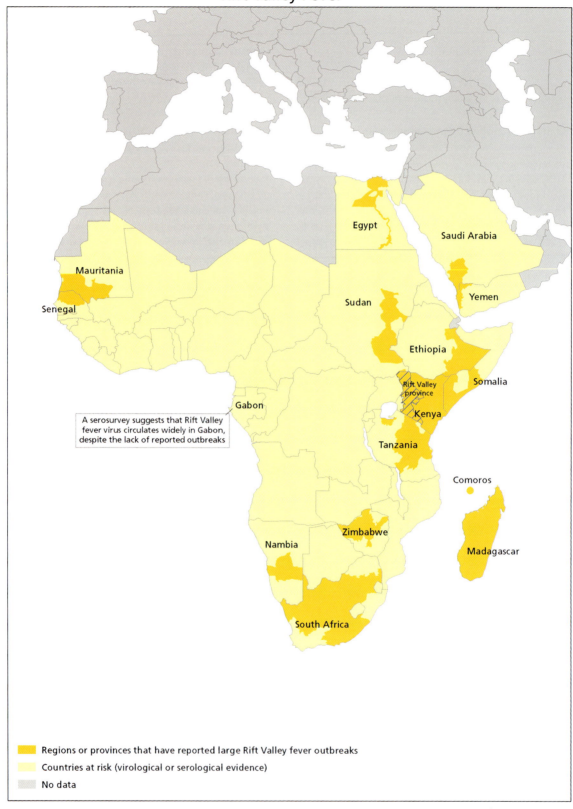

A serosurvey suggests that Rift Valley fever virus circulates widely in Gabon, despite the lack of reported outbreaks

Regions or provinces that have reported large Rift Valley fever outbreaks

Countries at risk (virological or serological evidence)

No data

Disease: Rift Valley Fever

Classification: ICD-9 066.3; ICD-10 A92.4

Syndromes and synonyms: None.

Agent: Rift Valley fever virus (RVFV), an enveloped, single-stranded tripartite RNA virus, belonging to the genus *Phlebovirus* of the family Bunyaviridae. There are three lineages: Egyptian, West African, and East-Central African. Zinga virus, isolated in 1982 in Madagascar, was later found to be a strain of RVFV.

Reservoir: Livestock (cattle, camels, goats, sheep), wild buffalo, waterbuck, some rodents.

Vector: Mosquitoes of the genera *Aedes, Culex, Mansonia* and others. There is transovarian transmission of RVFV in mosquitoes. Dried mosquito eggs can remain viable and infected for years. Originally, the eggs are laid in the damp soil above the water line and hatch when flooded.

Transmission: Human infections occur via two main transmission routes: (1) mosquito bite, and (2) direct or indirect contact with the blood or organs of infected animals (e.g. slaughtering, butchering, veterinary procedures, animal births, disposing of carcasses or fetuses) by percutaneous inoculation or inhaling aerosols. Transmission may be possible via consumption of raw milk of an infected animal. Person-to-person transmission has not been described. However, humans develop high viral loads in the blood, and may transmit virus to contacts.

Cycle: Animal–mosquito–animal with spillover to humans in epidemics via direct/indirect contact to infected animal tissue or mosquito bite.

Incubation period: 2–6 days.

Clinical findings: A self-limiting disease that lasts for about 4 to 7 days. Patients usually experience dengue-like illness with fever, muscle pain, headache, and joint pain. The disease may progress in some cases to one or more of three distinct syndromes: ocular (eye) disease (0.5–2% of patients) with retinitis and possible blindness; meningoencephalitis (about 1%), patients usually recover; or acute hepatitis and hemorrhagic fever (about 1%) with a CFR of 50%. Some patients are misdiagnosed as meningitis.

Diagnostic tests: Serology (IgM ELISA or EIA); RT-PCR on blood in early phase of disease; virus isolation in specialized laboratories.

Therapy: Supportive, there is no specific treatment.

Prevention: An inactivated virus vaccine (not licenced) is limited available to protect laboratory workers, veterinarians and others 'at risk.' Livestock vaccines are available, but are not licenced in Europe or the USA. Animal movement should be banned during outbreaks. Protective clothing worn by those exposed to infected animals/tissue. All animal products (blood, meat and milk) should be thoroughly cooked before eating. Infection control for those taking care of severe human cases. Personal anti-mosquito precautions. Larviciding at mosquito-breeding sites. Early warning systems for RVF are in place that use satellite images and weather/climate forecasting data.

Epidemiology: RVFV primarily causes disease in animals in Africa and Middle East, with human cases occurring during animal epidemics. Humans that regularly work with animals (farmers, herders, veterinarians, slaughterhouse workers) are at increased risk of infection. Epidemics in animals occur when mosquito populations dramatically increase after periods of heavy rainfall or the production of wetlands behind man-made dams. RVF was initially confined to Sub-Saharan Africa, but appeared in Egypt in 1977 and was discovered on the Arabian Peninsula (Saudi Arabia and Yemen) in 2000 and later also on the Comoros Islands. As RVFV epidemics are closely associated with above-average rainfall, outbreaks can be forecasted upon which preventive measures can be implemented.

Map source(s): The Rift Valley Fever map is modified from A. Clements et al. (2007), with permission, and updated with medical literature up to 2010.

Key references

Bouloy M (2001) In Service MW (ed.) Rift Valley fever virus. *The Encyclopedia of Arthropod-transmitted Infections*. CAB International, pp. 151–159.

Clements ACA, et al. (2007) A Rift Valley fever atlas for Africa. *Prevent Vet Med* **8B2**:72–82.

World Health Organization (2010) Rift Valley Fever. *Factsheet* Nr 207. Geneva.

Rotaviral Enteritis

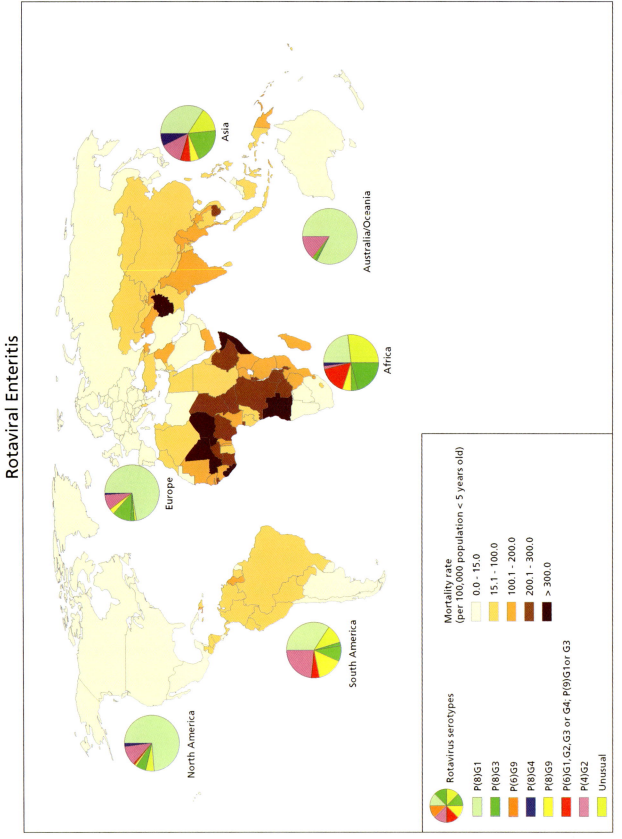

Asia

Australia/Oceania

Africa

Europe

North America

South America

Mortality rate
(per 100,000 population < 5 years old)

	0.0 - 15.0
	15.1 - 100.0
	100.1 - 200.0
	200.1 - 300.0
	> 300.0

Rotavirus serotypes

	P(8)G1
	P(8)G3
	P(6)G9
	P(8)G4
	P(8)G9
	P(6)G1,G2,G3 or G4; P(9)G1or G3
	P(4)G2
	Unusual

Last update on: 02/11/2010

Disease: Rotaviral Enteritis

Classification: ICD-9 008.61; ICD-10 A08.0

Synonyms: Rotavirus diarrhea, acute viral gastroenteritis, severe viral gastroenteritis.

Agent: Rotavirus, a non-enveloped double-stranded RNA virus within the Reoviridae family, is classified into 7 rotavirus groups (A–G) as determined by the antigenic properties of the VP6 capsid protein. Group A is most common in human disease, with B and C to a lesser extent. Subgroups and serotypes are determined by sero- and genotyping the epitopes P and G, of the VP4 and VP7 outer capsid proteins, respectively. These proteins are relevant for vaccine efficacy.

Reservoir: Humans. Rotaviruses in animals are distinct from those causing disease in humans.

Vector: None

Transmission: Direct fecal–oral transmission and via contaminated surfaces. Rotavirus has also been detected in repiratory secretions.

Incubation period: 1 to 3 days.

Clinical findings: Fever, vomiting, and watery diarrhea, and signs of dehydration in severe cases (mainly in young children). In adults the disease is often subclinical. Symptoms last for about one week.

Diagnostic tests: Rotavirus antigen detection by EIA and other serological techniques; RT-PCR.

Therapy: Supportive, including rehydration.

Prevention: Two licensed oral live attenuated rotavirus vaccines are available. Surveillance is needed to collect data on the burden of rotaviral disease and the circulating strains to assess the potential impact of vaccine introduction. Virus is shedded before and until ~1 week after onset of illness and can survive for a prolonged period of time on hard surfaces, hands, and in water. Improved sanitation, access to clean water, and hygiene have not yet shown to reduce rotavirus disease incidence.

Epidemiology: Group A rotaviruses have been established as the single most important cause of severe acute gastroenteritis in young children in developed and developing nations. Rotavirus is estimated to cause 138 million diarrheal episodes per year with 2 million requiring hospitalization and 440,000 deaths in children of <5 years. The incidence of rotavirus disease is similar in developed and developing countries, but deaths mainly occur in poverty stricken nations due to poor health infrastructure. Control is likely not achieved by improvements in clean water access, hygiene, and sanitation. Rotavirus vaccines are recommended to prevent severe and fatal rotavirus disease. For vaccine introduction, knowledge of the regional circulating rotavirus serotypes is needed. The epidemiology of rotavirus serotypes has substantial temporal and geographic variability and multiple serotypes may cocirculate within the same region and fluctuates each year within the same region. The 5 most common rotavirus serotypes (G1–G4 and G9) were responsible for approximately 95% of infections world wide with G1[P8] responsible for more than 70% of infections in North America, Australia, and Europe but only 30% of infections in South America, Asia, and Africa.

Map sources: The Rotavirus Enteritis map was made with data obtained from M. O'Ryan (2009) and WHO, available at: www.who.int/immunization_monitoring/burden/rotavirus_estimates/en/.

Key references

O'Ryan M (2009) The ever-changing landscape of rotavirus serotypes. *Ped Infect Dis J* **28**(3):S60–S62.

Parashar UD, et al. (2006) Rotavirus and severe childhood diarrhea. *Emerg Infect Dis* **12**(2):304–306.

MMWR (2008) Rotavirus surveillance – Worldwide, 2001–2008. *MMWR* **57**(46):1255–1257.

Atlas of Human Infectious Diseases, First Edition. Heiman F.L. Wertheim, Peter Horby and John P. Woodall.
© 2012 Blackwell Publishing Ltd. Published 2012 by Blackwell Publishing Ltd.

Rubella

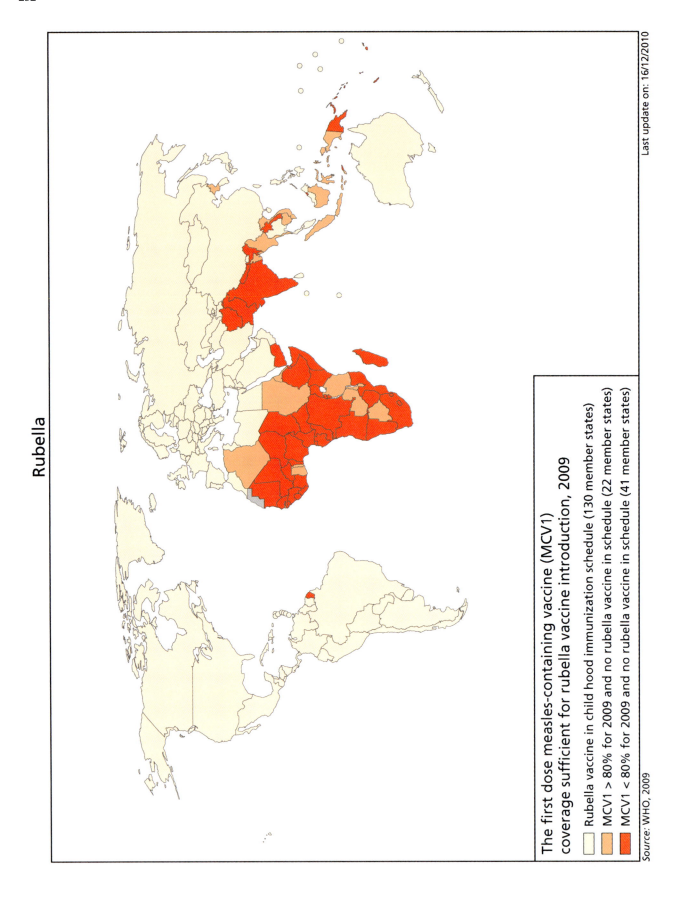

The first dose measles-containing vaccine (MCV1)
coverage sufficient for rubella vaccine introduction, 2009

Rubella vaccine in child hood immunization schedule (130 member states)

MCV1 > 80% for 2009 and no rubella vaccine in schedule (22 member states)

MCV1 < 80% for 2009 and no rubella vaccine in schedule (41 member states)

Source: WHO, 2009

Last update on: 16/12/2010

Disease: Rubella

Classification: ICD-9 056; ICD-10 B06

Synonyms: German measles

Agent: Rubella virus, a single-stranded RNA positive-sense rubivirus of the family Togaviridae.

Reservoir: Humans.

Vector: None.

Transmission: By airborne droplets from respiratory secretions of infected persons. Subclinical cases can transmit infection. Rubella virus may be transmitted to the fetus if the mother is infected during pregnancy.

Incubation period: 16–18 days (range 12–24 days)

Clinical findings: A generally mild and short-lived illness with fever, coryza, conjunctivitis, lymphadenopathy, and a fine maculopapular rash beginning on the face later spreading to the trunks and limbs. Postauricular, occipital or posterior cervical lymphadenopathy may precede the rash by 5–10 days. Around half of rubella infections are subclinical and constitutional symptoms may be minimal in children. Arthropathy may occur, especially in young women. The most important clinical consequence of rubella is congenital rubella syndrome (CRS), which may result from intra-uterine infection in the first 16 weeks of pregnancy. CRS is a severe disease characterized by deafness, cataract, cardiac abnormalities, and a range of neurological impairments.

Diagnostic tests: Rubella specific IgM or significant rise in antibody titer in paired samples; RT-PCR or virus isolation from throat swab, or other specimens in CRS.

Therapy: Supportive only. Human immunoglobulin has been given to pregnant women exposed to rubella and infected with rubella in an attempt to prevent infection or CRS, but its efficacy is not proven.

Prevention: Live attenuated virus vaccine, usually in combination with measles and mumps virus vaccine, at 12–18 months with a pre-school booster.

Epidemiology: World wide, but close to elimination in the Americas and targeted for elimination in Europe by 2015. In the absence of vaccination the prevalence of rubella infection by the age of 13 years ranges from 20 to 95%, but is most often over 50%. Reported data on clinical rubella are a vast underestimate since it is a mild disease with a clinical picture similar to several other infections. CRS is also grossly underreported. For example, it is estimated that over 45,000 CRS cases occur annually in Southeast Asia yet only an average of 13 CRS cases per year were reported to WHO between 2000 and 2009. Rubella is a public health concern because of CRS and in 1996 it was estimated that 110,000 CRS cases occurred annually in developing countries. Paradoxically, a poor rubella immunization program may actually increase the incidence of CRS if the burden of illness is shifted to young adults, where pregnancy is common. Therefore rubella immunization programs must achieve and maintain high immunization rates (>80%) or be supplemented by the immunization of women of childbearing age. In 2009 two-thirds of countries included a rubella containing vaccine in their national immunization schedule yet in many developing countries rubella vaccine has not been included because of lack of information on the burden of CRS, costs, and concerns about causing a paradoxical increase in CRS cases.

Map source: The Rubella map was made with data obtained from WHO, available at: www.who.int/immunization_monitoring/en/.

Key references

Brown DW, et al. (2004) Rubella. *Lancet* **363**(9415):1127–1137.

Centers for Disease Control and Prevention (2010) Progress toward control of rubella and prevention of congenital rubella syndrome - Worldwide, 2009. *MMWR* **59**(40): 1307–1310.

Cutts FT, et al. (1999) Modelling the incidence of congenital rubella syndrome in developing countries. *Int J Epidemiol* **28**(6):1176–1184.

World Health Organization (2009) *State of the World's Vaccines and Immunization*, 3rd edn. WHO, UNICEF, World Bank. Geneva.

Atlas of Human Infectious Diseases, First Edition. Heiman F.L. Wertheim, Peter Horby and John P. Woodall.
© 2012 Blackwell Publishing Ltd. Published 2012 by Blackwell Publishing Ltd.

254

Severe Acute Respiratory Syndrome (SARS)

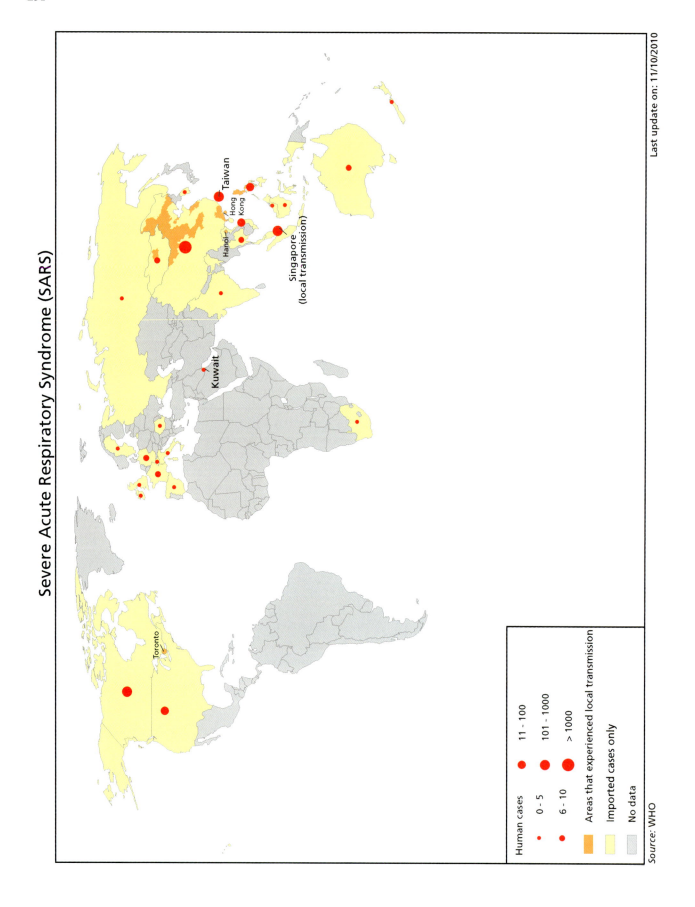

Last update on: 11/10/2010

Source: WHO

Disease: Severe Acute Respiratory Syndrome

Classification: ICD-10 J12.81

Synonyms: SARS

Agent: SARS coronavirus (SARS-CoV) is a positive-sense, single-stranded, enveloped RNA virus of the family Coronaviridae. The viral membrane contains a transmembrane (M) glycoprotein, spike (S) glycoprotein, and envelope (E) protein. Coronaviruses derive their name from the crown-like (corona-like) morphology on electron microscopy.

Reservoir: Although SARS-like coronaviruses with very high genetic homology to SARS-CoV have been identified in masked palm civets, civets are thought to be a non-reservoir, spillover species. Horseshoe bats are thought to be the natural reservoir of the progenitor of the SARS virus.

Vector: None.

Transmission: Direct person-to-person transmission, usually following close contact with a symptomatic case or the respiratory secretions or body fluids of a symptomatic case. Healthcare facilities were key in amplifying the transmission of SARS in 2003. Respiratory droplets or contaminated surfaces are thought to be the principal routes of transmission, although one outbreak in a residential block in Hong Kong was attributed to aerosol spread.

Incubation period: 4–5 days.

Clinical findings: SARS presents initially with fever, headache, myalgia, and a non-productive cough that may progress to dyspnoea with pulmonary infiltrations on chest x-ray. Gastrointestinal symptoms may also be present in early SARS illness. Case fatality is around 10%, and is higher in older adults than in children and young adults.

Diagnostic tests: Detection of virus in respiratory specimens, stool or blood by RT-PCR; virus isolation; serology by IFA or ELISA. Specimen processing and testing should be performed under strict biosafety measures (BSL-3).

Therapy: Supportive, no specific treatment is available.

Prevention: The control of wildlife farms and markets to reduce the risk of transmission from bats to humans through an intermediate species. Rapid case detection and isolation, contact tracing and quarantine, and stringent hospital infection control effectively controlled the SARS outbreak.

Epidemiology: SARS is thought to have emerged in Guangdong Province, China, in November 2002 and within 6 months cases were detected in 26 countries, with local transmission occurring in 6. In total over 8,000 cases and almost 800 deaths were recorded and, remarkably, much of the global transmission of SARS can be traced to a single individual who disseminated infection at a hotel in Hong Kong. 'Super spreading' events (where one person infects an unusually large number of people), such as occurred at the Hong Kong Hotel, appear to be an important feature of SARS epidemiology. The precise circumstances and timing of the interspecies transfer of SARS-CoV remains unknown. Many of the early cases in Guangdong had epidemiological links to the wild animal trade but later the transmission of SARS was exclusively person-to-person with a large nosocomial element. Laboratory-accident associated cases in late 2003 and April 2004, and a cluster linked to the wild animal trade in January 2004, highlight the potential for the re-emergence of SARS.

Map sources: The Severe Acute Respiratory Syndrome map is reproduced from WHO, available at: www.who.int/csr/disease/en/.

Key references

Anderson RM, et al. (2004) Epidemiology, transmission dynamics and control of SARS: the 2002–2003 epidemic. *Philos Trans R Soc Lond B Biol Sci* **359**(1447):1091–1105.

Poon LL, et al. (2004) The aetiology, origins, and diagnosis of severe acute respiratory syndrome. *Lancet Infect Dis* **4**(11):663–671.

Wanh LG, et al. (2006) Review of bats and SARS. *Emerg Infect Dis* **12**(12):1834–1840.

Atlas of Human Infectious Diseases, First Edition. Heiman F.L. Wertheim, Peter Horby and John P. Woodall.
© 2012 Blackwell Publishing Ltd. Published 2012 by Blackwell Publishing Ltd.

Sindbis Fever

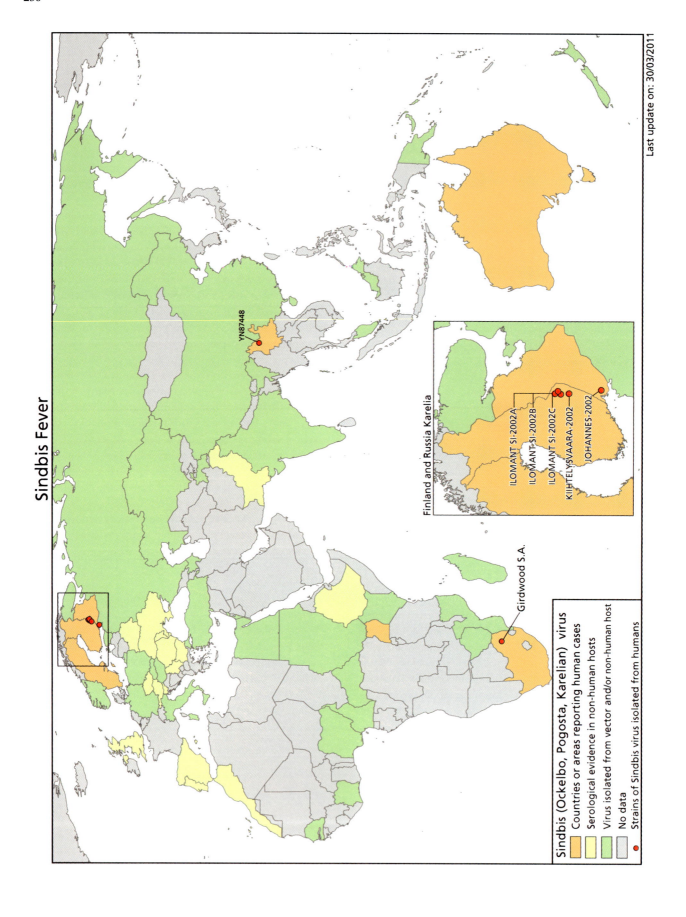

YN87448

Finland and Russia Karelia

ILOMANT SI-2002A
ILOMANT SI-2002B
ILOMANT SI-2002C
KIIHTELYSVAARA-2002
JOHANNES-2002

Girdwood S.A.

Sindbis (Ockelbo, Pogosta, Karelian) virus
Countries or areas reporting human cases
Serological evidence in non-human hosts
Virus isolated from vector and/or non-human host
No data
Strains of Sindbis virus isolated from humans

Last update on: 30/03/2011

Disease: **Sindbis Fever**

Classification: ICD-9 066.3; ICD-10 A92.8

Syndromes and synonyms: Ockelbo disease, Pogosta disease, Karelian fever

Agent: Sindbis virus (SINV), a single-stranded, positive sense, enveloped RNA alphavirus, with 5 genotypes: SIN I (European/African), SIN II and III (Asian/Australian), SIN IV (Azerbaijan/China), and SIN V (New Zealand). The first Sindbis virus isolated was cultured in 1952 from a mosquito near Sindbis village in the Nile Delta (Egypt). Almost 10 years later the first human case was detected in Uganda in 1961 and in Europe in 1971.

Reservoir: Wild, migratory birds of the order Passeriformes (mainly fieldfare, redwing, and songthrush) and Anseriformes (ducks, geese and swans). Tetraonid birds (grouse) population size changes coincide with SINV epidemics in Finland. Larger passerine species have higher prevalences of infection as compared to smaller species.

Vector: Mosquitoes: *Culex* and *Culiseta* spp. between birds, *Aedes* spp. from bird to human.

Transmission: By mosquito bite.

Cycle: Probably bird–mosquito–bird. Mosquitoes become infected when feeding on viremic reservoir birds. This is followed by an extrinsic cycle of a few days in the mosquito, with subsequent transmission to birds or humans by bite. Humans are a dead-end host. There is evidence for vertical (transovarial) transmission in mosquitoes.

Incubation period: Varies from a few days to just over a week, depending on infectious dose.

Clinical findings: The majority of infections are subclinical (~95%). Those with disease have mild fever, maculopapular rash often involving the palms and soles, which may be hemorrhagic and may recur, polyarthritis of both large and small joints, occasionally swollen extremities, anorexia, and lymphadenopathy. The disease is more severe in Scandinavia and South Africa than elsewhere. The disease is non-fatal, but moderate residual pain and stiffness in the joints may persist for years.

Diagnostic tests: Detection of viral RNA in blood by RT-PCR; serology (IgM ELISA); virus culture.

Therapy: Symptomatic, there is no specific treatment.

Prevention: Anti-mosquito precautions; there is no vaccine available.

Epidemiology: SINV has been isolated from Africa, Eurasia, and Australia. The highest disease burden is in northern Europe (approximately between 60 and 64°N) and South Africa. Evolutionary studies show that SINV likely originated from South America, with subsequent spread to North America, Asia, and Australia, with later spread to Europe and Africa. Intererestingly, there are high levels of gene sequence similarities of SINV isolates within the same north–south axis, which correlates with major bird migration patterns (see Bird Migration map). Preferred habitat is a wetland ecosystem. The disease is seasonal, coinciding with the period of mosquito abundance and reservoir presence. Overwintering in the northern hemisphere may be by vertical transmission in the vectors. In Scandinavia, most cases occur in July through September, when there is plenty of vector species. Peak incidence in Karelia is about one month after the peak in Finland. Highest attack rates in Finland are in the eastern parts, and mainly in the age group 45 to 65 years. Epidemics tend to occur every 7 years in Finland, with the last epidemic in 2002. No epidemic occurred in 2009, probably due to a decline in the grouse population.

Map source: The Sindbis Fever map was made with data on human Sindbis virus isolations obtained from S. Kurkela et al. (2004).

Key references

Hubalek Z (2008) Mosquito-borne viruses in Europe. *Parasitol Res* **103**(Suppl 1):S29–S43.

Kurkela S, et al. (2004) Causative agent of Pogosta disease isolated from blood and skin lesions. *Emerg Infect Dis* **10**(5):889–894.

Lundstrom JO, et al. (2010) Phylogeographic structure and evolutionary history of Sindbis virus. *Vector Borne Zoonotic Dis* **10**(9):899–907.

Sane J, et al. (2010) Epidemiological analysis of mosquito-borne Pogosta disease in Finland, 2009. *Euro Surveill* **15**(2) pii:19462.

Atlas of Human Infectious Diseases, First Edition. Heiman F.L. Wertheim, Peter Horby and John P. Woodall.
© 2012 Blackwell Publishing Ltd. Published 2012 by Blackwell Publishing Ltd.

Tacaribe Complex Virus Disease

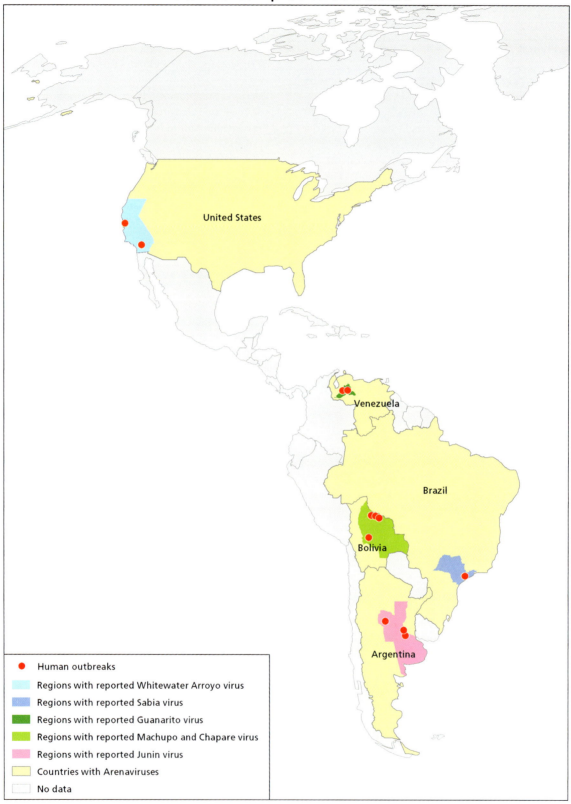

Last update on: 13/01/2011

Disease: Tacaribe Complex Virus Disease

Classification: ICD-9 078.7; ICD-10 A96

Syndromes and synonyms: Argentinian (Junin virus), Bolivian (Machupo virus), Brazilian (Sabiá virus), and Venezuelan (Guanarito virus) hemorrhagic fevers.

Agent: Tacaribe complex viruses are spherical or pleomorphic, enveloped arenaviruses containing two single-stranded RNA molecules, with four distinct lineages (A, B, C, and a recombinant RecA). Out of more than 20 known arenaviruses, only the following have been associated with human disease: Chapare, Guanarito, Junin, Machupo, Sabiá, and Whitewater Arroyo viruses. All South American hemorrhagic fever viruses, except Whitewater Arroyo virus, are classified as high-priority bioterrorism pathogens. Other Tacaribe complex arenaviruses are capable of infecting humans and possibly cause disease.

Reservoir: Each virus is associated with either one or a few closely related species of rodents, which constitute the virus's natural reservoir. Tacaribe complex viruses in the New World are generally associated with rats and mice (family Muridae, subfamily *Sigmodontinae*). The reservoir rodents are chronically infected, and the virus is transmitted among them, leading to lifelong viremia and virus excretion, and they do not die. The reservoir for Junin virus is *Calomys musculinus* and *C. laucha*, for Machupo virus, *C. callosus*, for Guanarito virus *Zygodontomys brevicauda*, and for Whitewater Arroyo virus *Neotoma albigula*. For Sabiá and Chapare viruses the reservoir host is unknown.

Vector: None.

Transmission: By contact with the excretions, or materials contaminated with the excretions, of an infected rodent, such as ingestion of contaminated food or by direct contact of abraded or broken skin with rodent excrement. Infection can also occur by inhalation of minute particles soiled with rodent urine or saliva (aerosol transmission). Person-to-person transmission is rare and known only for Machupo virus.

Incubation period: 5–21 days; usually 7–14 days.

Clinical findings: Gradual onset of malaise, headache, and retro-orbital pain, conjunctivitis, fever, and sweats, followed by prostration. Petechiae on the soft palate are frequent, on the body with ecchymoses less frequent. In severe cases: epistaxis, hematemesis, melena, hematuria, and gingival hemorrhage. Enceplalopathy, intention tremors, depressed deep tendon reflexes, bradycardia, and hypotension with shock are common. Infection during pregnancy can result in abortion. Convalescence may be prolonged. CFR due to these viruses, even after intensive hospital treatment, can be as high as 33%.

Diagnostic tests: Virus detection in blood or tissue by culture or RT-PCR; serology (IgM ELISA, IFA). Virus isolation should be done in a BSL-4 laboratory.

Therapy: Supportive treatment; ribavirin. Junin convalescent serum reduces the CFR of Argentinian hemorrhagic fever to <1%.

Prevention: There is a vaccine against Junin virus only. Targeted rodent control in houses, except for Junin virus, which is spread by rodents in the fields. Barrier nursing of cases.

Epidemiology: Junin virus is spread annually around harvest time by rodents to farmers. The range of Junin virus is extending to the north, putting an estimated 5 million people at risk. The other viruses are brought into villages and houses by peridomestic rodents, causing sporadic outbreaks with intervals of several years. Deforestation and human invasion into rodent habitat may have resulted in increased human exposure to infected rodents and a concomitant increase in human illnesses (see Forest Cover map). Only single cases of an infection by Sabiá and Chapare viruses have been recorded. Pathogenicity of Whitewater Arroyo virus remains to be confirmed since there was no virus isolation from the Californian cases.

Map source(s): The Tacaribe Complex Virus Disease map was made by geolocating reported human outbreaks in the medical literature between 1960 and 2008.

Key references

Bowen MD, et al. (1996) The phylogeny of New World (Tacaribe complex) arenaviruses. *Virology* 219:285–290.

Charrel RN, et al. (2010) Zoonotic aspects of arenavirus infections. *Vet Microbiol* 140(3–4):213–220.

Centers for Disease Control and Prevention (2005) Arenavirus. *CDC factsheet*.

Delgado S, et al. (2008) Chapare virus, a newly discovered arenavirus isolated from a fatal hemorrhagic fever case in Bolivia. *PLoS Path* 4(4):e1000047.

Jay MT, et al. (2005) The arenaviruses. *J Am Vet Med Assoc* 227 (6):904–915.

Atlas of Human Infectious Diseases, First Edition. Heiman F.L. Wertheim, Peter Horby and John P. Woodall.
© 2012 Blackwell Publishing Ltd. Published 2012 by Blackwell Publishing Ltd.

Tick-borne Encephalitis

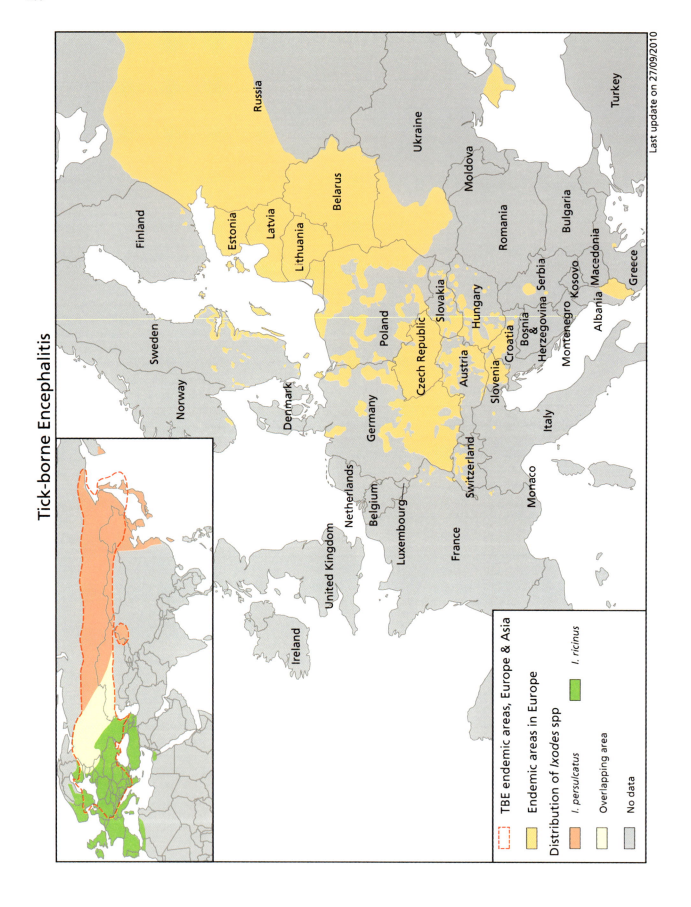

Last update on 27/09/2010

TBE endemic areas, Europe & Asia
- Endemic areas in Europe

Distribution of Ixodes spp
- *I. persulcatus*
- *I. ricinus*
- Overlapping area
- No data

Disease: Tick-borne Encephalitis

Classification: ICD-9 063; ICD-10 A84.0, A84.1

Synonyms: TBE, Western, European or Central European tick-borne encephalitis, Siberian tick-borne encephalitis, Far Eastern tick-borne encephalitis (formerly known as Russian Spring Summer encephalitis), diphasic milk fever, diphasic meningoencephalitis

Agent: Tick-borne encephalitis (TBE) virus, an enveloped RNA virus with three subtypes: European (EUR), Siberian (SIB), and Far-Eastern (FE).

Reservoir: The only real reservoir is the tick. Viremia persists only for a few days in transmission competent vertebrates, rodents (mainly *Apodemus* spp.). Deer, birds, possibly marmots are not competent to transmit to ticks.

Vector: Hard ticks, with *Ixodes ricinus* as the most important vector of the European subtype and *I. persulcatus* for the other subtypes.

Transmission: Via tick bite. Or consumption of raw milk or dairy products from infected animals. For EUR, rarely, by blood transfusion and breast milk.

Cycle: Wildlife–tick–wildlife. The tick ingests infected blood of reservoir host, virus passes from gut to hemocoele to salivary glands and is transmitted to a new host at the next feed. The virus is transmitted from tick to tick trans-stadially and transovarially. Trans-stadial transmission is key to tick-borne infections.

Incubation period: 4–28 days (median 8 days).

Clinical findings: TBE causes acute meningitis, encephalitis, or meningoencephalitis with or without myelitis. Severity of disease increases with age, with an excess of males and is highest in adults, of whom half develop encephalitis. It begins with fever (99%), fatigue, and general malaise (62%), headache and body pain (54%). In diphasic infections (EUR), neurological symptoms appear 4–10 days after apparent recovery. FE disease is often severe with signs of encephalitis, focal epilepsy and flaccid paralysis of the shoulder girdle (CFR: 5–40%); EUR is a milder disease, with death and severe sequelae less frequent than in FE. Long-lasting or permanent neuropsychiatric sequelae are observed in 10–20% or more of infected patients. Infections with the European and Siberian subtypes are less severe (CFR: 1–3%).

Diagnostic tests: IgM serology on paired sera; specific identification to subtype by virus isolation; RT-PCR.

Therapy: Supportive, there is no specific treatment.

Prevention: Avoid tick bites, use repellent on skin and repellent or acaricide on clothing, check body daily for ticks after exposure, boil or pasteurize milk from cows, sheep, and goats in endemic areas. An inactivated vaccine is available. Specific hyperimmune globulin used in the past as prophylaxis after tick-bite may worsen the disease.

Epidemiology: The disease is seasonal, generally coinciding with tick activity; there are peaks of incidence every 5–7 years in China. Europe and Russia have an estimated 12,000 cases per year (2007). In eastern regions the disease coincides with tick habitat in cold, moist forest, but tick ranges extend well beyond reported disease at both eastern and western geographical extremes. During the past two decades, new endemic foci and an increase in cases have been reported in many European countries, in spite of widespread vaccination of at-risk populations. In 1989, FE virus was isolated from *Ixodes ovatus* ticks and the blood of a febrile patient in Yunnan province, southwestern China. The virus may have completely different rodent hosts and tick vectors from those in northern China.

Map sources: The Tick-Borne Encephalitis map is modified from the maps produced by Baxter (http://www.baxter.com/press_room/factsheets/vaccines/tick-borne_encephalitis.html) and L. Lindquist et al. (2008). Baxter produces a TBE vaccine and for this purpose keeps track of the TBE distribution.

Key references

Dumpis U, et al. (1999) Tick-borne encephalitis. *Clin Infect Dis* **28**(4):882–890.

Lindquist L, et al. (2008) Tick-borne encephalitis. *Lancet* **371**(9627):1861–1871.

Mansfield KL, et al. (2009) Tick-borne encephalitis virus – a review of an emerging zoonosis. *J Gen Virol* **90**(Pt 8):1781–1794.

Lu Z, et al. (2008) Tick-borne encephalitis in mainland China. *Vector Borne Zoonotic Dis* **8**(5):713–720.

Atlas of Human Infectious Diseases, First Edition. Heiman F.L. Wertheim, Peter Horby and John P. Woodall.
© 2012 Blackwell Publishing Ltd. Published 2012 by Blackwell Publishing Ltd.

Variant Creutzfeldt - Jakob Disease

Last update on: 21/03/2011

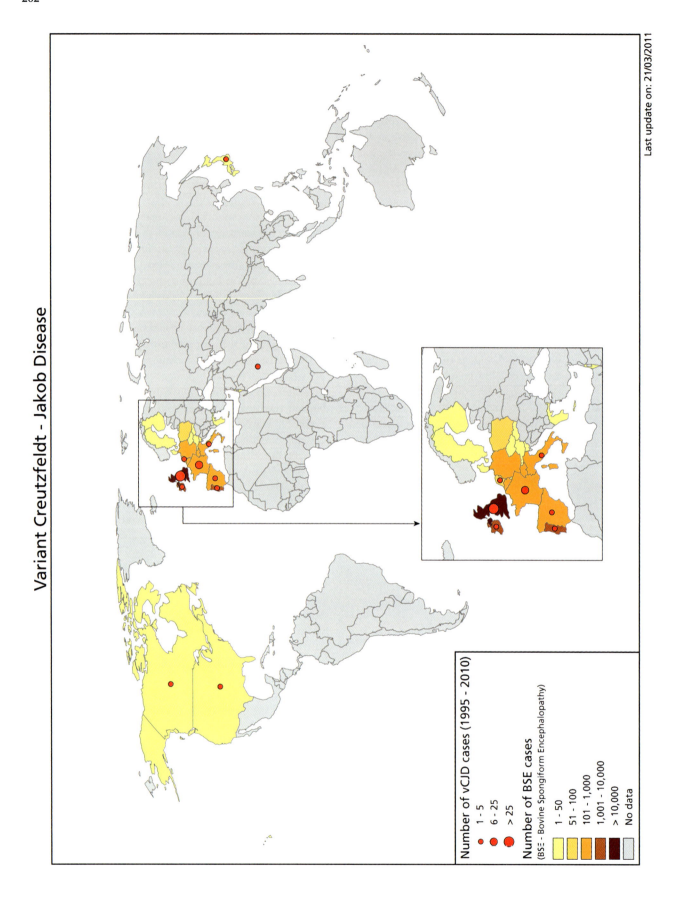

Number of vCJD cases (1995 - 2010)

- 1 - 5
- 6 - 25
- > 25

Number of BSE cases
(BSE - Bovine Spongiform Encephalopathy)

- 1 - 50
- 51 - 100
- 101 - 1,000
- 1,001 - 10,000
- > 10,000
- No data

Disease: Variant Creutzfeldt–Jakob Disease

Classification: ICD-9 046.1; ICD-10 A81.0

Synonyms: vCJD, mad cow disease, transmissible spongiform encephalopathy, prion disease.

Agent: The etiological agent of variant Creutzfeldt–Jakob Disease (vCJD) is thought to be an abnormal form of a naturally occurring host protein, which is transmissible and can transform normal host protein into the pathogenic form, known as 'prions.' vCJD refers specifically to the neurodegenerative prion disease of humans and is associated with Bovine Spongiform Encephalopathy (BSE), a prion disease of cows. vCJD is clinically and neuropathologically distinct from sporadic CJD, which is endemic throughout the world and has no known association with BSE.

Reservoir: Cattle with Bovine Spongiform Encephalopathy.

Transmission route: Thought to be acquired primarily through ingestion of infected tissue from cattle with BSE. Iatrogenic transmission has occurred through blood transfusion. To date there have been no known transmissions of vCJD by tissue or organ transplantation from infected people, or through contaminated surgical instruments.

Cycle: The protein concentrates in tissues of the central nervous system. Prions are resistant to normal cooking temperatures and humans are thought to be infected by ingesting contaminated food. In contrast to other forms of human prion diseases, in vCJD significant levels of infectivity are found in the lymphoreticular system (lymph nodes, spleen, tonsil, and appendix).

Incubation period: Uncertain; the mean incubation period is likely to be 10 to 20 years, but shorter periods have been observed in transfusion-associated cases.

Clinical findings: vCJD is characterized by a relatively early age of onset (28 years) and prominent early psychiatric symptoms: anxiety, depression, agitation, delusions, and unpleasant sensory symptoms. Neurological features are: unsteadiness, difficulty walking, and involuntary movements. Memory loss progresses to severe cognitive impairment and, at the time of death, patients have become unable to move or speak. The median duration of illness is 14 months.

Diagnostic tests: Compatible clinical features, a characteristic MRI (pulvinar sign) and the exclusion of other neurological diseases, are usually sufficient to diagnose 'probable vCJD.' Definitive diagnosis of vCJD is by neuropathological examination of the brain, usually at postmortem.

Therapy: No proven treatment available.

Prevention: Prevention is focused on eliminating BSE in cattle, preventing infected bovine material entering the animal and human food chain, and reducing the risk of secondary transmission to humans in the healthcare setting. To this end many countries have banned bovine meat and bone meal from livestock feed, slaughtered infected herds, and taken other precautions to prevent infected cattle from entering the human food chain. Measures to reduce the risk of transmission of vCJD through blood products include low-risk sourcing and leucodepletion. Further precautionary methods to reduce the risk of transmission through contaminated surgical instruments.

Epidemiology: There is strong epidemiological and laboratory evidence for a causal relation between vCJD and the BSE agent. In the UK, the primary epidemic has been associated with dietary exposure to BSE-infected bovine material during the BSE epidemic in the late 1980s to mid-1990s, before effective controls to prevent the BSE agent entering the human food supply were put into place. Most people who have developed vCJD have lived in or visited the UK during this time period. The behavior of the vCJD agent under laboratory conditions is also very like that of BSE. There is a strong host genetic component, with certain variants of the prion protein gene being much more susceptible to vCJD

Map sources: The Variant Creutzfeldt–Jakob Disease map was made with data from the European Creutzfeldt–Jakob Disease Surveillance Network (EUROCJD) and the World Organization for Animal Health (OIE), available at: www.eurocjd.ed.ac.uk and www.oie.int/eng/info/en_esbmonde.htm

Key references

Heath CA, et al. (2010) Validation of diagnostic criteria for variant Creutzfeldt–Jakob disease. *Ann Neurol* **67**(6):761–770.

Hilton DA (2006) Pathogenesis and prevalence of variant Creutzfeldt–Jakob disease. *J Pathol* **208**(2):134–141.

Will RG (2003) Acquired prion disease: iatrogenic CJD, variant CJD, kuru. *Br Med Bull* **66**:255–265.

Atlas of Human Infectious Diseases, First Edition. Heiman F.L. Wertheim, Peter Horby and John P. Woodall.
© 2012 Blackwell Publishing Ltd. Published 2012 by Blackwell Publishing Ltd.

Venezuelan Equine Encephalitis (VEE)

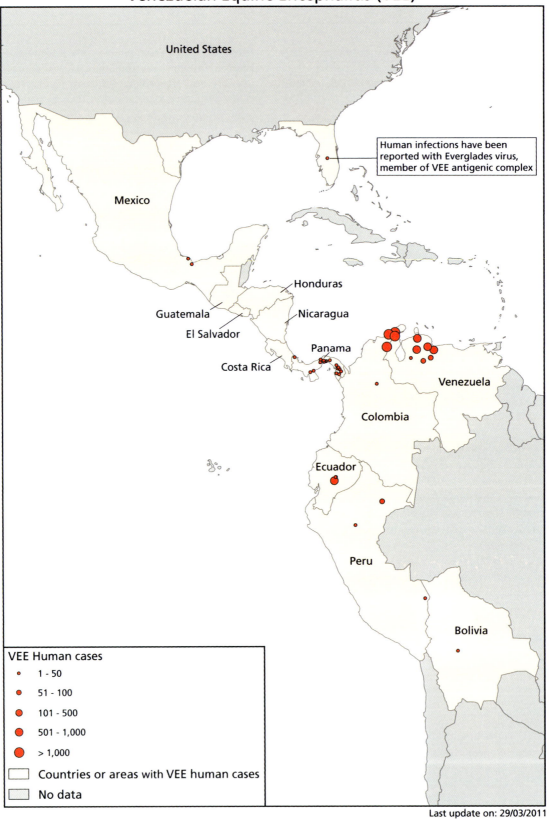

Human infections have been reported with Everglades virus, member of VEE antigenic complex

United States

Mexico

Honduras

Guatemala

El Salvador

Nicaragua

Panama

Costa Rica

Venezuela

Colombia

Ecuador

Peru

Bolivia

VEE Human cases

- · 1 - 50
- ● 51 - 100
- ● 101 - 500
- ● 501 - 1,000
- ● > 1,000

☐ Countries or areas with VEE human cases

☐ No data

Last update on: 29/03/2011

Disease: Venezuelan Equine Encephalitis

Classification: ICD-9 066.2; ICD-10 A92.2

Syndromes and synonyms: Venezuelan equine encephalomyelitis, Venezuelan equine fever, Mucambo virus fever.

Agents: Venezuelan equine encephalitis virus (VEEV), an enveloped, spherical, single-stranded positive-sense RNA virus, genus *Alphavirus* in the family Togaviridae. Epizootic or epidemic VEE viruses belong to subtypes IAB and IC. Enzootic VEE complex viruses belong to subtypes II to VI and ID, IE, and IF. With the exception of IE strains, these do not cause disease in equids, but can cause sporadic disease in humans. VEEV is considered a potential biological warfare agent.

Reservoir: Principally sylvatic rodents; also marsupials, bats, and shore birds may be involved in the enzootic virus cycle.

Vector: Mosquitoes. The main vector of enzootic VEEV is the *Culex (Melanoconion)* spp. (Spissipes group). During VEEV outbreaks, *Ochlerotatus taeniorhynchus* is often the main vector in coastal regions. Epizootic/epidemic subtypes of VEEV are transmitted by mosquitoes of many different genera.

Transmission: Mosquito bite. Direct person-to-person transmission has not been documented.

Cycle: Mosquito–reservoir animal–mosquito. Humans are dead-end hosts. Equines (horses, mules, and donkeys) are amplifying hosts for the epidemic subtypes of VEEV, with high viremias that can infect a wide range of mosquitoes. Half of infected equids die from VEEV. Viremia lasts 2–5 days in birds and 3 days in equids. Extrinsic cycle in the mosquito lasts up to 7 days but transmission can occur in as little as 4 days.

Incubation period: Usually 2–3 days.

Clinical findings: Infections are often mild, with more severe neurologic disease in 4–14% of the cases that may progress to death. VEEV infection often presents like an influenza-like illness. Severe encephalitis is less common in adults as compared to children. Absence of a rash distinguishes it from dengue and Mayaro fevers. About 30% of survivors have neurological sequelae. CFR for VEE is <1%. VEEV infection may cause stillbirths.

Diagnostic tests: Serology or RT-PCR on blood or CSF; virus isolation.

Therapy: Supportive, there is no specific treatment.

Prevention: Personal anti-mosquito precautions. Inoculation of equids with live, attenuated TC-83 VEE vaccine blocks amplification; this vaccine is available to laboratory personnel but not to the public. VEE is infectious if airborne and can cause infections in laboratory staff.

Epidemiology: VEEV was isolated for the first time in 1938 from a diseased horse in Venezuela. The VEEV distribution is limited to the Americas, and predominantly in Central and South America. In 1995, a large outbreak with approximately 100,000 human cases, of which 300 were fatal, happened in Colombia and Venezuela. The Guajira peninsula (region in northern Colombia and northwest Venezuela) has the highest disease burden, probably due to a large donkey population that serves as an amplifying host. In 2005, human VEE cases were detected for the first time in Bolivia, cause by a new Bolivia–Peru ID genotype. Typical VEEV enzootic habitats are lowland forests and swamps in (sub)tropical areas of the Americas, from northern Argentina up to southern USA (Florida and Colorado). Enzootic subtype distribution generally does not overlap, except in the Amazon regions.

Map sources: The Venezuelan Equine Encephalitis map was made with data from the Pan-American Health Organization (www.paho.org/english/sha/epibul_95-98/be954out.htm), CDC (www.cdc.gov) and medical literature.

Key references

Aguilar PV, et al. (2009) Genetic characterization of Venezuelan equine encephalitis virus from Bolivia, Ecuador and Peru: identification of a new subtype ID lineage. *PLoS Negl Trop Dis* **3**(9):e514.

Ventura AK, et al. (1974) Human Venezuelan equine encephalitis virus infection in Florida. *Am J Trop Med Hyg* **23**(3):507–521.

Weaver SC (2001) Venezuelan equine encephalitis. In Service MW (ed.) *The Encyclopedia of Arthropod-transmitted Infections*. CAB International, pp. 539–548.

Zacks MA, et al. (2010) Encephalitic alphaviruses. *Vet Microbiol* **140**(3–4):281–286.

Atlas of Human Infectious Diseases, First Edition. Heiman F.L. Wertheim, Peter Horby and John P. Woodall.
© 2012 Blackwell Publishing Ltd. Published 2012 by Blackwell Publishing Ltd.

Western Equine Encephalitis (WEE)

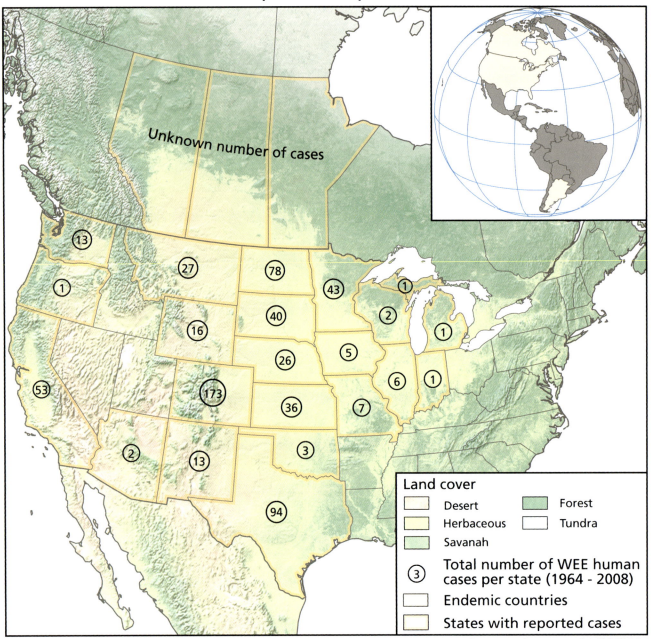

Unknown number of cases

Land cover

☐ Desert		☐ Forest	
☐ Herbaceous		☐ Tundra	
☐ Savanah			

③ Total number of WEE human cases per state (1964 - 2008)

☐ Endemic countries

☐ States with reported cases

Last update on: 31/03/2011

Disease: Western Equine Encephalitis

Classification: ICD-9 062; ICD-10 A83.1

Syndromes and synonyms: None.

Agents: Western equine encephalitis virus (WEEV), an enveloped, spherical, single-stranded positive-sense RNA virus, genus *Alphavirus* in the family Togaviridae. WEEV is believed to have descended from an ancestral recombinant derived from eastern equine encephalitis virus and Sindbis virus.

Reservoir: Principally birds, secondarily rabbits, poultry.

Vector: Mosquitoes. In North America, the primary vector of WEEV for the enzootic cycle is *Culex tarsalis*. WEEV is transmitted to humans and horses by bridging mosquitoes (e.g. *Ochlerotatus melanimon* and *Aedes* species).

Transmission: Mosquito bite. There is no direct person-to-person transmission.

Cycle: Mosquito to reservoir animal to mosquito. There is an enzootic cycle, mainly between *C. taralsis* and passerine birds. There is a secondary cycle that involves rabbits. Viremia lasts 2–5 days in birds. Extrinsic cycle in the mosquito lasts up to 7 days but transmission can occur in as little as 4 days. Humans and horses are dead-end hosts for WEEV because their viremia is generally not high enough to infect mosquitoes.

Incubation period: Usually 2–7 days.

Clinical findings: Infections are generally asymptomatic to mild. WEE can present as an influenza-like illness with sudden onset fever, severe headache, chills, and myalgia. Other symptoms are: retro-orbital pain, nausea, vomiting, and diarrhea. The disease can progress to more severe disease with encephalitis and death. Encephalitis occurs in about 13% of infected cases. Absence of a rash distinguishes it from dengue and Mayaro fevers. Younger children with WEE are more severely affected neurologically and fatally. About 30% of infants develop serious neurologic sequelae. The overall CFR for WEE is 3–7%.

Diagnostic tests: Serology or RT-PCR on blood or CSF; virus isolation.

Therapy: Supportive, there is no specific treatment.

Prevention: Personal anti-mosquito precautions; there is no vaccine for WEE.

Epidemiology: WEEV was first isolated during an equine epizootic in California in 1930. Eight years later WEEV was isolated from a fatal human WEE case in California. The WEEV distribution is limited to the Americas with human epidemics occurring in North America west of the Mississippi river and Brazil. WEEV does not occur at higher altitudes in the Rocky Mountains. In the USA it overlaps with eastern equine encephalitis virus (EEEV) in Texas, Indiana, Wisconsin, Tennessee, and Michigan. It is absent from Central America (except Veracruz, Mexico). In South America, WEEV epizootics occur periodically in northern Argentina. The WEEV vector, *Culex tarsalis*, is associated with irrigated agriculture and stream drainages. The WEEV cycle in warmer regions is maintained and in colder areas it can be reintroduced by migratory birds or remain in an unknown reservoir host species. Between 1964 and 2005, there were 639 confirmed human WEE cases in the USA. In temperate regions the disease is seasonal with cases appearing during the warmer summer months. The incidence declined to less than 10 cases per year since 1988.

Map sources: The Western Equine Encephalitis map was made with data from the Pan-American Health Organization (www.paho.org/english/sha/epibul_95-98/be954out.htm), CDC (www.cdc.gov) and the medical literature.

Key references

Reisen WK (2001) Western equine encephalitis. In Service MW (ed.) *The Encyclopedia of Arthropod-transmitted Infections*. CAB International, pp. 558–563.

Weaver SC, et al. (2010) Present and future arboviral threats. *Antiviral Res* **85**(2):328–345.

Zacks MA, et al. (2010) Encephalitic alphaviruses. *Vet Microbiol* **140**(3–4):281–286.

Atlas of Human Infectious Diseases, First Edition. Heiman F.L. Wertheim, Peter Horby and John P. Woodall.
© 2012 Blackwell Publishing Ltd. Published 2012 by Blackwell Publishing Ltd.

268

West Nile Fever

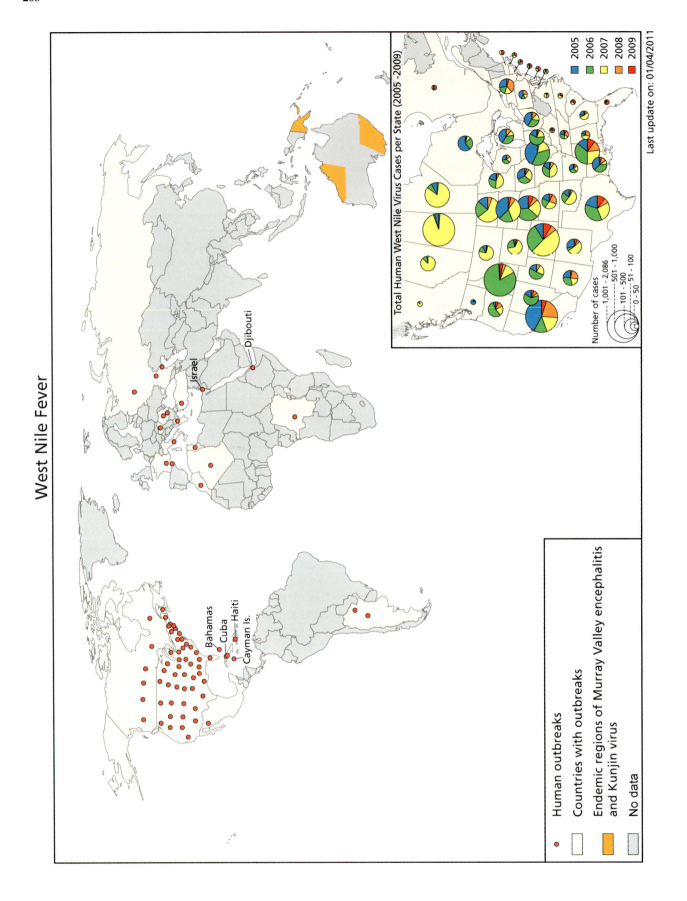

Last update on: 01/04/2011

Total Human West Nile Virus Cases per State (2005 -2009)

2005
2006
2007
2008
2009

Number of cases
1,001 - 2,086
501 -1,000
101 - 500
51 - 100
0 - 50

Djibouti

Israel

Bahamas
Cuba
Haiti
Cayman Is.

Human outbreaks

Countries with outbreaks

Endemic regions of Murray Valley encephalitis
and Kunjin virus

No data

Disease: West Nile Fever

Classification: ICD-066.3; ICD-10 A92.3

Syndromes and synonyms: None.

Agent: West Nile virus (WNV), a flavivirus, with an envelope and RNA plus-strand genome. Sequencing and phylogenetic analysis of full-length genomes has resulted in a division of WNV strains into four distinct lineages, with lineage 1 strains further separated into three clades (1a, 1b, and 1c). Kunjin virus and Murray Valley encephalitis virus are subtypes of WNV that are endemic in parts of Oceania.

Reservoir: Wild birds. Over 100 bird species can be infected by WNV infection. Many birds get infected and amplify the virus but do not die. The robin is probably the main amplifying host, and rarely has overt disease. American crows, blue jays, and hawks are susceptible to death. The number WNV bird deaths can predict subsequent disease severity in humans and equines.

Vector: Mosquitoes of more than 40 species, principally of the genus *Culex*, but also *Anopheles, Aedes* and others. Some vector species can shift their feeding preference from birds to humans, depending on the season (e.g. *Culex pipiens*). The main vectors in the USA are: *Culex pipiens* (Eastern), *Culex tarsalis* (Midwest and West), and *Culex quinquefasciatus* (Southeast). In Europe two populations of *Culex pipiens* exist: one that feeds on birds and the other on humans.

Transmission: By mosquito bite. Transfused red cells, platelets, and fresh-frozen plasma from infected donors can transmit WNV; transmission has also been reported more rarely through organ transplantation, blood transfusion, and mother-to-child. Laboratory infections have occurred from aerosols and percutaneous exposures.

Cycle: Bird–mosquito–bird, with accidental dead-end infections in humans, equines, and other vertebrate animals.

Incubation period: Typically from 2 to 14 days, longer in immunocompromised persons.

Clinical findings: The majority of the cases (70–80%) are asymptomatic. Sudden onset of fever, headache, malaise, myalgia, arthralgia, abdominal pain and upset, nausea, sore throat, conjunctivitis, lymphadenopathy, and frequently a maculopapular rash. Less than 1% of infected persons develop neuroinvasive disease. Neurological disorders are more frequent in the elderly and immunocompromised, and may be fatal, with the exception of the Kunjin strain. After 5 years 60% of patients who presented with neuroinvasive disease continued to report weakness, fatigue, memory loss, and ataxia.

Diagnostic tests: Serology (IFA, ELISA) or RT-PCR on blood or CSF. Serology may cross-react with other flaviviruses and lead to false-positives. Plaque Reduction Neutralization Tests (PRNT) and virus isolation are only done in specialized laboratories.

Therapy: Supportive, there is no specific treatment.

Prevention: Personal anti-mosquito precautions; vector control; screening blood and transplant products. There is no vaccine approved for human use. There are several veterinary vaccines.

Epidemiology: WNV was cultured for the first time from a woman with a fever of unknown origin in the West Nile district of Uganda in 1937. Molecular studies suggest that WNV emerged in Africa and spread through migrating waterbirds. Until the introduction of WNV in New York in 1999, WNV infections usually caused mild disease outbreaks and episodes of neuroinvasive disease in the old world. Since the introduction to northeast America, the virus has spread to most regions in North America, Canada, Mexico, the Caribbean and several cases in South America. The national average annual incidence of neuroinvasive disease in the USA during 1999 to 2008 was 0.40 per 100,000 population (range: 0.01–1.02). In that time period in the USA, 28,961 cases were confirmed, including 1,131 deaths. Neuroinvasive disease incidence is higher among males, especially among persons aged ≥ 60 years. The highest incidence of neuroinvasive disease occurred in the West Central and Mountain regions, probably resulting from the high efficiency of *Cx. tarsalis* as both an epizootic and epidemic WNV vector in those areas. Most US cases occur in the late summer, when Culex mosquitoes are more active and after WNV amplification in the bird reservoir. In warm climates year-round transmission is seen.

Map sources: The West Nile Fever map was made with data from CDC (www.cdc.gov/ncidod/dvbid/westnile/surv&control.htm#maps), the Canadian public health agency (www.eidgis.com/wnvmonitorca/) and reported outbreaks in ProMED mail and medical literature.

Key references

Hayes EB, et al. (2005) Virology, pathology, and clinical manifestations of West Nile virus disease. *Emerg Infect Dis* **11**(8):1174–1179.

Lindsey NP, et al. (2010) Surveillance for Human West Nile Virus Disease – United States, 1999–2008. *CDC/MMWR Surveill Sum* **59**(02):1–17.

Murray KO, et al. (2011) The virology, epidemiology, and clinical impact of West Nile virus. *Epidemiol Infect* **23**:1–11.

Atlas of Human Infectious Diseases, First Edition. Heiman F.L. Wertheim, Peter Horby and John P. Woodall.
© 2012 Blackwell Publishing Ltd. Published 2012 by Blackwell Publishing Ltd.

Yellow Fever

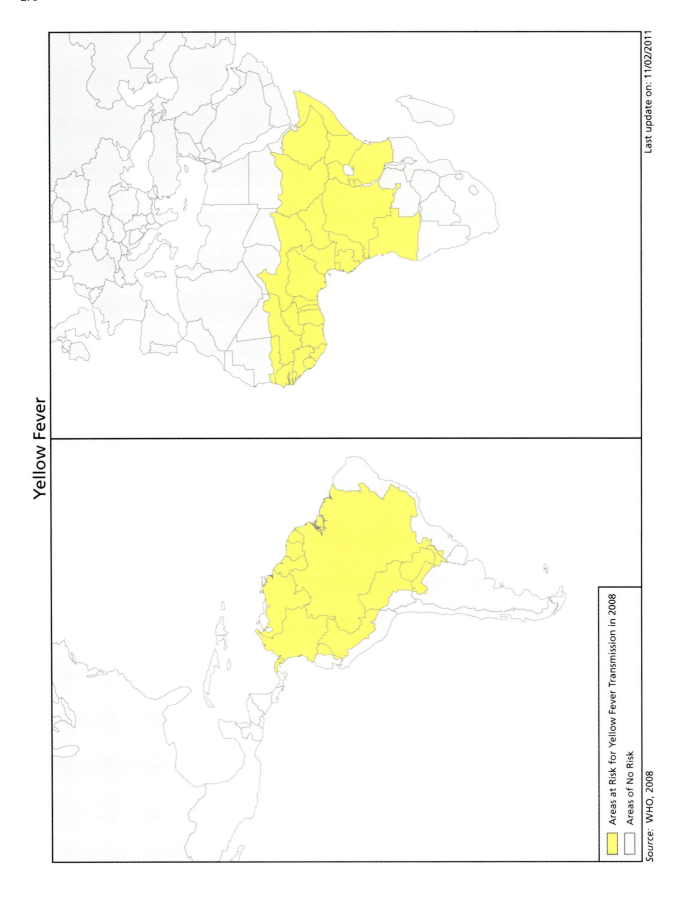

Areas at Risk for Yellow Fever Transmission in 2008

Areas of No Risk

Source: WHO, 2008

Last update on: 11/02/2011

Disease: Yellow Fever

Classification: ICD-9 060; ICD-10 A95

Syndromes and synonyms: Hemorrhagic fever, jungle yellow fever, urban yellow fever.

Agent: Yellow fever virus (YFV) is an enveloped single-stranded positive-sense RNA virus that belongs to the genus *Flavivirus*. YFV is genetically more heterogeneous in Africa than in America, suggesting it originated in Africa.

Reservoir: Humans and non-human primates are the main reservoirs.

Vector: Tree-hole-breeding forest mosquitoes: *Aedes* spp. in Africa, and *Haemagogus* and *Sabethes* spp. in South America. Transovarian transmission occurs in the mosquito and may be the way the virus survives in the years between cycles. The urban vector on both continents is *Aedes aegypti*.

Transmission: By mosquito bite.

Cycle: There are three transmission cycles: (1) sylvatic or jungle, (2) intermediate or savannah, and (3) urban. All three cycles exist in Africa and the sylvatic and urban yellow fever occur in South America. The sylvatic cycle happens in tropical rainforests where monkeys are infected by mosquitoes, and pass the virus onto other mosquitoes that feed on them; sporadically humans can become infected when entering the forest for work. The intermediate cycle is present in the savannahs of Africa, resulting in small outbreaks in rural settlements. Urban yellow fever can lead to large outbreaks in humans when infected individuals introduce the virus to the urban mosquito population (mainly *Aedes aegypti*), that subsequently can transmit to other humans.

Incubation period: 3–6 days.

Clinical findings: Sudden onset of fever, chills, headache, and can progress with signs of myalgia, photophobia, arthralgia, nausea, vomiting, jaundice, and congestion of conjunctivae. After 3–4 days there can be a remission phase leading to either recovery or more severe disease with hemorrhagic signs (epistaxis, gingival bleeding, hematemesis, melena) and hepatorenal syndrome, multi-organ failure and death. CFR in severe cases is 15 to 50%.

Diagnostic tests: Early phase: RT-PCR on blood; serology (IgM and IgG), but there is cross-reactivity with other flaviviruses; positive serology requires confirmation by more specific tests, like plaque-reduction assay.

Therapy: Supportive, there is no specific treatment. Aspirin should be avoided.

Prevention: The 17D live, attenuated vaccine is protective after 10 days; revaccination is recommended every 10 years. Anti-mosquito precautions. Prevent infected individuals from mosquito exposure to break the transmission cycle.

Epidemiology: An estimated 200,000 yellow fever cases occur annually with 30,000 deaths. The disease is present in the jungles of South America and in the jungles and Savannahs of Sub-Saharan Africa. On both continents it is endemic in various species of forest monkey, transmitted among them by mosquito bite. The disease is more common in West Africa as compared to East Africa. In Africa, mainly children acquire infection as older persons have acquired immunity. In South America, yellow fever is mainly an occupational disease of men who work in forests and can carry the infection back home, causing urban epidemics. The yellow fever virus is thought to have originated in Africa and to have been carried to the Americas in slave ships. Due to the relatively recent introduction (about 500 years ago) in the Americas, the virus has not yet adapted to the reservoir, explaining why South American monkeys become diseased, but not African monkeys. All countries with urban dengue are at risk of the introduction of yellow fever, including Asia and Australasia, because the vector is the same (see *Aedes egypti* and *Aedes albopictus* map). Why Asia has remained free from yellow fever is not understood.

Map sources: The Yellow Fever map is reproduced from WHO, at: http://gamapserver.who.int/mapLibrary/ (accessed June 2010)

Key references
Barrett AD, et al. (2007) Yellow fever: a disease that has yet to be conquered. *Ann Rev Entomol* **52**:209–229.

Ellis BR, et al. (2008) The enigma of yellow fever in East Africa. *Rev Med Virol* **18**(5):331–346.

Staples JE, et al. (2010) Yellow fever vaccine: recommendations of the Advisory Committee on Immunization Practices (ACIP). *MMWR Recom Rep* **59**(RR-7):1–27.

Atlas of Human Infectious Diseases, First Edition. Heiman F.L. Wertheim, Peter Horby and John P. Woodall.
© 2012 Blackwell Publishing Ltd. Published 2012 by Blackwell Publishing Ltd.

272

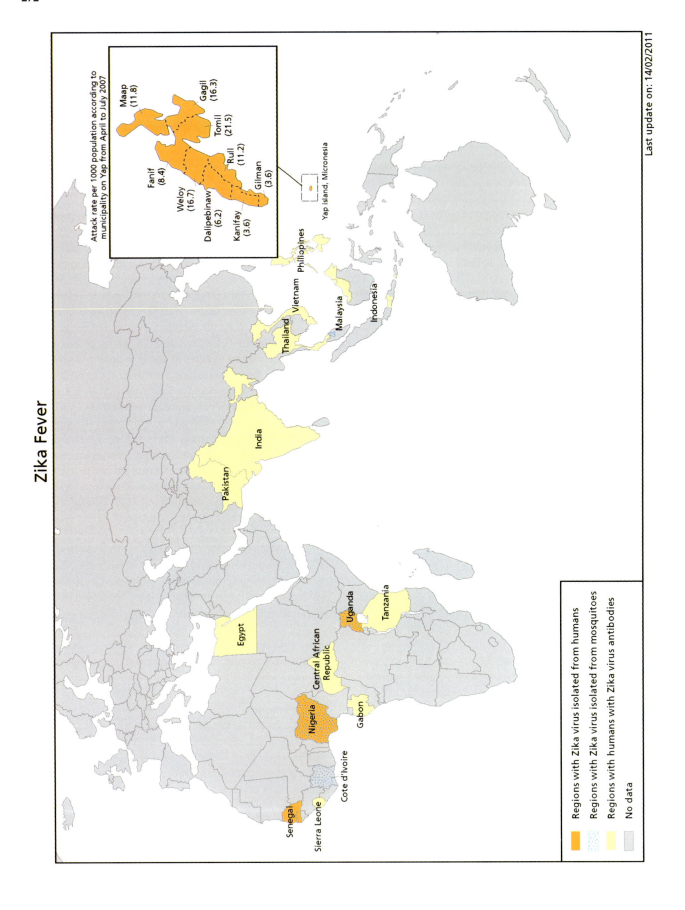

Zika Fever

Attack rate per 1000 population according to municipality on Yap from April to July 2007

Maap (11.8)
Gagil (16.3)
Tomil (21.5)
Rull (11.2)
Gilman (3.6)
Kanifay (3.6)
Dalipebinaw (6.2)
Weloy (16.7)
Fanif (8.4)

Yap Island, Micronesia

Philippines
Vietnam
Indonesia
Malaysia
Thailand
India
Pakistan

Egypt
Uganda
Tanzania
Central African Republic
Gabon
Nigeria
Cote d'Ivoire
Senegal
Sierra Leone

Regions with Zika virus isolated from humans
Regions with Zika virus isolated from mosquitoes
Regions with humans with Zika virus antibodies
No data

Last update on: 14/02/2011

Disease: Zika Fever

Classification: ICD-10 A92.9

Synonyms: Zika virus fever.

Agent: Zika virus, an enveloped RNA flavivirus; closely related to Spondweni virus.

Reservoir: Monkeys, possibly rodents.

Vector: In Africa, isolated from *Aedes africanus, Ae. apicoargenteus, Ae. luteocephalus, Ae. aegypti, Ae. Vitattus,* and *Ae. furcifer* mosquitoes; probably *Ae. Hensilii* on Yap island.

Transmission: By mosquito bite. There is no person-to-person transmission.

Cycle: Reservoir host to mosquito to reservoir host; 2–5 days viremia in host, 5–7 days in mosquito, then back into host.

Incubation period: 3–12 days.

Clinical findings: Mild self-limiting dengue-like febrile illness, with headache, malaise, arthralgia, myalgia, nausea, vomiting, photophobia, maculopapular rash, and conjunctivitis. Other symptoms may include anorexia, diarrhea, constipation, and abdominal pain.

Diagnostic tests: Virus detection in the blood by RT-PCR or virus isolation; IgM ELISA is available, cross-reactivity may occur with other flaviviruses.

Therapy: Supportive.

Prevention: Anti-mosquito precautions.

Epidemiology: Zika virus is present in the tropical regions in the Old World and is absent from the Americas (a single case in the USA was imported from Yap island). The competence of mosquitoes on the American continent for Zika virus is unknown. The geographic distribution is confirmed by virus isolation from cases, mosquitoes and sentinel monkeys. Positive results in serosurveys are not conclusive, because of extensive cross-reactions among flaviviruses. In 2007 a virgin soil epidemic affected 73% of the population of Yap island. There were no hospitalizations or deaths during this outbreak. Due to intense air travel in the Pacific region and presence of competent vectors, there is concern that the disease will spread to other islands and even beyond. Adult females have higher attack rates and few cases are found above the age of 60 years. Approximately 18% of individuals infected by the Zika virus develop symptoms; this is similar to that reported for West Nile virus infection.

Map sources: The Zika Fever map was made with data obtained from M.R. Duffy et al (2009) and E.B. Hayes et al (2009).

Key references

Duffy MR, et al. (2009) Zika virus outbreak on Yap island, Federated States of Micronesia. *New Engl J Med* **360**(24):2536–2543.

Hayes EB, et al. (2009) Zika virus outside Africa. *Emerg Infect Dis* **15**(9):1347–1350.

Index

Achatina fulica, 145
acute flaccid paralysis (AFP), 245
acute hemolytic anemia (AHA), 29
Aedes aegypti, 33, 205, 273
Aedes africanus, 273
Aedes albopictus, 33, 199, 205
   global distribution, 32, 33
   spread of infection, 33
   temperate strains of, 33
Aedes apicoargenteus, 273
Aedes camptorhynchus, 191
Aedes furcifer, 273
Aedes hensilli, 273
Aedes luteocephalus, 273
Aedes nivaeus, 205
Aedes normanensis, 191
Aedes notoscriptus, 191
Aedes scutellaris, 205
Aedes triseriatus, 197
Aedes furcifer-taylori complex spp, 205
Aedes vigilax, 191
Aedes vittatus, 273
African tick bite fever (ATBF), 95
air travel routes, 8, 9
A/H1N1 subtype, novel influenza, 9
Ajellomyces dermatitidis, 113
Amblyomma africanum, 95
Amblyomma americanum, 93
Amblyomma cajennense, 93
Amblyomma hebraeum, 95
Amblyomma maculatum, 93
amebiases, 17, 127
Ancylostoma duodenale, 153
ancylostomiasis, 153
Angiostrongylus cantonensis, 145
anisakiasis, 129
anisakidosis, 129
Anopheles dirus, 35
anthrax, 7, 13, 37, 43
antibiotics, 27
   in agriculture, 27
   usage, 26, 27
antimicrobial resistance, 7, 27
arbovirus, 33

ascariasis, 17
Astrakhan fever (AF), 95
Avian influenza (A/H5N1), 7, 39, 189

Babesia divergens, 131
Babesia duncani, 131
Babesia microti, 131
Babesia venatorum, 131
babesiosis, 131
Bacillus anthracis. See Anthrax
Barmah forest, 191
Barmah forest virus (BFV), 191
Bartonella bacilliformis, 45
Bartonella quintana, 47
bartonellosis, 45, 47
   oroya fever cases, 44
BCG vaccination, 105
biodiversity, 3
bird migration, 39
black flies, 23
Blastomyces dermatitidis, 113
blastomycosis, 113
blood-borne viruses, 7, 13
Bordetella parapertussis, 81
Bordetella pertussis, 81
Borrelia burgdoferi, 39
Borrelia burgdorferi, 73
Borrelia lusitaniae, 73
Borrelia recurrentis, 91
Borrelia spielmanii, 73
botulinum toxin, 49
botulism, 49
Boutonneuse fever, 95
Bradypus tridactylus, 243
brucellosis, 37, 51
Brugia malayi, 151
Brugia timori, 151
bulbar polio, 245
Bundibugyo virus (BDBV), 209
Bunyamwera viral fever, 193
Bunyavirus group C disease, 195
Burkholderia mallei, 75
Burkholderia pseudomallei, 21, 75
Buruli ulcer, 53

Atlas of Human Infectious Diseases, First Edition. Heiman F.L. Wertheim, Peter Horby and John P. Woodall.
© 2012 Blackwell Publishing Ltd. Published 2012 by Blackwell Publishing Ltd.

California group virus disease, 197
Calodium hepaticum, 133
Calymmatobacterium granulomatis, 59
Campylobacter, 17, 37
Cannomys badius, 123
Capillaria aerophila, 133
Capillaria hepatica, 133
Capillaria philippinensis, 133
capillariasis, 133
carbapenem-resistant bacteria (NDM-1), 27
Chagas disease, 23, 185
chikungunya fever, 33, 199
chikungunya virus (CHIKV), 199
childhood nutrition, 19
child mortality, 14. *See also* life expectancy
Chlamydia trachomatis, 103
cholera, 13, 17, 55
chronic war, adverse effects of, 15
Chrysops dimidiata, 161
Chrysops distinctipennis, 161
Chrysops silacea, 161
clean water, access to, 16
climate change, 17, 21
    Köppen classification, 21
climate-dependent pathogen, 21
clonorchiasis, 135
Clonorchis sinensis, 135
Clostridium barati, 49
Clostridium botulinum, 49
Clostridium tetani, 101
coccidioidomycosis, 115
Coccidioides immitis, 21, 115
Coccidioides posadasii, 115
cod worm disease, 129
Colorado tick fever, 201
Colorado tick fever virus (CTFV), 201
Coquillettidia linealis, 191
Corynebacterium diphtheriae, 57
Corynebacterium ulcerans, 57
Coxiella burnetii, 37
Crimean–Congo hemorrhagic fever, 37, 203
Crimean-Congo hemorrhagic fever virus (CCHFV), 203
Cryptococcus gattii, 23
Cryptosporidiosis, 17
Culex annulirostris, 191
Culex tarsalis, 267
Culicoides paraensis, 243
Culiseta melanura, 207
cyclones, 25
cysticercosis, 137

deforestation, 23
dengue fever (DF), 21, 33, 205
dengue virus (DENV), 205
Dermacentor andersoni, 93, 201
Dermacentor variabilis, 93
diarrhea, 7, 17, 19
    deaths, of young children, 17

diphtheria, 13, 57
diphtheria, tetanus, and pertussis vaccine
    (DTP3), 31
diphyllobothriasis, 139
donovanosis, 59
dracunculiasis, 17, 141
Dracunculus medinensis, 141
drinking water, 7
    source, 17
    target, 17
droughts, 25
drug-resistance in bacteria, 27
drug-resistant tuberculosis, 105
Duffy antigen, 29
dysentery, 13

earthquakes, 25
eastern equine encephalitis, 207
eastern equine encephalitis virus (EEEV), 207
Ebola hemorrhagic fever, 13, 209
Ebola viruses, 23, 209
echinococcosis, 143
Echinococcus multilocularis, 143
E. coli., 17, 37
economic development, 11
education, 7
ehrlichioses, 61
El Niño Southern Oscillation (ENSO), 21
emerging infectious diseases (EIDs), 2, 3
endemic treponematosis, 62, 63
Entamoeba dispar, 127
Entamoeba histolytica, 127
Entamoeba moshkovskii, 127
eosinophilic meningitis, 144, 145
European Antimicrobial Resistance Surveillance
    (EARSS), 27
European Surveillance of Antimicrobial Consumption (ESAC)
    project, 27
extrapulmonary tuberculosis, 105

Falciparum, 163
Fasciola gigantica, 147
Fasciola hepatica, 147
fascioliasis, 37, 147
fasciolopsiasis, 149
Fasciolopsis buski, 149
filariasis, 151
Flinders Island spotted fever (FISF), 95
floods, 25
food-borne infections, 7
forest-adapted malaria vectors, 35
forest associated infections, 23
forest cover change, 22, 23
forest resources assessment (FRA), 23
Francisella novicida, 107
Francisella tularensis, 107
Fusobacterium necrophorum, 79
Fusobacterium nucleatum, 79

G6PD. *See* glucose-6-phosphate dehydrogenase deficiency

Gambian trypanosomiasis, 183

German measles, 253

Giardiasis, 17

Gilchrist disease, 113

Global Alliance for Vaccines and Immunization (GAVI), 31

global burden of infectious diseases, 11

global conflict, 13

global connectivity, 8, 9

  major air travel routes, 8, 9

globalization, 9

global peace index (GPI), 12, 13

Glossina. *See* Tsetse fly

Glossina fuscipes, 183

Glossina morsitans, 183

Glossina pallidipes, 183

Glossina palpalis, 183

Glossina swynnertoni, 183

Glossina tachinoides, 183

glucose-6-phosphate dehydrogenase (G6PD) deficiency, 29

Gnathostoma spinigerum, 145

GPI. *See* global peace index (GPI)

gross domestic product (GDP), 10, 11

Guaroa virus (GROV), 197

Guinea worm disease, 141

Haemophilus influenzae type b, 65

Hantaviral disease, 211, 212, 213

Hantavirus pulmonary syndrome (HPS), 211

HDI. *See* human development index (HDI)

healthcare-associated infections, 7

hemorrhagic fever with renal syndrome (HFRS), 213

Hendra virus, 214, 215

Hendra virus disease, 215

hepatitis A, 17

  HAV seroprevalence, 216

hepatitis A virus (HAV), 217

hepatitis B

  distribution of HBV genotypes, 218

hepatitis B virus (HBV), 219

hepatitis C, 220, 221

hepatitis C virus (HCV), 221

hepatitis E, 17, 223

hepatitis E virus (HEV), 223

Herring worm disease, 129

Histoplasma capsulatum, 117

Histoplasma capsulatum var. *duboisii*, 117

histoplasmosis, 116, 117

HIV/AIDS epidemic, 15

hookworm. *See* Ancylostomiasis

hookworm disease, 17

HTLV-1. *See* human T-lymphotropic virus 1

human development index (HDI), 10, 11

human granulocytic anaplasmosis (HGA), 61

human immunodeficiency virus (HIV), 224, 225

  M-subtypes and recombinants, 224

human monocytic ehrlichiosis (HME), 61

human pathogen diversity, 21

human T-lymphotropic virus 1 (HTLV-1), 227

hydrophobia, 247

hygiene, 17

IBDs. *See* inherited blood disorders (IBDs)

immunity, 19, 21

immunization, 9, 31

  coverage

    Hib3, 64

    measles, 234

    mumps, 238

    rubella, 252

    tetanus, 101

  programs, 13

indian tick typhus (ITT), 95

indoor residual insecticide spraying (IRS), 35

infantile paralysis, 245

infectious parotitis, 239

influenza, 7, 13, 37

  avian, 189

inherited blood disorders (IBDs), 29

  Duffy antigen, 28, 29

Inkoo virus (INKV), 197

insecticide-treated mosquito nets (ITNs), 35

Israeli spotted fever (ISF), 95

Ixodes dammini, 73

Ixodes persulcatus, 73, 261

Ixodes ricinus, 73, 261

Ixodes scapularis, 73

Jamestown Canyon virus (JCV), 197

Japanese B encephalitis, 33, 37, 39, 229

Karelian fever, 257

Katayama syndrome, 177, 179

Klebsiella granulomatis, 59

Knowlesi malaria, 165

Kyasanur forest virus, 23

LaCrosse virus (LACV), 33, 197

Lassa fever, 231

Lassa fever virus (LFV), 231

Leishmania chagasi, 159

Leishmania donovani, 159

Leishmania infantum, 159

leishmaniasis

  cutaneous and mucosal, 154–157

  visceral, 158, 159

leprosy, 66, 67

Leptospira interrogans, 69

leptospirosis, 37, 69

Leptotrombidium, 97

life expectancy, 14, 15

Listeria monocytogenes, 37, 71

listeriosis, 37, 71

livestock density, 37

Lloviu virus (LLOV), 209

Loa loa, 161

loiasis, 161
louse-borne relapsing fever (LBRF), 91
Lutzomyia verrucarum, 45
lyme disease, 39, 73

malaria, 13, 19, 21, 23, 25, 167, 169. *See also* Falciparum malaria;
      Knowlesi malaria
malaria vectors, 35
malnutrition, 19
Marburg hemorrhagic fever, 209
Marburg virus, 23, 209
Mayaro virus (MAYV), 233
measles, 13, 19, 235
measles virus, 235
Medina worm disease, 141
Mediterranean spotted fever (MSF), 95
melioidosis, 75
meningococcal meningitis. *See also* eosinophilic meningitis, 77
micronutrient deficiency, 19
monkeypox, 23, 237
monkeypox virus (MPV), 237
mucocutaneous leishmanisasis, 23
mumps, 239
mumps virus, 239
mycetoma, 119
Mycobacterium africanum, 105
Mycobacterium bovis, 105
Mycobacterium canetti, 105
Mycobacterium leprae, 67
Mycobacterium tuberculosis, 105
Mycobacterium ulcerans, 53

Nantucket fever, 131
natural disasters, 25
    global cyclone hazard distribution, 24
    global drought hazard distribution, 24
    global earthquake hazard distribution, 24
    global flood hazard distribution, 24
    infectious diseases, significance for, 25
natural hazards. *See* natural disasters
Necator americanus, 153
necatoriasis, 153
Neisseria meningitidis, 77
neurocysticercosis, 137
Nipah virus, 23, 37, 215
noma, 79
non-communicable diseases, 11

Ochlerotatus melanimon, 267
Ochlerotatus vigilax, 191
Ockelbo disease, 257
Onchocerca volvulus, 171
onchocerciasis, 23, 171
o'nyong-nyong virus (ONNV), 241
o'nyong-nyong virus disease, 241
opisthorchiasis, 173
Opisthorchis felineus, 173

Opisthorchis viverrini, 173
Orf virus, 37
Orientia tsutsugamushi, 97
Oropouche virus (OROV), 243
Oropouche virus disease, 243
overnutrition, 19

paludism, 167
Paracoccidioides brasiliensis, 121
paracoccidioidomycosis, 121
paragonimiasis
Pediculus humanus corporis, 47
penicilliosis, 123
Penicillium marneffei, 123
pentavalent botulinum toxoid (PBT) vaccine, 49
pertussis, 13, 81
Pharaoh worm disease, 141
pharyngeal fascioliasis, 147
piroplasmosis, 131
plague, 83
Plasmodium falciparum, 29, 163
Plasmodium knowlesi, 23, 29, 165
Plasmodium ovale, 167
Plasmodium vivax, 29, 169
    chloroquine-resistant, 168
    Duffy-negativity prevalence, 168
pneumococcal disease, 85
pneumococcal vaccine, immunization program, 84
pneumonia, 17, 19, 25
Pogosta disease, 257
polio, 13
poliomyelitis, 13, 245
political stability, 13
Pomacea canaliculata, 145
population density, 4, 5
    urban growth, 7
population in urban slums, 6
poverty, 11
pseudaterranovosis, 129
public health surveillance systems, 13
purchasing power parity (PPP), 11

Q fever, 37, 87
Queensland tick typhus (QTT), 95

rabies, 247
rabies virus, 247
rat bite fever, 89
Ravn virus (RAVV), 209
relapsing fever, 91
Reston virus (RESTV), 209
Rhipicephalus sanguineus, 93, 95
Rhizomys pruinosus, 123
Rhizomys sinensis, 123
Rhizomys sumatrensis, 123
Rhodesian trypanosomiasis, 183

Rickettsia africae, 93, 95
Rickettsia australis, 95
Rickettsia conorii caspia, 95
Rickettsia conorii conorii, 95
Rickettsia conorii indica, 95
Rickettsia conorii israelensis, 95
Rickettsia aeschlimannii, 95
Rickettsia helvetica, 95
Rickettsia honei, 95
Rickettsia japonica, 95
Rickettsia massiliae, 95
Rickettsia parkeri, 93
Rickettsia rickettsii, 92, 93, 94
Rickettsia sibirica, 95
Rickettsia tsutsugamushi, 97
Rickettsioses, 92–95
Rift Valley fever, 21, 37, 249
Rift Valley fever virus (RVFV), 249
Rocky Mountain spotted fever (RMSF), 93
Ross river virus (RRV), 191
rotaviral enteritis, 251
rotavirus, 17
rubella, 253
rubella virus, 253
rural areas, 7
rural populations, 5

Salmonella enterica enterica serovar
        Typhi (S. Typhi), 109
sanitation, 7, 17
    access to, 16
SARS coronavirus (SARS-CoV), 255
scabies, 17
Schistosoma guineensis, 177
Schistosoma haematobium, 109, 177
Schistosoma intercalatum, 177
Schistosoma japonicum, 179
Schistosoma malayensis, 179
Schistosoma mansoni, 177
Schistosoma mekongi, 179
schistosomiasis, 17, 177
    Africa & Americas, 177
    Asia, 179
scrub typhus, 97
sealworm disease, 129
Semliki forest virus, 23
Sennetsu fever, 61
serpent worm disease, 141
severe acute respiratory syndrome (SARS), 7, 9, 255
sexually transmitted infections, 13
sickle cell disease, 29
sickle hemoglobin (HbS), 29
simian variola, 237
Sindbis fever, 257
Sindbis virus (SINV), 257
sleeping sickness, 183

slum dwelling, increased risks of diseases, 7
smallpox, 13
snowshoe hare virus (SSHV), 197
social disruption, 11
socioeconomic development, 21
soil-transmitted helminths (STHs), 153
St Louis encephalitis, 39
Streptococcus pneumoniae, 85
Streptococcus suis, 37, 99
strongyloidiasis, 181
Strongyloides fuelleborni, 181
Strongyloides stercoralis, 181
Sudan virus (SUDV), 209

tacaribe complex virus disease, 259
Taenia saginata, 137
Taenia solium, 137
Tahyna virus (TAHV), 197
Taï forest virus (TAFV), 209
tetanus, 101
thalassemia, 29
tick-borne encephalitis (TBE), 261
tick-borne relapsing fever (TBRF), 91
trachoma, 17, 103
trichuriasis, 17
tropical fever, 167
Trypanosoma brucei, 183
Trypanosoma brucei gambiense, 183
Trypanosoma brucei rhodesiense, 183
Trypanosoma cruzi, 23, 185
trypanosomiasis, 37, 183
    African, 183
    American, 185
Tsetse fly, 183
tsutsugamushi disease, 97
tuberculosis, 7, 19, 25, 105
tularemia, 107
typhoid fever, 7, 17, 109

uncinariasis, 153
undernutrition, 19
urbanization, 6, 7, 17, 37
    significance for infections, 7
    trends, 7
uruma fever, 233

vaccination, 25, 30, 31
    coverage, 30, 31
variant Creutzfeldt–Jakob disease, 263
vector-borne diseases, 7, 13, 25
vector control, 13
Venezuelan equine encephalitis, 264, 265
Venezuelan hemorrhagic fever, 23

water-based infections, 17
water-borne infections, 17, 25

Western equine encephalitis, 39, 267
Western equine encephalitis virus (WEEV), 267
West Nile fever, 269
West Nile virus (WNV), 39, 269
whaleworm disease, 129
world climate zones, 20
world population, 4, 5

world's urban population, 7
Wucheraria bancrofti, 151

yellow fever, 13, 23, 33, 271
Yersinia pestis. See plague

Zika fever, 273